Essentials of
FACIAL
GROWTH

Essentials of
FACIAL GROWTH

DONALD H. ENLOW, M.S., PH.D.
Thomas Hill Distinguished Professor Emeritus
Department of Orthodontics
Case Western Reserve University
Cleveland, Ohio

MARK G. HANS, D.D.S., M.S.D.
Associate Professor and Chairman
Department of Orthodontics
Case Western Reserve University
Cleveland, Ohio

W. B. SAUNDERS COMPANY
A Division of Harcourt Brace & Company
Philadelphia, London, Toronto, Montreal, Sydney, Tokyo

W. B. SAUNDERS COMPANY

A Division of Harcourt Brace & Company

The Curtis Center
Independence Square West
Philadelphia, Pennsylvania 19106

Library of Congress Cataloging-in-Publication Data

Enlow, Donald H.
    Essentials of facial growth / Donald H. Enlow, Mark G. Hans.
      p.   cm.
    ISBN 0–7216–6106–8
    1. Face—Growth.   I. Hans, Mark G.   II. Title.
    [DNLM: 1. Maxillofacial Development—physiology.   2. Face—
physiology.   3. Skull—growth & development.   WE 705 E58e 1996]
QM535.E469   1996
611′.92—dc20
DNLM/DLC
for Library of Congress   96-16720

ESSENTIALS OF FACIAL GROWTH   ISBN 0–7216–6106–8

Printed in the United States of America.

Last digit is the print number: 9   8   7   6   5   4   3   2   1

To
Martha (DHE)
and
Gunther and Ruth (MGH)

CONTRIBUTORS

DAVID S. CARLSON, Ph.D.
Robert E. Gaylord Professor of Orthodontics
Chairman, Department of Biomedical Sciences
Baylor University of Dentistry
Dallas, Texas
Maturation of the Orofacial Neuromusculature

ROBERT E. MOYERS, D.D.S., Ph.D.*
Professor Emeritus, School of Dentistry and
Director Emeritus, Center for Human Growth and Development
University of Michigan
Ann Arbor, Michigan
Maturation of the Orofacial Neuromusculature

B. HOLLY BROADBENT, JR., D.D.S.
Director, Bolton-Brush Growth Study Center
Case Western Reserve University
Cleveland, Ohio
Cephalometrics

*Deceased.

PREFACE

Radiographic cephalometry was a pioneering advance introduced decades ago that led to many fundamental insights into the behavior of the face and neurocranium during growth. It remains to this day a basic tool in research and diagnosis. The techniques were necessarily formulated before present-day understanding of the actual biology underlying craniofacial morphogenesis, and thus could not incorporate today's biologic concepts. *This biology is the particular subject of the pages that follow.* The purpose is to outline in *abridged format* the enormous range of morphogenic information dealing with key craniofacial growth concepts. *The biological grounding for basic clinical theory is highlighted.* Just as an understanding of the basics of cephalometry remains essential to academic researchers as well as clinicians, so now certainly is the biological aspect as well. Meaningful insight into diagnosis, treatment planning, treatment selection, treatment effects, and rebound is not possible without the latter. These considerations, without contradiction, are the near and long-term clinical craniofacial future. The predoctoral dental curriculum and, importantly, graduate dental and medical training programs touching this biology only lightly or not at all are seriously incomplete. The present condensed version of previous editions is an attempt to distill details down into the "essentials". An all-new introductory chapter has been added that presents a panorama of the craniofacial growth process as a whole. It emphasizes the developmental interplay among all tissues, soft as well as hard. In effect, this section is a "short course" of facial growth, summarizing highlights and key concepts of the chapters that follow. For teachers and speakers needing to present core material in a limited time frame, these new pages can be useful. The format and selection of content for all the other chapters have been refined, extensively re-organized for teaching and for an interested professional's reading, and the text has been updated and clinically tuned throughout.

The preparation of this extensively revised edition has been strengthened by the talents and gracious tolerance of our office secretary, Mrs. LaVerne Vogel. We are grateful indeed. We all value and appreciate the professional expertise and helpful collaboration provided by the editors and production staff of W.B. Saunders Company.

CONTENTS

PROLOGUE

HISTORICAL PERSPECTIVE

The morphogenic *interrelationships* among the diverse families of soft tissues and the growth and development of the craniofacial skeleton are highlights of the present monograph. However, the early historical story of "bone" is especially interesting because of bone's unusual "oxymoron" character. That is, how in the world can this unique rock-like substance actually grow and develop into constantly changing shapes and sizes *perfectly* matching the developing soft tissues it serves. This question festered in early scholars' minds and has been a particular wonderment since Biblical times. In the book of Ecclesiastes (11:5), for example, it was said that "As thou knowest not the way of the spirit, nor how the bones do grow in the womb of her that is with child, even so thou knowest not the works of God who maketh all." Many Old and New Testament passages make frequent reference to bone in health and disease. That bone is actually a living substance is certainly not a modern notion at all. Greek philosophers and physicians, including Hippocrates (*De carnibus*), Aristotle (*De generatione animalium*), Galen (*Opera omnia*), and Plato (*Timaeus*), all recorded allegories on bone formation, describing how the earthy, less fluid, and thicker seminal parts become solidified by internal body heat, comparable to the manner in which moist clay (i.e., cartilage) is kiln-fired (endochondral ossification) into earthenware. A reasonable analogy at the time, considering that microscopes, histology textbooks, and the Cell Doctrine were in the distant future. Arnobius accounted for the control of childhood bone formation by a goddess "who hardens and solidifies the bones in infants." Then, century by century, many, many of the great names in the anatomy and medicine Hall of Fame assembled our foundations of bone knowledge in a long series of plateaus, each following some technological advance or conceptual breakthrough. These familiar names include Albinus, Vesalius, Bartholin, Harvey, Sue, Havers, Nesbitt, Monro, Leewenhoek (who observed canals in bone years before Havers, but that doesn't detract from the latter's classic monograph "*Osteologia Nova*"), Todd, Bowman, Tomes, Demorgan, Von Ebner, Gagliardi, Malpighi, Bell, Howship, Belchier, Hales, Hunter, Volkmann, Wolff, Hassall, Meckel, Virchow, Purkinje, Sharpey, and Schwann. All, and many more, were directly involved in the quest. (See Enlow, 1963, for a more extensive historical review, including the specific landmark contributions of these early scholars.)

Overview of Craniofacial Growth and Development

"Growth" is a general term implying simply that something changes in magnitude. It does not, however, presume to account for **how** it happens. For the professional clinician, such a loose meaning is often used quite properly. However, to try to understand "how" it works, and what actually happens, the more descriptive and explanatory term "development" is added. This connotes a maturational process involving progressive differentiation at the cellular and tissue levels, thereby focusing on the actual biologic mechanism that accounts for growth.

"Growth and development" is an essential topic in many clinical disciplines and specialties, and the reason is important. Morphogenesis is a biologic process having an underlying **control** system at the cellular and tissue levels. The clinician intervenes in the course of this control process at some appropriate stage and substitutes (augments, overpowers, or replaces) some activities of the control mechanism with calculated clinical regulation. It is important to understand that the actual biologic process of development itself is the same. That is, the histogenic functioning of the cells and tissues still carry out their individual roles, but the **control signals** that selectively activate the composite of them are now clinically manipulated. It is the rate, timing, direction, and magnitude of cellular divisions and tissue differentiation that become altered when the clinician's signals modify or complement the body's own intrinsic growth signals. The subsequent course of development thus proceeds according to a programmed treatment plan by "working with growth" (an old clinical tenet). Of course, if one does not understand the workings of the underlying biology, any real grasp of the actual basis for treatment design and results, and why, is an illusion. Importantly, craniofacial biology is independent of treatment intervention strategy. Therefore, some clinicians may argue about the relative merits of different intervention strategies (e.g., headgear versus Frankel appliance therapies). The biologic rules of the game are the same.

Morphogenesis works constantly toward a state of composite, architectonic **balance** among all of the separate growing parts. This means that the various parts developmentally merge into a functional whole, with each part complementing the others as they all grow and function together.

During development, balance is continuously transient and can never actually be achieved because growth itself constantly creates ongoing, normal regional imbalances. This requires other parts to constantly adapt (develop) as they all work toward composite equilibrium. It is such an imbalance itself that fires the signals which activate the interplay of histogenic responses. Balance, when achieved for a time, turns off the signals, and regional growth activity ceases. The process recycles throughout childhood, into and through adulthood (with changing magnitude), and finally on to old age sustaining a changing morphologic equilibrium in response to ever-changing intrinsic and external conditions.

For example, as a muscle continues to develop in mass and function, it would outpace the bone to which it inserts, both in size and in mechanical capacity. However, this imbalance signals the osteogenic, chondrogenic, neurogenic, and fibrogenic tissues to immediately respond, and the whole bone with its connective tissues, vascular supply, and innervation develops (remodels) to work continuously toward homeostasis.

By an understanding of how this process of progressive morphogenic and histogenic differentiation operates, the clinical specialist thus selectively augments the body's own intrinsic activating signals using controlled procedures to jump-start the remodeling process in a way that achieves an intended treatment result. For example, rapid palatal expansion separates the right and left halves of the maxilla (displacement) and initiates a period of increased remodeling in the midpalatal suture.

The genetic and functional **determinants** of a bone's development (i.e., the origin of the growth-regulating signals) reside in the composite of soft tissues that turn on or turn off, or speed up or slow down, the histogenic actions of the osteogenic connective tissues (periosteum, endosteum, sutures, periodontal membrane). Growth is not "programmed" within the bone itself or its enclosing membranes. The "blueprint" for the design, construction, and growth of a bone thus lies in the muscles, tongue, lips, cheeks, integument, mucosae, connective tissues, nerves, blood vessels, airway, pharynx, the brain as an organ mass, tonsils, adenoids, and so forth, all of which provide information signals that pace the histogenic tissues producing a bone's development.

A major problem in orthodontics and orthognathic surgery can be *relapse* (rebound subsequent to treatment). The potential for relapse exists when the functional, developmental, or biomechanical aspects of growth among key parts are clinically altered to a physiologically imbalanced state. The possibility of instability exists because clinicians strive to bring about a state of aesthetic balance that at times produces physiologic imbalance. The underlying conditions that led to the pretreatment dysplasia can still exist and thus trigger the growth process to rebound in response to those conditions. The "genic" tissues (see below) are brought into play in a way attempting to restore balance,* thereby returning in a developmental direction toward the pretreatment state or some combination between. It is, in effect, a built-in protective mechanism but, again, is the same growth process working toward physiologic, biomechanical, and developmental equilibrium. (See Fig. 1–1.)

The evolutionary design of the human head is such that certain regional clinical situations naturally exist. For example, variations in headform design establish natural tendencies toward different kinds of malocclusions. The growth process, in response, develops some regional imbalances, the aggregate of which serves to make corrective adjustments. A

---

*A malocclusion or other dysplasia (including congenital malformations), although clinically abnormal, is nonetheless in a "balanced" state.

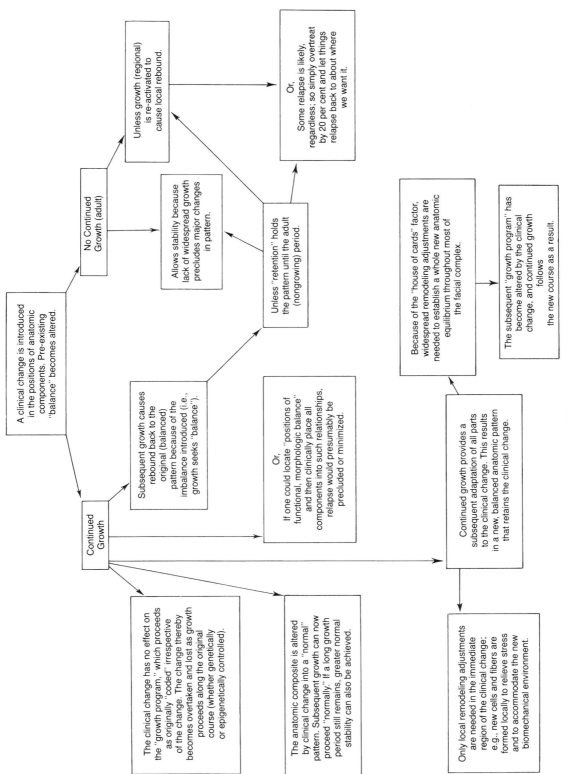

FIGURE 1–1

Class I molar relationship with an aesthetically pleasing face is the common result in which the underlying factors that would otherwise have led to a more severe Class II or III malocclusion still exist but have been "compensated for" by the growth process itself. The net effect is an overall, composite balance.

As pointed out above, clinical treatment can disturb a state of structural and functional equilibrium, and a natural rebound can follow. For example, a premature fusion of some cranial sutures can result in growth-retarded development of the nasomaxillary complex because the anterior endocranial fossae (a template for midfacial development) are foreshortened, as in the Crouzon or Apert syndromes. The altered nasomaxillary complex itself nonetheless has grown in a balanced state proportionate to its basicranial template, even though abnormal in comparison with a population norm for esthetics and function. Craniofacial surgery has disturbed the former balance, and some degree of natural rebound can be expected. The growth process attempts to restore the original state of equilibrium, since some extent of the original underlying conditions (e.g., the basicranium) can still exist that were not, or could not be, altered clinically. These are examples in which the biology of the growth process is essentially normal, either with treatment or without, but is producing abnormal results because of altered input control signals.

The Big Picture

The following paragraph outlines a growth concept basic to the overall developmental process. It deals with the separate but **interrelated** and **interdependent** nature of the assembly of all the regional parts comprising the neurocranium (for the brain and associated sensory organs) and viscerocranium (face). It underscores the variety of developmental conditions in any given local region, but at the same time points to the necessary morphogenic and functional interplay among them.

No craniofacial component is developmentally self-contained and self-regulated. Growth of a component is not an isolated event unrelated to other parts. Growth is the composite change of all components. While this seems self-evident, it might be perceived, for example, that the developing palate is essentially responsible for its own intrinsic growth and anatomic positioning, and that an infant's palate is the same palate in the adult simply grown larger. The palate in later childhood, however, is not composed of the same tissue (but with more simply added), and it does not occupy the same actual position. Many factors influence (impact) that growing palate from without, such as developmental rotations, displacements in conjunction with growth at sutures far removed, and multiple remodeling movements that relocate it to progressively new positions and adjust its size, shape, and alignment continuously throughout the growth period. Similarly, for the mandible, the multiple factors of middle cranial fossa expansion; anterior cranial fossa rotations; tooth eruption; pharyngeal growth; bilateral asymmetries; enlarging tongue, lips, and cheeks; changing muscle actions; headform variations; an enlarging nasal airway; changing infant and childhood swallowing patterns; adenoids; head position associated with sleeping habits; body stance; and an infinite spread of morphologic and functional variations, all have input in creating constantly changing states of structural balance. As emphasized above, **development** is an architectonic process leading to an aggregate state of structural and functional equilibrium, with or without an imposed malocclusion or other morphologic dysplasia. Very little, if anything, can be exempted from the "big picture" of factors affecting the operation of the growth control process, and no region can be isolated. Meaningful insight into all of this underlies the basis for clinical diagnosis and treatment planning. The direct target for clinical intervention must be the control process regulating the biology of growth and development.

A Cornerstone of the Growth Process

A grasp of how facial growth operates begins with distinction between the two basic kinds of **growth movement**. These are (1) remodeling and (2) displacement (Fig. 1–2). Each category of movement involves virtually all developing hard and soft tissues.

For the bony craniofacial complex, the process of growth **remodeling** is paced by the composite of soft tissues relating to each of the bones. The functions of remodeling are to (1) progressively create the changing **size** of each whole bone; (2) sequentially **relocate** each of the component regions of the whole bone to allow for overall enlargement; (3) progressively **shape** the bone to accommodate its various functions; (4) provide progressive fine-tune **fitting** of all the separate bones to each other and to their contiguous, growing, functioning soft tissues; and (5) carry out continuous structural adjustments to **adapt** to the intrinsic and extrinsic changes in conditions. Although these remodeling functions relate to childhood growth, most also continue on into adulthood and old age in reduced degree to provide the same ongoing functions. This is what in freshman histology is meant when it is stated that bones "remodel throughout life," but without an explanation of the reasons. Added to this, now, is that all soft tissues *also* undergo equivalent remodeling and for all of the same reasons.

In Figures 1–3 and 1–4, note that many external (periosteal) surfaces are actually resorptive. Opposite surfaces are depository. This is required in order to sculpture the complex configurations involved.

As a bone enlarges, it is simultaneously carried away from other bones in direct articulation with it. This creates the "space" within which bony enlargement takes place at the interface between bone-to-bone joint contacts. The process is termed **displacement** (also called "translation"). It is a physical movement of a whole bone and occurs while the bone simultaneously remodels by resorption and deposition (to an equivalent extent).

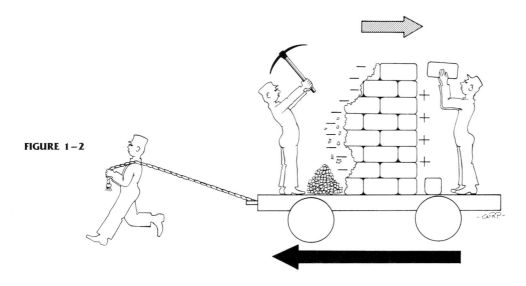

FIGURE 1–2

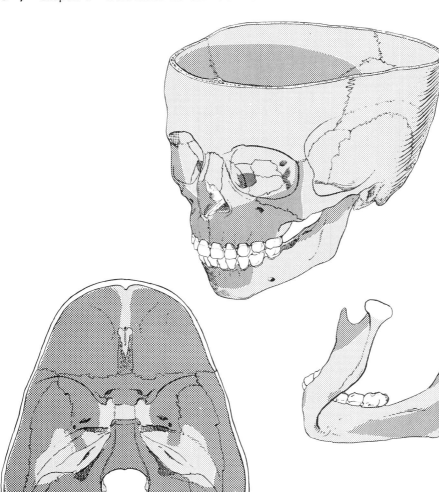

FIGURE 1–3. Summary diagram of the resorptive (darkly stippled) and depository (lightly stippled) fields of remodeling (From Enlow, D. H. T. Kuroda, and A. B. Lewis: The morphological and morphogenetic basis for craniofacial form and pattern. Angle Orthod., 41:161, 1971, with permission.)

As the bone enlarges in a given direction within the joint, it is simultaneously displaced in the **opposite** direction (Fig. 1–5). The relationships underscore why facial articulations (sutures and condyles) are important factors; they are direct clinical targets.

The process of new bone deposition does not cause displacement by **pushing** against the articular contact surface of another bone. Rather, the bone is **carried** away by the expansive force of all the growing soft tissues surrounding and attached to it by anchoring fibers. As this takes place, new bone is added immediately (remodeling), the whole bone enlarges, and the two separate bones thereby remain in constant articular junction. The nasomaxillary complex, for example, is in sutural contact with the floor of the cranium. The whole maxillary region, **in toto**, is **displaced** downward and forward away from the cranium by the expansive growth of the soft

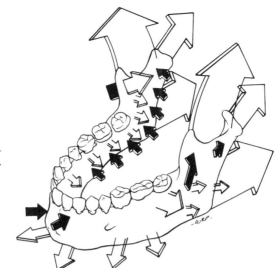

FIGURE 1–4. Black arrows are surface resorptive, and white arrows are depository.

tissues in the midfacial region (Fig. 1–6A). This then triggers new bone growth at the various sutural contact surfaces between the nasomaxillary composite and the cranial floor (Fig. 1–6B). Displacement thus proceeds downward and forward an equivalent amount as maxillary remodeling simultaneously takes place in an opposite upward and backward direction (i.e., **toward** its contact with the cranial floor).

Similarly, the whole mandible (Fig. 1–5) is **displaced** "away" from its articulation in each glenoid fossa by the growth enlargement of the composite of soft tissues in the developing face. As this occurs, the condyle and ramus grow upward and backward (relocate) into the "space" created by the displacement process. Note that the ramus also remodels in shape and size as it relocates posterosuperiorly. It becomes longer and wider to accommodate (1) the increasing mass of masticatory muscles inserted onto it, (2) the enlarged breadth of the pharyngeal space, and (3) the vertical lengthening of the nasomaxillary part of the growing face.

A beginning student is always confused because it is repeatedly heard and read that the face "grows forward and downward." It would seem reasonable, then, that the growth activity of the mandible or the maxilla would be in their anterior, forward-facing parts. However, it is mostly the displacement movement that is forward and downward, thereby complementing the predominantly posterosuperior vectors of remodeling. This is one fundamental reason, as mentioned above, that all joint contacts and bone ends are of basic significance in the growth picture. They are the points away from which displacement proceeds and, at the same time, the sites where remodeling lengthens a given bone. Thus, they are key locations where certain clinical procedures affect the growth process.

Note this significant point. If a non-biologic material, such as a metal or plastic plate or other prosthetic appliance, is implanted within the developing craniofacial complex, it lacks both of these two systems of growth movement! It cannot (1) move by patterns of REMODELING since resorptive and depository fields do not exist. It (2) cannot become moved by DISPLACEMENT through traction growth forces because the enlarging soft tissues are not anchored into its substance by Sharpey's fibers. The

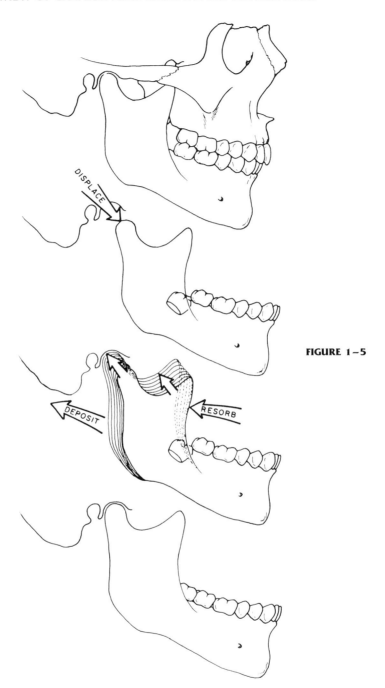

FIGURE 1–5

growing bone contiguous with any non-biologic material, thus, simply grows away from it as they become progressively disjoined. The skeletal as well as soft tissue parts previously around it when originally implanted thereby continue to (1) remodel and (2) displace, while the non-biologic material itself remains behind without dual biologic growth movement capacity. It now becomes a developmental block against any advancing tissues behind.

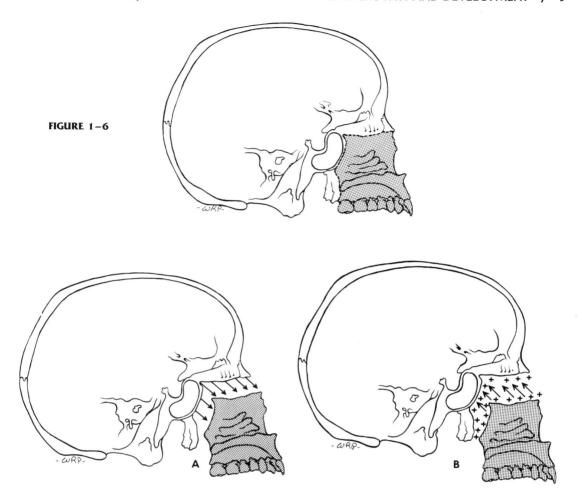

FIGURE 1-6

The "Genic" Tissues

The histogenic "blast" cells and tissues are activated by a shower of intercellular signals targeted toward the signal-sensitive cell membrane receptors of each cell type, including chondroblasts, osteoblasts, myoblasts, fibroblasts, neuroblastic (satellite) cells, and any other progenitor or undifferentiated cellular types. Signals include mechanical forces, bioelectric potentials, hormones, enzymes, oxygen tension, and other similar agents. Within each cell, a chain of reactions then passes through the cytoplasm to and from the nucleus, endoplasmic reticulum, or organelles such as lysosomes and mitochondria, ending either in (1) output of secretions such as alkaline and acid phosphatase, ground substance (protein mucopolysaccharides), and collagen; or (2) differentiation by cell divisions and maturation into specific tissue types comprising cartilage, bone, periosteum, muscle, epithelia, blood vessels, and lengthening nerves. Ongoing activating signals are "intrinsic" during development, but, as emphasized herein, are subject to clinical modification that then alters regulation of the same underlying biology. This affects the **timing** and **duration** of the cellular activity, and the growth **vectors** (magnitude and direction). It is the selective nature of the signals that governs the pattern of developmental activity that leads to variations in morphology, not any real change in the growth biology itself.

Regional Control of Development

Replacing the archaic notion of "master growth control centers" of yes-teryear, is the understanding that tissues within each **local** area contain an array of cell types carrying out the specific developmental requirements of that area. Sensitive to the play of "primary messengers" (activating signals) relating to particular localized **functions** and structural relation-ships, each and every location has a developing size and shape that is custom-made by its own "genic" cells receiving the local information that determines it. Because the local signals continuously change, regional size and shape correspondingly and progressively adapt. Complex architectonic combinations of regional parts, such as those comprising the mandible and maxilla as a whole and all of the soft tissues associated with them, achieve their differentiating morphology by continuous adjustments among the de-veloping local parts (condyles, coronoid processes, tuberosities, alveolar sockets, tubercles, etc.). This provides a precise and ongoing "fit" among all of them. Everything continues to function all the while.

With regard to the "goodness of fit" of separate bones, muscles, teeth, blood vessels, and all other such anatomic parts to each other, consider several examples illustrating the remarkable developmental interplay characterizing "growth." This interplay is a key factor that makes the whole thing work. When dealing with the growth process, we sometimes forget to appreciate this, or, actually, don't even think of it at all.

For example, a tooth **precisely** matches its alveolar socket in shape, size, and the timing of developmental changes and movements during growth. The osteogenic and fibrogenic periodontal connective tissue (1) shapes and progressively reshapes the bony socket, (2) moves the tooth (drift and eruption) by mechanical traction forces mediated by the collag-enous fibers of the periodontal connective tissue, (3) moves the socket by remodeling, and (4) remodels its own periodontal connective tissue (fibro-genic) to sustain continuous attachment and to move itself in precise lock step with the moving tooth and bone.[†]

Another example of "goodness of fit" is a cranial nerve with its sheath of vascular connective tissue passing through a basicranial foramen. The configurational and dimensional fit and the positioning of the foramen must be absolutely perfect. As the nerve constantly moves with the grow-ing brain, the remodeling of the bony passage precisely conforms. If such were not the case, development itself would reach a dead end. (See page 103 Chapter 6 for further phylogenic insight.) Another example is the pre-cise match of a bony tuberosity to which a muscle inserts. There can be no misfit whatever between the two. The match is perfect because of their constant histogenic interplay. Also, any given bone fits precisely within its articular joint. Actually, tissues everywhere throughout the whole body involve virtually limitless adaptive interactions as a part of the growth process, and function continues all the while it happens.

Figure 1−7 schematizes this process. Although the growth activities involved are separated into little boxes, in real life such isolation of rela-tionships, of course, is not possible because of the interdependence among them. This is one basic reason why so many laboratory experiments ad-dressing the "determinants of growth" have historically yielded equivocal results: either (1) **all** of the categories were not taken into account (almost always), or (2) the experimental design often calls for separation of the

[†]It is this same histogenic ("growth") process that is utilized in orthodontic tooth move-ment. Only the signals are changed in order to alter the directions and amounts of tooth movement.

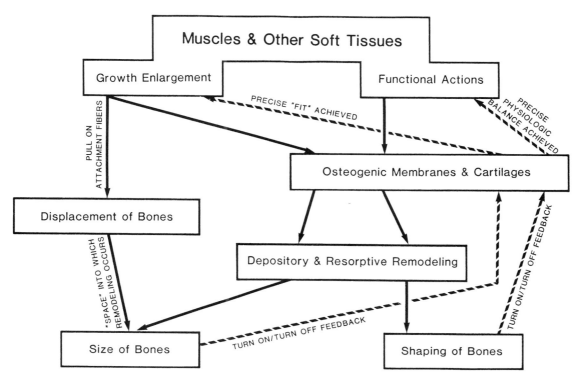

FIGURE 1–7. See text for discussion. (From Enlow, D. H.: Structural and functional "balance" during craniofacial growth. In: *Orthodontics: State of the Art, Essence of the Science*. Ed. by L. W. Graber, St. Louis, C. V. Mosby, 1986, with permission.)

categories in order to attempt to control variables, but which simply cannot be done. (See also later chapters.)

THE THREE PRINCIPAL REGIONS OF FACIAL AND NEUROCRANIAL DEVELOPMENT

The major but mutually interrelated form/function components involved in development are the brain with its associated sensory organs and basicranium, the facial and pharyngeal airway, and the oral complex. Although discussed below separately, they are, of course, developmentally inseparable. This interrelation factor is important in the clinical application of growth concepts since the developmental factors underlying most craniofacial dysplasias involve all three.

The Brain and Basicranium

The configuration of the neurocranium (and brain) determines a person's headform type which, in turn, sets up many of the proportionate and topographic features characterizing facial type. A long and narrow basicranium (dolichocephalic) with its more elongate and open-angle configuration, for example, programs the developmental process so that it characteristically leads to an anteroposteriorly and vertically elongate facial pattern and a more frequent built-in tendency for mandibular retrusion (Fig. 1–8, top).

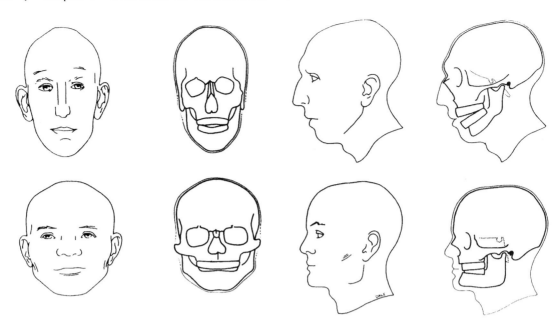

FIGURE 1–8. (From Enlow, D. H., and J. Dale: In: *Oral Histology*, 4th Ed. Ed. by R. Ten Cate, St. Louis, C. V. Mosby, 1994, with permission.)

A rounder basicranium (brachycephalic) is characterized by a proportionately wider but anteroposteriorly shorter configuration, a more obtuse basicranial flexure, and a vertically and protrusively shorter but wider midface (nasomaxillary complex). These features generally underlie a more orthognathic (or less retrognathic) profile or, in the extreme, a tendency for mandibular or bimaxillary protrusion (Fig. 1–8, bottom).

These characteristic features exist because the basicranium is the template that establishes the shape and perimeter of the facial growth field. The mandible attaches by its condyles onto the ectocranial side of the middle endocranial fossae, and the bicondylar dimension is thus determined by this part of the cranial floor. The nasomaxillary complex is suspended from the anterior endocranial fossae, and the width of the facial airway, the configuration of the palate and maxillary arch, and the placement of all these parts are thus established by it.

The Airway

The facial and pharyngeal airway is a space determined by the multitude of separate parts comprising its enclosing walls. The configuration and dimensions of the airway are thus a product of the composite growth and development of many hard and soft tissues along its pathway from nares to glottis.

Although determined by surrounding parts, those parts in turn are dependent upon the airway for maintenance of their own functional and anatomic positions. If there develops any regional childhood variation along the course of the airway that significantly alters its configuration or size, growth then proceeds along a different course, leading to a variation in overall facial assembly that may exceed the bounds of normal pattern. The airway functions, in a real sense, as a keystone for the face. A keystone, as you know, is that part of an arch which, if of proper shape and size, stabilizes the positions of the remaining parts of the arch. In Figure

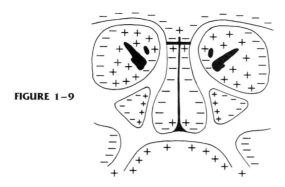

FIGURE 1–9

1–9 a few of the many "arches" in a face can be recognized, and the bony remodeling (+ and −) producing them. Horizontally and vertically, the archform of the orbits, the nasal and oral sides of the palate, the maxillary arch, the sinuses, the zygomatic arches, and so forth are all subject to airway configuration, size, and integrity. Note that the airway is strategically pivotal to all of them.

Two easy personal tests can be performed illustrating the airway as a significant factor in programming the developmental course of the facial "genic" tissues. This is useful in explanations of malocclusion etiology for patients or their parents.

First, starting with an open mouth, close the lips and jaws, noticing that you likely raise the tongue against the palate and, momentarily, swallow. This evacuates the oral air into the pharynx, creating an oral vacuum. The effect is to stabilize the mandible and hold it in a closed position with minimal muscle effort. Now, open the jaws and lips, feeling a rush of air into the mouth. To hold the lower jaw in this "mouth breathing" posture requires a different pattern of muscle activity, and the osteogenic, chondrogenic, periodontal, fibrogenic, and other histogenic tissues thereby receive a correspondingly different pattern of signals. This causes different developmental responses to a different functional morphology adapted to the conditions. As emphasized before, the operation of the growth process itself functions normally. It is the nature of the **activating signals** that produces emerging deviations in the course of development that results in any morphologic variation and perhaps malocclusion.

Another test is similar. With closed jaws and lips compared to open, try swallowing. Open-jawed swallows are possible, but can be difficult when one is accustomed to a closed mouth. Note the very different pattern of masticatory and hyoid muscle actions required. As with the mouth-breathing test outlined above, altered signals are generated, and the genic tissues work toward a different balance combination, producing a variation in facial morphology. A factor often overlooked by clinicians is that these altered signals may result in different treatment responses to the same intervention. For example, a patient's response to a Frankel appliance may vary dramatically based upon the patient's mode of breathing.

The Oral Region

In addition to the basicranial and airway factors described above affecting mandibular and maxillary shape, size, and positioning, other basic considerations are involved. If a brain and basicranial asymmetry exists, this condition can either be (1) passed on to cause a corresponding facial asymmetry, or (2) compensated by the facial developmental process to either offset or reduce its magnitude. For the latter, remodeling adjustments produce an actual opposite asymmetry in the nasomaxillary complex and/or mandible that counteracts the basicranial condition.

For the maxilla, if not developmentally compensated or only partially so, the maxillary arch can become deviated laterally, matching the lateral asymmetry of the anterior endocranial fossae. (See Thimaporn et al., 1990.) Or, vertically, one side can become lowered or elevated relative to the other, including the orbits, palate, and maxillary arch. For the mandible, the middle endocranial fossae determine the placement of the temporomandibular joints and, if asymmetric, one or the other will be lower or higher, forward or back. Whole-mandible alignment necessarily follows if not fully or partially adjusted by remodeling during development.

Many other such compensatory adjustments by the remodeling process occur throughout growth and development in many ways, as discussed in subsequent chapters. It involves the development of certain regional imbalances to offset others, resulting in a composite overall structural and functional equilibrium.

Craniofacial Levels

There exists a descending, cause-and-effect stratographic arrangement of structural **levels** in the design of the face. Beginning with the frontal lobes of the cerebrum, the floor of the anterior endocranial fossae become adapted in size and shape during their interrelated development. The ectocranial side of this floor is the roof of the nasal chambers, thus programming the perimeter of that key facial part of the airway. This configuration, in turn, is projected inferiorly to the next level, establishing the proportions and configuration of the nasal side of the palate. Then, the perimeter of the apical base of the maxillary dental arch is set by the oral side of the hard palate, all representing configurational projections from the anterior endocranial fossae. The next level following is the maxillary cuspal arch, and then the mandibular bony and dental arches, all preprogrammed in configuration and proportions in descending order from the basicranium.

The mandible has a component not represented in the maxilla, and that is its **ramus**. The anteroposterior size of the ramus develops by an amount approximating the horizontal span of the pharynx, which has a programmed anteroposterior dimension established by **its** ceiling, which is the ectocranial side of the middle endocranial fossae underlying the temporal lobes of the cerebrum. The ramus, thus, places the mandibular arch in occlusion with the maxillary arch following a pattern set up by the basicranium. Vertically, the developing ramus lowers the corpus by progressive amounts, adapting to the vertical growth of the middle cranial fossae (clivus) as well as the vertical expansion of the nasal airway and developing dentition.

The face, thus, is a stratified series of vertical levels all sharing a common developmental template. This makes possible a workable morphogenic system having a structural design allowing large numbers of separate parts to develop together in harmony and to carry out respective functions while it happens.

The Two Basic Clinical Targets

There is one developmental concept that needs to be addressed with particular emphasis because of its great significance to the old clinical axiom "working with growth." While a factor such as the basicranium can prescibe and determine a "growth field" in the contiguous facial complex, as described above, it is within the boundaries of that field that **remodeling** then engineers the **shape and size and functional fit** of all parts and develops them through time. However, it can be misunderstood if one presumes that all "local growth" is regulated solely by a single local, intrinsic growth system. Remember, there are **two** kinds of growth activity: (1) localized, regional **remodeling** ("genic" tissues), and (2) the **displacement** movements of all the separate parts as they remodel. Thus, there are two corresponding histogenic recipients of clinical intervention.

To illustrate this fundamental concept, the incisor and premaxillary alveolar region of the maxilla develops into its adult shape and dimensions by the local remodeling process. But the principal source of the considerable extent of its downward-and-forward growth movement is by displacement, and **that** comes from biomechanical forces of growth enlargement occurring **outside** the premaxillary region itself. Thus, most of the growth movements responsible for the anatomic **placement** of this region, along with, passively, its teeth, are not controlled within its own tissues or any genetic blueprint therein, even though this might be a natural presumption. **Two** clinical targets thereby exist for orthodontists: local remodeling and, separately, the displacement of some whole part produced by the sum of developmental expansions occurring everywhere. There are certain clinical procedures that relate specifically to one or the other target, and some that involve both. For example, rapid palatal expansion mimics displacement; incisor retraction primarily involves remodeling of the anterior portion of the alveolar arch, and Bionator treatment involves both remodeling of the alveolar process and displacement via changes in the ramus.

These two basic growth movements are often not separated in the clinical literature. Unfortunately, this historical oversight severely limits the clinician's ability to provide a biologic explanation of how any given treatment procedure actually operates.

Child-to-Adult Changing Proportions

The three principal craniofacial growing parts (brain and basicranium, airway, oral region) each has its own separate timetable of development even though all are inseparately bound as an interrelated whole. Some body systems, such as the nervous and cardiovascular systems, develop earlier and faster compared to others, including the airway and oral regions. The reason is that airway growth is proportionate to growing body and lung size, and the oral region is linked to developmental stages involving the fifth and seventh cranial nerves and associated musculature, the suckling process, dental eruption stages, and masticatory development.

The infant and young child are characterized by a wide-appearing face because of the precociously broad basicranial template, but the face otherwise is vertically short (Fig. 1–10). This is because the nasal and oral regions are yet diminutive, matching the smallish body and pulmonary parts and with masticatory development in a transitory state. The mandibular ramus is vertically yet short because it is linked in developmental feedback with the shorter, later-maturing nasal and dental regions. Masticatory musculature is proportionately sized and shaped to progressively match increasing function and to interplay developmentally with the ramus.

During later childhood and into adolescence, vertical nasal enlargement keeps pace with growing body and lung size, and dental and other oral components have approached adult sizes and configuration. The mandibular arch is lowered by increasing vertical ramus length. Overall, the early

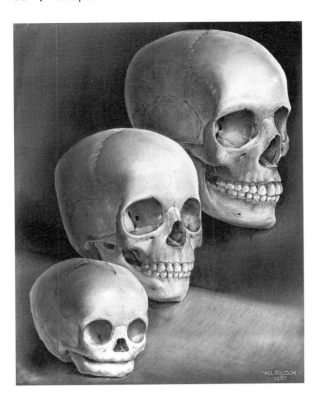

FIGURE 1–10. (Courtesy of William L. Brudon. From Enlow, D. H.: *The Human Face.* New York, Harper & Row, 1968, with permission.)

wide face has become altered in proportion by the later vertical changes. The end effect is particularly marked in the dolichocephalic long-headed and long-face pattern, and less so in the brachycephalic headform type.

Tooth Movement

As with all other sections of this introductory chapter, the subject of how a tooth undergoes intrinsic growth or clinical movements is elaborated in subsequent pages.

To begin, a tooth is moved by either or both of two developmental means: (1) by becoming actively moved in combination with its own remodeling periodontal connective tissue and alveolar socket; and (2) by being carried along passively as each entire maxilla or mandible becomes displaced anteroinferiorly during facial morphogenesis. A second basic and clinically significant concept is that **bone and connective tissues** (such as the periodontal connective tissue, periosteum, endosteum, and submucosa, all of which participate directly and actively in a tooth's movement) have an intrinsic remodeling process that, when activated, move themselves as a growth function. When a tooth is moved, these other contiguous parts move with it by their own "genic" remodeling process to sustain relationships. A tooth, however, **cannot move itself** in a comparable manner by its own remodeling. It is mobile, but not motile. A tooth is **moved** by a biomechanical force external to the tooth itself, and there is an elaborate "biology" in the composite process that produces a tooth's growth movements. A tooth must move (drift, erupt, etc.) during maxillary and mandibular growth in order to become properly placed in progressively changing anatomic positions (see Chapters 3, 4, and 5). Whether the force producing the tooth's change in position is intrinsic *or clinically induced*, the actual biology is the same. As mentioned again because the point is important, it is the nature of the activating **signals** that is different, and this causes (1) the multiple array of genic tissues to alter the course of remodeling or (2) the displacement process of a whole bone to become altered in direction or magnitude.

Drift

A worthy advance was made when it was realized that teeth undergo a process of *drift*. For many years this fundamental concept was limited to horizontal (mesial and distal) movements, and the essential function was held to be a stabilization of the dental palisade to compensate for interproximal attrition. Added to this, now, is that drift has a basic **growth** function. It serves to anatomically place the teeth as the maxilla and mandible enlarge. Such movements are significant considering that a jawbone lengthens considerably from prenatal to adult sizes. Also, the original drift concept was for horizontal movement. Important to the clinician, now, is awareness that teeth, especially maxillary, have a marked **vertical** extent of drift. This is in addition to "eruption" and should not be so termed. **Vertical drift** is a basic growth movement the clinician "works with" because it can be modified by clinical intervention (i.e., orthodontic treatment).

Just as teeth undergo a drifting movement, the bone housing them also moves. Unlike a tooth, however, bone moves by the remodeling action of its enclosing osteogenic membranes, and this is also a direct target for clinical intervention. The intrinsic coordination of these bone-tooth movements is remarkable.

A Fundamental Principle of Growth

It has been emphasized in the preceding pages that facial growth is a process requiring intimate morphogenic **interrelationships** among all of its component growing, changing, and functioning soft and hard tissue parts. No part is developmentally independent and self-contained. This is a fundamental and very important principle of growth. As underscored earlier, the growth process works toward an ongoing state of composite functional and structural equilibrium. In clinical treatment, no key anatomic part can be fully segregated and altered without affecting "balance" with other parts and their state of physiologic equilibrium as well.

In essence, orthodontic treatment seeks to maximize the effectiveness of anatomic compensations to achieve an aesthetically harmonious masticatory system.

2

Basic Growth Concepts

An in-depth understanding of facial morphogenesis is essential so that the clinician as well as the research biologist can properly grasp (1) differences between "normal" and ranges of abnormal; (2) biologic reasons for these differences and the virtually limitless variations involved; (3) reasons for rationales utilized in diagnosis, treatment planning, and selection of appropriate clinical procedures; and (4) the biologic factors underlying the important clinical problems of retention, rebound, and relapse after treatment.

It was emphasized in the previous chapter that one of the most important elements of the facial growth process is that two separate but closely interrelated systems of **movement** exist—remodeling and displacement. For remodeling, a bone (or any other kind of organ or tissue composite) is not simply "modeled" when it first appears prenatally. It cannot simply grow by new additions keeping the same form. That is not possible given the architectonically complex designs involved. Because some areas of any given part grow faster or to a greater extent than others, *re*modeling is a necessary growth function. Then, when bones and all other kinds of organs enlarge, they must necessarily all move away from each other to allow for the enlargement. Because these movements are primary clinical targets, **how** it actually works is a fundamental consideration. Historically, there have been spirited arguments over the underlying theory. Surprisingly, however, even to this day, the rationale of many clinical procedures (e.g., Frankel function regulators, bionators and activators) seldom takes the remodeling and displacement factor fully into account. This is one of the basic reasons why the actual biology of these procedures remains incompletely understood.

The following pages will address the remodeling process first. The craniofacial skeleton initially is emphasized because the bones represent the head as a whole as seen in radiographs. This displacement process is then described, and a developmental merger of the two is presented in the following chapter.

REMODELING

A lay person's natural perception of "growth" is often quite incorrect. A bone such as the mandible **does not** grow simply by generalized, uniform

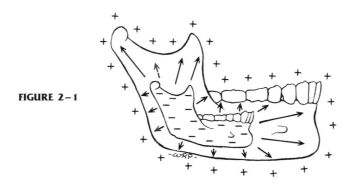

FIGURE 2-1

deposition of new bone (+) on all outside surfaces (Fig. 2-1), with corresponding resorption (-) from all inside surfaces, as one might erroneously presume (and as has often been incorrectly taught). It is not possible for bones having the complex morphology of, for example, the mandible or the maxilla to increase in size by such a growth process. Because of the topographically complex nature of each bone's shape, the bone must have a **differential** mode of enlargement, in which some of its parts and areas grow much faster and to a much greater extent than others. Many of the **external** surfaces of most bones are actually **resorptive** in nature. In Figure 2-2, **fields** of surface resorption (darkly shaded) and deposition (lightly shaded) blanket the whole bone. How can a bone increase in size, even though many outside (periosteal) surfaces undergo resorptive removal as the bone grows? Keep this question in mind as the processes of facial growth are explained in the pages that follow.

The reason a bone must remodel* during growth is because its regional parts must become **moved** (Fig. 2-3). This calls for sequential remodeling changes in the shape and size of each region. The mandibular ramus, for example, moves progressively posteriorly by a combination of deposition and resorption. As it does so, the anterior part of the ramus becomes **remodeled** into a new addition for the mandibular corpus. This produces a growth elongation of the corpus. This progressive, sequential movement of component parts as a bone enlarges is termed **relocation**. The whole ramus is thus relocated posteriorly, and the posterior part of the lengthening corpus becomes relocated into the area previously occupied by the ramus. Structural remodeling from what **used to be** part of the ramus into what then **becomes** a new part of the corpus takes place. The corpus grows longer as a result.

The mandible remodels differentially in directions that are predominantly posterior and superior. Even though successive remodeling of one part into another constantly takes place as the whole bone enlarges, the form of the bone as a whole is sustained (with some characteristic age changes in shape). It is remarkable that the external morphologic characteristics of any given bone are relatively constant, even though its sub-

---

*Four different kinds of remodeling occur in bone tissues. One is biochemical remodeling, taking place at the molecular level. This involves the constant deposition and removal of ions to maintain blood calcium levels and carry out other mineral homeostasis functions. Another type of remodeling involves the secondary reconstruction of bone by haversian systems and also the rebuilding of cancellous trabeculae. A third kind of remodeling relates to the regeneration and reconstruction of bone during or following disease and trauma. The remodeling process that we are dealing with in facial morphogenesis, however, is **growth remodeling**. In order for a bone to grow and enlarge, it must also undergo a simultaneous process of remodeling.

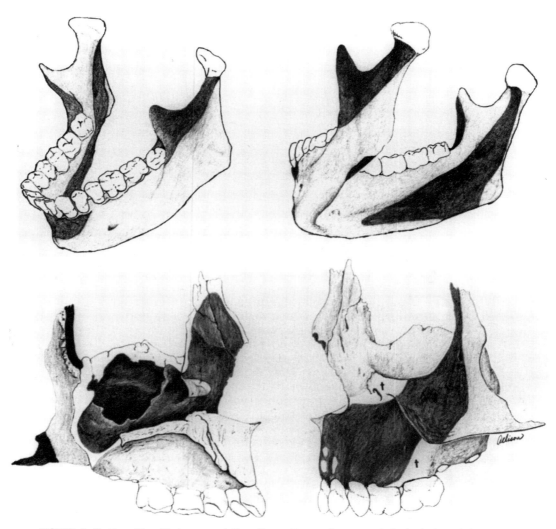

FIGURE 2–2. *Top,* Mandibular remodeling. Resorptive surfaces are dark shaded, and depository surfaces are unshaded. *Bottom,* Maxillary remodeling. (From Moyers, R., and D. Enlow. Growth of the craniofacial skeleton. In: *Handbook of Orthodontics,* 4th Ed. Chicago, Mosby-Year Book, Inc. 1988, with permission.)

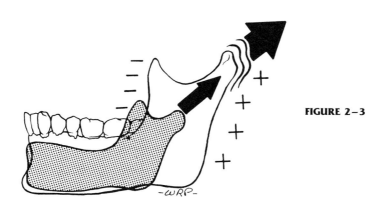

FIGURE 2–3

stance undergoes massive internal changes and all its parts experience widespread alterations in regional shape and size as they are relocated. This is the special function of growth remodeling; it **maintains** the form of a whole bone while providing for its enlargement at the same time. Thus, remodeling is not a process that functions essentially to alter overall shape, although some degree of this is also involved. Although the term "remodeling" implies such change, the actual changes produced by growth remodeling are mostly those that deal with the sequential **relocation** of the bone's component parts.

Bone produced by the covering membrane ("periosteal bone") constitutes about half of all the cortical bone tissue present; bone laid down by the lining membrane ("endosteal bone") makes up the other half (Fig. 2–4). In this diagram, note how the cortex on the right was formed by the periosteum and the cortex on the left by the endosteum as both sides shifted (drifted) in unison to the right.

The surface that faces **toward** the direction of movement is depository (+). The opposite surface, facing away from the growth direction, is resorptive (−). If the rates of deposition and resorption are equal, the thickness of the cortex remains constant. If deposition exceeds resorption, overall size and cortical thickness gradually increase. In Figure 2–5, the pattern of growth fields results in a **rotation** of the skeletal part shown. Such rotations are a significant part of the developmental process of the face and cranium, as will be seen later. See also page 34.

The operation of the remodeling fields covering and lining the surfaces of a bone is actually carried out by the osteogenic **membranes** and other surrounding tissues, rather than by the hard part of the bone. The bone does not "grow itself"; growth is produced by the **soft tissue matrix** that encloses each whole bone. The genetic and functional determinants of bone growth reside in the composite of soft tissues that turn on and turn off, or speed up and slow down, the histogenic actions of the osteogenic connective tissues (periosteum, endosteum, sutures, periodontal membrane, etc.). Growth is not "programmed" within the calcified part of the bone itself. The "blueprint" for the design, construction, and growth of a bone thus lies in the muscles, tongue, lips, cheeks, integument, mucosae, connective tissues, nerves, blood vessels, airway, pharynx, the brain as an organ mass, tonsils, adenoids, and so forth, all of which provide information signals that pace a bone's development by its osteogenic tissues.

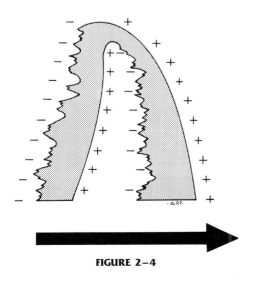

FIGURE 2–4

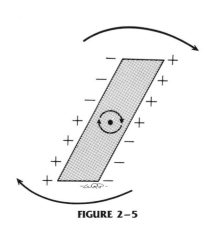

FIGURE 2–5

Fields that have some special significance or noteworthy role in the growth process are often called growth **sites**. The mandibular condyle, for example, is such a growth site (Fig. 2–6). Remember, however, that growth does not occur just at such special growth sites, as is sometimes presumed. The entire bone participates. **All** surfaces are, in fact, sites of growth, whether specially designated or not. The old term "condylar growth" is still often used. It is misleading, however, because it mistakenly implies that the condyle is **the** growth center largely responsible for overall mandibular growth and development. If only condylar growth were operative, the condyle would sit on an elongated neck as a giraffe's head perches high on its neck. The **entire** ramus, together with its condyle, participates actively and directly. Clinical interventions designed to manipulate mandibular growth must necessarily achieve therapeutic effects by altering the entire ramus and not merely by affecting "condylar growth."

In Figure 2–7, the osteogenic connective tissue overlying field a moves to a^1. The underlying area of bone beneath it is remodeled and moves under its control. This remodeling field is thus relocated to occupy the region located just posteriorly. A **reversal line** (x) separates field a from the area of the ramus behind it, and moves to x^1. The resorptive field in the larger mandible (a^1) occupies the same **relative** position as when it was smaller during the former growth stage (a). The overlying osteogenic field, however, is now larger and has moved to a new location, relocating its underlying bone with it by continuous bone deposition and resorption (i.e., remodeling growth). Remember, the osteogenic connective tissue of the field moves by its own remodeling; the bone deep to it moves by remodeling (deposition and resorption) produced by this connective tissue. The actual bone tissue present in the ramus of the smaller stage has been replaced by a whole new generation of bone in the location occupied by the ramus of the larger stage following relocation. The **patterns of distribution** of all the various resorptive and depository fields, however, have not changed; the fields have only moved from one position to another as the whole bone enlarged. This requires sequential remodeling as any one field expands into areas previously occupied by other fields which, in turn, have moved on to hold successively new locations. The same developmental process continues, over and over again.

Although these growth movements are carried out by the osteogenic membranes and cartilages, the bone itself contributes feedback information to them so that as the size, shape, and biomechanical properties of the bone come into equilibrium with functional requirements, the histogenetic activity then becomes adjusted. Removable orthopedic devices such as the bionator seek to modify this biomechanical equilibrium to achieve a specified orthodontic treatment goal.

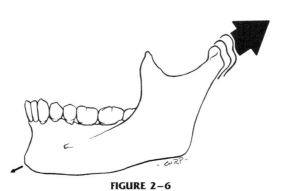

FIGURE 2–6　　　　　　　　　　　　　　　　**FIGURE 2–7**

Fields of Remodeling

As already seen, resorptive and depository **fields** of growth blanket all of the outside and inside surfaces of a bone (Fig. 2–2). This mosaic pattern is more or less constant for each bone throughout the growth period, unless a major change in the shape of a region becomes involved. As the perimeter of each of these growth fields enlarges, the parts of the bone associated with them correspondingly increase in size. As emphasized earlier, of course, the actual operation of these fields of growth is performed by the enclosing osteogenic connective tissues. The bone itself is the product of this field activity. Thus, during the operation of the relocation process, it is the growth fields formed by the "genic" connective tissues that first move and control the relocation movements of the underlying bony parts associated with each field. The growth movement of the bone **follows** the pace-setting movement of the overlying growth field. There is virtually no lag time, however, between the two.

Variations in facial configuration are always the rule. No two faces are quite alike. Morphologic variations, normal and abnormal, are produced by corresponding developmental variations that take place during the growth process. Some can be genetically established by characteristic soft tissue relationships that are hereditary determinants of bone growth. Other variations are largely determined by functional changes in soft tissue relationships during an individual's own development. The results, however, are all based on the following factors that establish the nature of anatomic variations in an individual person:

1.   Fundamental differences in the **pattern** of the fields of resorption and deposition, that is, the distribution of the growth fields in an individual person.
2.   The specific placement of the **boundaries** between growth fields; that is, the size and shape of any given growth field.
3.   The differential **rates** and **amounts** of deposition and resorption throughout each field.
4.   The **timing** of the growth activities among the different fields.

Understanding the regional growth field concept and the operation of the remodeling process is basic for the clinician. Clinicians must also understand how the complementary process of displacement operates (described later), and how an individual's growth variations can occur. The question can be one of working "with" or "against" the intrinsic morphogenic processes in the use of different orthodontic procedures. Does a given procedure, for example, harness the same intrinsic regional remodeling or displacement direction, but with alteration of magnitude? For example, the use of extra oral forces to distalize the maxillary molars moves these teeth into an area of depository growth activity. Such tooth movement may favorably augment the remodeling pattern in the tuberosity area, resulting in a more stable orthodontic correction. Or, is a direction actually changed, perhaps with severe violations of remodeling field boundaries and balance, leading to rebound? For example, labial movement of lower incisors to reduce crowding places those teeth in an area of bone normally undergoing resorption. This creates the potential for biologic failure because normally new bone is not forming in this area.

As mentioned, the mandibular condyle is a specially recognized growth **site**. The condyle and some other special sites have sometimes been termed growth **centers**. This label has come into disfavor, however, because it is now understood that such a site does not actually control the growth processes of the bone as a whole. They are not "master centers" that directly regulate the overall morphogenic process of the entire bone and all its regional parts. Although developmentally unique (see Chapter 4), they represent only regional fields of growth adapted to the localized morphogenic circumstances in their own particular areas, just as all other regional developmental sites are locally adapted. Growth "centers" are a conceptual anachronism.

Routine headfilms, of course, are **two-dimensional,** and this is a limitation that presents many troublesome problems. Only the anterior and posterior **edges** of the ramus, for example, can be visualized (as at *A* and *B*) in lateral cephalograms (Fig. 2–8). Important changes on surfaces in the span **between** these edges (*C*) cannot be visualized. This is all the more reason for the clinician and researcher to thoroughly understand what happens when such areas grow in a **three-dimensional** manner not representable by the headfilm itself.

Implant Markers

Metallic implants (tiny pieces of tantalum or some other appropriate metal) are often used as radiographic markers in clinical and experimental work to study bone remodeling and displacement in headfilms. Using the markers as registration points when superimposing serial headfilm tracings, one can readily determine the amount and direction of remodeling as well as displacement movements.

If a metallic marker is implanted on the depository side of a cortex, it becomes progressively more deeply embedded in the cortex as new bone continues to form on the surface and as resorption takes place from the other side. Eventually, the marker would become translocated from one side of the cortex to the other, not because of its own movement (the marker itself is immobile), but because of the "flow" of the drifting bone around it.

If two implants are placed across from each other on the two sides of a joint (suture, synchondrosis, temporomandibular joint [TMJ]), the distance of their separation, subsequent to a period of growth, indicates the direction and amount of displacement as well as the total extent of bone deposition on these two joint surfaces. Vital dyes (alizarin, procion, tetracycline, etc.) can also be used to determine the sequence and amount of new bone formation as well as specific locations utilizing histologic sections.

The "V" Principle

A most useful and basic concept in facial growth is the V principle (Fig. 2–9). Many facial and cranial bones, or parts of bones, have a V-shaped configuration (or a funnel-shape in three dimensions). Note that bone deposition occurs on the **inner** side of the V; resorption takes place on the outside surface. The V thereby **moves** from position *A* to *B* and, at the same time, **increases** in overall dimensions. The direction of movement is toward the wide end of the V. Thus, a simultaneous growth movement and enlargement proceeds by additions of bone on the inside with removal from the outside. The V principle will be referred to many times in later explanations of the facial growth process.

The Relocation Function of Remodeling

Why do bones remodel as they grow? The key factor is the process of **relocation**. To illustrate, in the stack of chips in Figure 2–10, the black

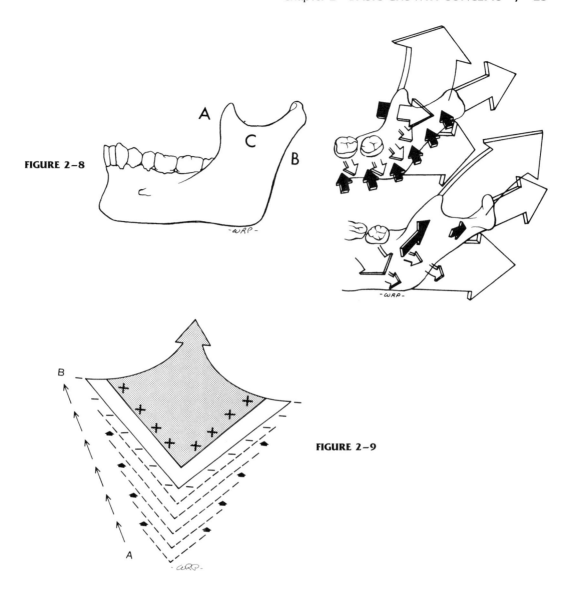

FIGURE 2–8

FIGURE 2–9

chip is at the right end in *a* at the level of the condyle in the smallest
mandibular stage. This location then becomes translocated "across" the
ramus to lie at the level of the anterior margin in the third stage. As
"growth" has continued to take place, the black chip became progressively
"relocated"—not by its own movement, but because new chips have been
added on one side and removed from the other. This changes the **relative
position** of the black chip within the stack, even though this chip itself
does not move. Let the stack of chips represent a whole growing area
having complex topographic shape, such as the ramus, rather than a perfectly cylindrical form. It is apparent that the changing relative positions
of the black chip would require continuous **remodeling** of the shape and
sectional dimensions to conform with each successive position the chip
comes to occupy. A **sequence** of continuous remodeling changes is required level by level. Remodeling is a process of **reshaping** and **resizing**
each level (chip) within a growing bone as it is relocated sequentially into

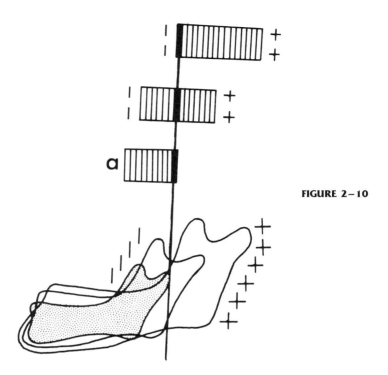

FIGURE 2–10

a succession of new levels. This is because additions and/or resorption in the various **other** parts cause changes in the relative positions of all levels. Note that the **position** of the condyle in the smallest mandibular stage becomes relocated into the middle of the ramus and then onto the anterior border of the ramus. Continuous remodeling is thus involved as this and all other areas change in relative position.

In the face of a young child, the levels of the maxillary arch and nasal floor lie very close to the inferior orbital rim. The maxillary arch and palate, however, **move** downward. This process involves (in part) an inferior direction of **remodeling** by the hard palate and the bony maxillary arch (Fig. 2–11). Bone deposition occurs on the downward-facing oral surface, together with resorption from the superior-facing nasal surface of the palate. The combination results in a downward **relocation** of the whole palate and maxillary arch composite into the progressively lower levels, so that the arch finally comes to lie considerably below the inferior orbital rim. The vertical dimension of the nasal chamber is greatly increased as a result.

About half of the external surfaces involved in these growth and remodeling examples are resorptive and half depository. About half of the bone tissue of the palate is thus endosteal and half periosteal. (The cortex on the nasal side of the palate is produced by the endosteum of the medullary cavity.)

Because of the **relocation** process, the inferior nasal region of the adult occupies an area where the bony maxillary arch **used to be** located during earlier childhood (Fig. 2–12). What was once the bony maxillary arch and palatal region has been converted into the expanded nasal region. This is "growth remodeling"; the basis for it is **relocation**.

As the palate and arch grow downward by constant deposition of new bone on one side and resorption of previously formed bone from the other, the bone tissue that comes to house the teeth at older age periods is not

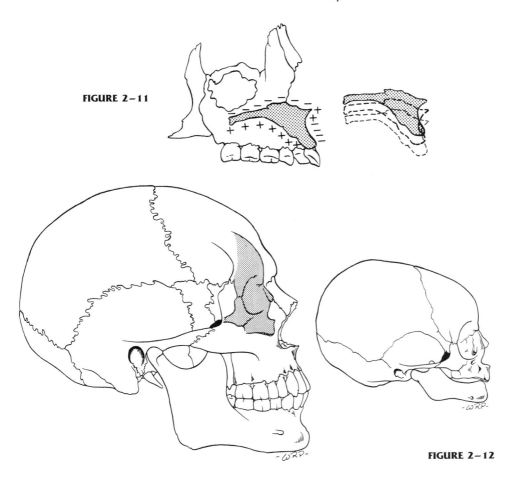

FIGURE 2–11

FIGURE 2–12

the same actual bone enclosing them during the succession of former growth levels. This is significant because the growth movement and the exchanges of bone involved are **used** by the orthodontist to "work with growth." (See "vertical drift" Chapter 3 and 5.)

It was shown above that as the mandible grows, the ramus moves in a backward direction by appropriate combinations of resorption and deposition. As the ramus is **relocated** posteriorly, the corpus becomes **lengthened by a remodeling conversion** from what was at one time the ramus during a former growth period (Fig. 2–3). During growth from the fetus to the adult, the "molar" region in the younger mandible, for example, undergoes relocation to occupy the "premolar" region of the larger, older mandible. It is apparent that remodeling is a process of relocation and that the same **deposition and resorption producing growth enlargement is the same that also carries out the growth remodeling process.** See page 5 for the multiple functions of remodeling.

A transverse section through the zygomatic arch in Figure 2–13 demonstrates how a bone relocates laterally as the whole bone simultaneously grows in length. The zygomatic arch is moving and enlarging laterally and also inferiorly as the entire face, brain, and cranium widen and expand into space formerly occupied by the zygomatic arch. It does this by progressive deposition on the lateral-facing and downward-facing periosteal and endosteal surfaces, with resorption from the opposite cortical sides. The remnants of the old cortical contours can be recognized in microscopic

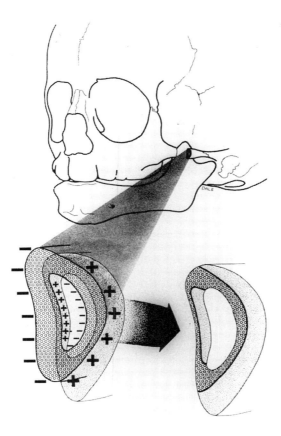

FIGURE 2-13. (From Enlow D., and J. Dale. Childhood facial growth and development. In: *Oral Histology*, 4th Ed. Ed. by R. Ten Cate. St. Louis, C. V. Mosby, 1990, with permission.)

sections. The right and left zygomatic arches thus grow out and away as the rest of the head enlarges between. The arches also increase in size to accommodate the growing muscles attached to them. (Note: Half of the bone tissue is endosteal in origin, and half is periosteal. Half of the inner and outer surfaces are resorptive, and half are depository.)

THE DISPLACEMENT PROCESS

In **remodeling**, the bone surface moves (relocates) by deposition on the side facing the direction of growth movements, as seen in Figure 2-13. In the process of **displacement**, however, the **whole** bone is **carried** by mechanical force as it simultaneously enlarges. Remodeling and displacement are separate processes, but always where **joints** (sutures, TMJ, synchondroses) are involved, they necessarily occur in conjunction with one another, since either one without the other is not possible. (See Fig. 1-5.)

The growth expansion of a single bone is a process by which its size, shape, and fitting develop in response to the composite of all the functional soft tissue relationships associated with that individual bone. The bone does not grow and enlarge in an isolated way, however. Its increases in size involve one or more articular contacts with **other** bones that are also enlarging at the same time. For this reason, as emphasized above, all articular contacts are important because they are the sites where displacement is involved. Articulations are the interface surfaces "away" from which the displacement movements proceed as each whole bones enlarges.

The amount of enlargement equals the extent of displacement. That is, a bone grows into the space being created as the whole bone is displaced by amounts determined by the extent of surrounding soft tissue enlargement. The enlargement of each bone thereby keeps pace with that of the soft tissues it serves in a mutually interrelated and controlled manner.

In the analogy shown in Figure 2–14, the expansion of a single balloon does not "compete" for space. However, if **two** enlarging balloons are in contact with each other, a displacing **movement** takes place until their positions become adjusted as either one or both expand. This movement proceeds away from the interface between the two balloons. What happens when the mandible, for example, grows in a direction **toward** its articular contact with the cranium? A "displacement" takes place in which the whole mandible moves **away** as it enlarges by an equal amount toward the temporal bone (Fig. 2–15).

Do the balloons **shove** each other apart **because** of the pushing force produced by the expansion? Or, are the balloons **carried** apart by other (outside) mechanical forces, with growth expansion **responding** by an equal amount to the separation, thereby maintaining the precise contact between them (Fig. 2–16)? In the first possibility, the extent of push (displacement) equals, but **follows**, the combined amount of expansion. In the second possibility, the extent of combined enlargement equals, but follows (virtually simultaneously), the amount of separation (displacement), with the balloons "growing" into the potential space being created. In other words, which is the primary (pacemaker) movement, displacement or remodeling enlargement? The question is more than academic; clinical treatment procedures utilize one or the other or both kinds of growth movements in response to clinical signals activating the appropriate "biology."

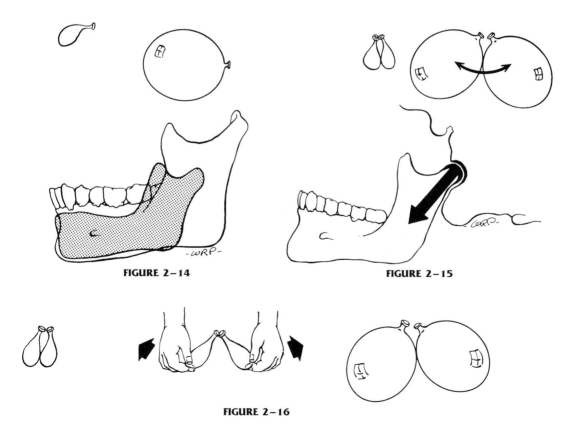

FIGURE 2–14   FIGURE 2–15

FIGURE 2–16

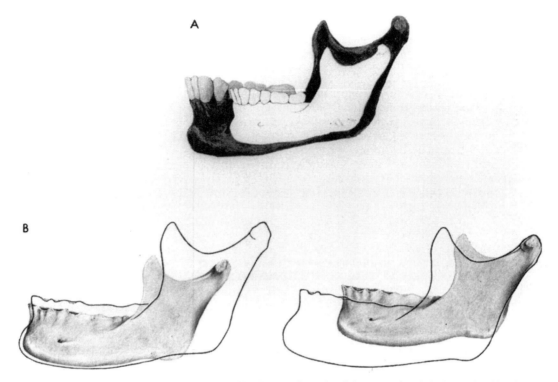

FIGURE 2–17. (From Moyers, R. E., and D. Enlow. Growth of the craniofacial skeleton. In: *Handbook of Orthodontics*, 4th Ed. Chicago, Mosby-Year Book, Inc., 1988, with permission.)

The above question has been, and still is, one of the great historical controversies in craniofacial biology. The mandible does not enlarge by simple, symmetrical expansion, as shown in Figure 2-17(A). Rather, it remodels by deposition and resorption in the manner shown in Figure 2–17(B). The predominant vectors (direction and magnitude) are posterior and superior. Thus, the condyle enlarges directly **toward** its articular contact in the glenoid fossa of the cranial floor.

As this takes place, the whole mandible is moved forward and downward by the same amount that it remodels upward and backward (Fig. 2–17 lower right). The direction of remodeling by new bone additions on the ramus and at the condyle and, separately, the direction of displacement are opposite to each other.

Is the forward and downward displacement movement of the mandible accomplished by a **shove** against the articular surface caused by the growth of the condyle, or conversely, by a **carry** of the entire mandible away from the basicranium[†] by mechanical forces (described in following chapters) extrinsic to the mandible itself (Fig. 2–18)? If the latter is true, bone remodeling follows secondarily (but virtually simultaneously) at the condyle and entire ramus to maintain constant contact with the temporal bone. As "force *a*" carries the mandible anteriorly and inferiorly, the con-

---

[†]The proper anatomic term in the context used here is **basicranium**, not "cranial base." The latter, more properly, is a radiographic term used in cephalometry and has a two-dimensional meaning with "collapse" to the midline. **Basicranium,** however, connotes the entire cranial floor, including the lateral parts where the condyles articulate, which is important to the present discussion.

dyle is **triggered to respond** in response to mutual developmental and functional signals by an equal amount of growth at *b*.

Is condylar growth thus the active cause of displacement (a "push" or "thrust") or the passive response to it? This was a heated controversy for many years. Current theory is outlined next.

In summary, two basic modes of skeletal movement take part in the growth of the face and neurocranium. **Remodeling** involves deposition of bone on any surface pointed toward the direction of enlargement of a given area; resorption usually occurs on the opposite side of that particular bony cortex (or cancellous trabecula). **Displacement** is a separate movement of the **whole bone** by some physical force that carries it, in toto, away from its contacts with other bones, which are also growing and increasing in overall size at the same time. This two-phase remodeling-displacement process takes place virtually simultaneously. The displacement movement is presently believed by many researchers to be the pacemaking (primary) change, with the rate and direction of bone growth representing a transformative (secondary) response. It can be argued, however, that the terms primary and secondary are biologically inappropriate for these two processes. Rather, they are each respondents to common signals that separately but simultaneously activate both to operate in unison. A widespread symphony of such interdependent movements proceeds throughout the craniofacial complex throughout growth.

There are, however, two different kinds of displacement that utilize these same two commonly used terms—primary and secondary. The word application here seems appropriate, since there is a basic difference in the source of movement. In **primary displacement**, the process of physical carry takes place in conjunction with a bone's **own** enlargement (Fig. 2–19). Two principal remodeling vectors in the maxilla, for example, are posterior and superior. As this occurs, the whole bone is displaced in opposite anterior and inferior directions. Primary displacement produces the "space" within which the bone continues to enlarge. The amount of this primary displacement exactly equals the amount of new bone deposition that takes place within articular contacts. The respective directions are always opposite in the primary type of displacement. Because primary displacement takes place at an interface with other, contiguous skeletal elements, **joint contacts** are thus important growth sites involved in this kind of remodeling change.

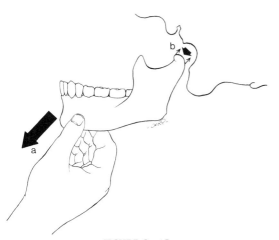

FIGURE 2–18

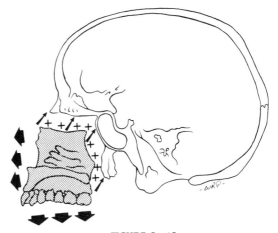

FIGURE 2–19

In **secondary displacement**, the movement of a bone and its soft tissues is not directly related to its own enlargement. For example, the anterior direction of growth by the middle cranial fossae and the temporal lobes of the cerebrum **secondarily** displaces the entire nasomaxillary complex anteriorly and inferiorly (Fig. 2–20). Midfacial growth and enlargement itself, however, is not "primarily" involved in this particular kind of displacement movement. Thus, as any bone develops, remodels, and becomes displaced in conjunction with its own growth process, it is also secondarily displaced, in addition, resulting from the growth of **other** bones and their soft tissues. This can have a "domino effect." That is, growth changes can be passed on from region to region to produce a secondary (spinoff) effect in areas quite distant. Such effects are cumulative.

Note that much of the anterior part of the midfacial region is **resorptive** in nature (see Fig. 1–3). Yet the face grows **forward**. How can this be? The face does not simply "grow" directly anteriorly. The forward movement is a **composite** result of growth changes (1) by resorption and deposition that cause the maxilla to **enlarge backward** and (2) by primary and secondary displacement movements that cause it to be **carried forward**. The resorptive nature of the anteriorly facing surface of the premaxilla is concerned primarily with its downward, not forward, remodeling, as explained in Chapter 5.

To illustrate the composite nature of these different growth processes, the growth of the arm is used as an analogy (Fig. 2–21). The tip of the finger moves away from the shoulder as the whole arms increases in length. Most of this growth movement of the finger, of course, is not a consequence of growth at the fingertip itself. The aggregate summation of linear growth increments by all the separate bones in the arm at each particular interface between the phalanges, carpals, metacarpals, radius, ulna, humerus, and scapula is involved. The contribution by the tip of the terminal phalanx is only a relatively small part of the total. It is the secondary displacement effect produced by all the **other** bones in the arm that causes most of the growth movement of the fingertip, not its own remodeling and primary displacement.

Similarly, the greater part of the growth movement of the tip of the premaxilla is produced by the growth expansion of all the bones behind and above it and by growth in other parts of the maxilla. The premaxillary tip itself contributes only a very small part of its own forward growth movement. The enlargement of the maxilla proper and the frontal, ethmoid, occipital, sphenoid, lacrimal, vomer, and temporal bones and all of

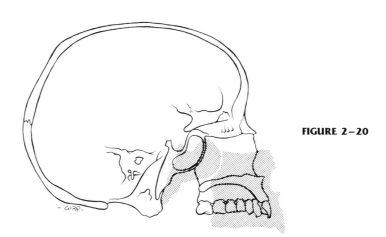

FIGURE 2–20

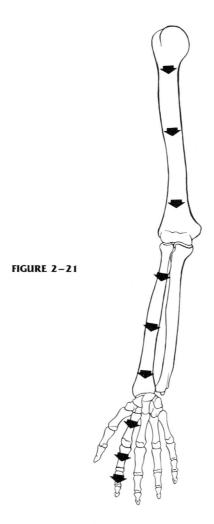

FIGURE 2-21

their soft tissues provides an aggregate expansion, the sum of which is the basis for most of the total forward movement of the premaxilla and its teeth. (It contributes somewhat more to its own downward movement, however, as illustrated in Chapter 5.) Keep in mind, also, that the biomechanical basis for these primary and secondary displacement growth movements is actually the "carry effect" produced by the expansion of the soft tissues associated with the bones, not a "pushing effect" of bones against bones.

Understanding of these concepts can be difficult for a beginning student. This is because it is natural to presume that (1) any given growing region is mostly responsible within itself for its own growth, and (2) since the maxilla "grows forward and downward," the forward/downward pointing area is where it should seem logically to "grow."

The points made in the previous paragraphs are basic and should be understood from day one in any postdoctoral specialty training program requiring an understanding of facial development. If one is to "work with growth" and has presumed that "growth" is exclusively within any given region itself rather than substantially elsewhere, a false start has been made that will seriously handicap the professional.

The factor of secondary displacement, as just seen, is a fundamental part of the overall process of craniofacial enlargement. Growth effects of skeletal parts far removed are passed on, bone by bone, to become expressed on the resultant topography of the face. Cranial floor–facial growth imbalances contribute materially to variable alignments and multitudes of positionings of the different facial bones. Secondary displacement is one of several basic factors involved in the developmental basis for malocclusions and most types of facial dysplasias. In Figure 2–22, note, for example, how a remodeling rotational alignment of the middle cranial fossae, in the manner shown, has the secondary displacement effect of maxillary retrusion and mandibular protrusion.

Growth Rotations

The subject of developmental **rotations** is a major consideration. Although confused by a jumble of terminologies in the literature, there are, simply, two basic categories of rotations: (1) remodeling rotations and (2) displacement rotations. Thus, rotational movements conform, understandably, to the same two categories of growth movements as described above.

While there are countless examples of **remodeling rotations** throughout the craniofacial complex, several in particular have considerable clinical significance. Refer to Figure 2–5.

A principal anatomic function of the mandibular ramus, in addition to providing insertion for masticatory muscles, is to properly position the lower dental arch in occlusion with the upper. To do this, it usually becomes more upright in alignment as development proceeds, closing the ramus-to-corpus ("gonial") angle. (See Chapter 4 for more details.) It is primarily remodeling of the ramus, not the corpus, that is responsible, and it is a combination of remodeling fields that carries out the **remodeling rotation** of the ramus, as illustrated in Figure 4–13. As this growth change proceeds, the entire mandible can also become rotated more downward and backward or upward and forward (as determined by the vertical height of the developing nasomaxillary complex. See Fig. 10–14). This is a **displacement rotation** of the mandible as a whole as its ramus simultaneously rotates to a (usually) more closed position by an adjustive **remodeling** rotation.

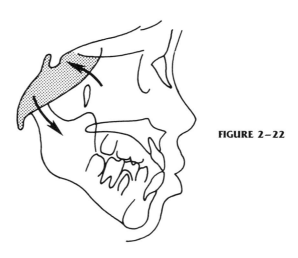

FIGURE 2–22

A second example is the maxilla and its palate. The whole nasomaxillary complex is rotated by **displacement** in either a clockwise or counterclockwise direction, depending on growth activities of the overlying basicranium and also the extent of growth by the sutural system attaching the midface to the cranial floor. This would result in a canting and misfit of the palate and maxillary arch into either open or deep bite positions. However, the remodeling fields pictured in Figure 2–11 can become modified to provide adjustment by producing a counter-direction palatal **remodeling** rotation. This involves either gradients of depository (+) and resorptive (−) activity or actual reversals of remodeling fields along the nasal and oral sides of the palate to offset and compensate for the direction and magnitude of the whole-maxilla displacement rotation. (Note: dental and alveolar adjustments are also involved, as explained in Chapter 10.)

REMODELING AND DISPLACEMENT COMBINATIONS

Both primary and secondary displacements as well as remodeling are involved in the multiple-direction growth movements of all bones. A great many different combinations of all three processes are found throughout the craniofacial complex. As schematized in Figure 2–23, it is seen that essentially comparable results can be produced by quite different developmental combinations. It is the task of diagnosis and treatment planning to determine just which combination is at issue in any given real-life situation. Bones X and Y are in articular contact (as by a suture, condyle, or synchondrosis). A growth increment by bone deposition at a produces a similar end-effect as deposition at b, with accompanying primary displacement of the whole bone to the right. Or increment c is added at the contact interface, with accompanying primary displacement of the whole bone to the right. Resorption at d occurs, however, producing an end-result equivalent to the two examples above. Or, secondary displacement of segment Y is caused by separate segment X, owing to growth addition e. Primary displacement accompanies growth at f. With resorption at g, it is thus seen that this combination also produces end-results similar to all the examples above.

The analysis of composite growth changes is always difficult in headfilm evaluation because, as just seen, the **same** growth results can be theoretically attained by many different combinations of remodeling and displacement. The purpose of Chapter 3 is to analyze just which of the many hypothetical combinations actually take place in each of the many regions of the face and cranium.

Note this important point. The word "growth" is a loose term that we all use, quite properly, when a more descriptive meaning is not needed.

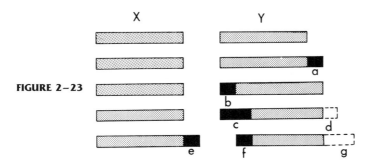

FIGURE 2–23

However, in many instances, a specific and precise meaning should indeed be used. For example, it is frequently heard that some given clinical procedure "stimulates growth." One should always attempt to specify, whenever appropriate, just what kind of "growth" is indeed involved. Remodeling? Primary or secondary displacement? A particular combination? The biologic reason is apparent. If one is to control the growth process, just what is to be controlled must be understood, and the specific local targets involved must be identified. Trying to understand, biologically, how a functional regulator or an activator actually works, explanations that take into account these different movement types, and the specific biologic targets of each, are seldom encountered in the literature.

Superimposing Headfilm Tracings

The conventional method used to show facial "growth" is to superimpose serial headfilm tracings on the cranial base, as shown in Figure 2–24. Sella and a plane from sella to nasion are usually used for registration of the superimposition. Tracings are ordinarily employed instead of the headfilms themselves because superimposed x-ray films pass insufficient light.

Superimposing on the midline cranial base demonstrates the "downward and forward" (one of the most common clichés in facial biology) expansion of the whole face relative to the cranial base. Great caution must be exercised, however; one must understand possible misrepresentations of just what this really shows, because multiple, complex combinations of regional remodeling and primary and secondary displacement are all involved. This is the subject of Chapter 3.

First this method of superimposition is appropriate and valid because we all naturally tend to visualize facial enlargement in **relation** to the

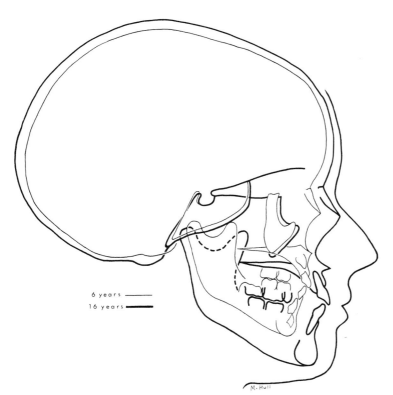

6 years ———
16 years ▬▬▬

FIGURE 2–24. (From Enlow, D. H.: *The Human Face.* New York, Harper & Row, 1968, with permission.)

M. Hull

neurocranium (and brain) behind and above it. That is, the characteristically small face and larger brain of early childhood **change** progressively in respective proportions. Then, as the facial airway and oral region progressively enlarge, the face grows and develops rapidly throughout the childhood period. The size and shape of the brain and the cranial vault also continue to develop, but at a much lesser pace and much less noticeably. The parent **sees** the structural transformations of the child's face, month by month, as it "catches up" with the earlier maturing calvaria and forehead (Fig. 2–25). Superimposing on the cranial base (sella, etc.) thereby represents what we all actually visualize by direct observation as the face progressively enlarges.

Superimposing headfilm tracings "on the cranial base" is not valid, however, if the following **incorrect** assumptions are made:

1.   The incorrect assumption that the cranial base is truly stable and unchanging. It is not. This notion has often mistakenly been made. The floor of the cranium continues to grow and undergo remodeling changes throughout the childhood period (although this is much more marked in some regions than others at different age levels). Properly taken into account, however, this is not necessarily a factor, since the purpose, really, is only to show facial growth changes **relative** to the cranial base, whether or not it is actually stable.

2.   The incorrect assumption that "fixed points" actually exist (i.e., anatomic landmarks that do not move or remodel). All surfaces, inside and out, undergo continued, sequential displacement movements and remodeling changes during morphogenesis (with the exception of no size changes by the ear ossicles once formed; see previous editions of the present book). Although the **relative** position of some landmarks can remain constant, the structures themselves actually experience significant growth movements and remodeling changes along with everything else. Sella has often been presumed to be a true "fixed" point or one that represents the "zero growth point" in the head. Of course, it is not. Sella changes during continued growth. This, however, does not invalidate the use of sella to represent a registration point on the cranial base **if** these various considerations are properly taken into account. *Nasion* is another such landmark. So many marked growth and remodeling variations are associated with this point relating to age, sex, headform types, and ethnic and individual

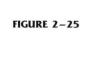

FIGURE 2–25

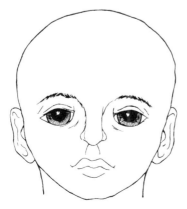

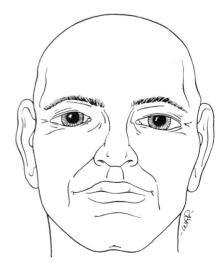

differences, however, that the use of nasion as a cephalometric landmark requires great caution. (Note: There are other basic reasons why points such as nasion and sella are misleading if improperly used, as explained in Chapter 5.)

3. The incorrect assumption that the traditional "forward and downward" picture of facial enlargement, seen when serial tracings are superimposed on the cranial base, represents the **actual mode of facial growth**. Many workers have believed, quite incorrectly, that this is how the face really grows, that is, the facial profile of the younger stage expands straight to the profile of the older stage by direct "growth" and expansion from one to the other. This has been one of our most common misconceptions and one of the most difficult to overcome. The face is a multifactorial, cumulative composite of diverse, multi-directional changes throughout the head, the summation of which produces the "forward and downward" expansion seen in the overlay.

As mentioned above, superimposing headfilm tracings on the cranial base shows the **combined** results of (a) deposition and resorption (remodeling) and (b) primary and secondary displacement **relative** to a common reference plane (such as sella-nasion). The superimposing procedure, however, does not provide an accurate representation for either remodeling or displacement in most facial regions. Note that the two placements of the mandible in the preceding Figure 2–24, for example, do not properly represent either its growth by deposition and resorption (B, left) or its primary displacement (right), as shown in Figure 2–17. The overlay positions for the mandible in Figure 2–24 (and all other facial bones as well) simply indicate their successive **locations** at the two age levels represented relative to the cranial base, not their actual modes of development. To presume the latter is to completely misunderstand how any treatment procedure actually works, and to miss as well the rationale for a true morphogenic diagnosis and treatment plan.

One basic problem always encountered with routine methods of superimposing headfilm tracings on the cranial base is that the **separate** effects of growth by disposition and resorption and by displacement are **not distinguishable.** This is an important consideration. The purpose of the following chapters is to demonstrate these separate effects and to explain how the process of craniofacial development is really carried out.

3

The Developmental Sequence

This short chapter is a condensed summary of the overall pattern of combined remodeling and displacement movements representing the essence of the "big picture." Keep in mind that, although only the bare bones are pictured, their actions are representative of all the other growing parts. Furthermore, it is the bones that are seen in headfilms used for diagnosis. Following chapters elaborate on the underlying biology.

The multiple growth processes in all the various parts of the face and cranium are described separately as individual "regions" or "stages." The sequence begins arbitrarily with the maxillary arch. Changes are then shown for the mandible, followed by growth changes in parts of the cranium and then those of the other regions, one by one. Keep in mind that these regional growth processes all take place simultaneously, even though they are presented here as a sequence of separate stages.

Growth increases are shown in such a way that the same craniofacial form and pattern are maintained throughout; that is, the proportions, shape, relative sizes, and angles are, purposely, essentially unaltered to the extent possible as each separate region enlarges. Thus, the geometric form of the whole face for the first and last stages is the same; only the overall **size** has been changed. Each sequential region incorporates all the changes that precede it. The final stage is a cumulative composite.

Facial and cranial enlargement, in which form and proportions remain constant, constitutes "balanced" growth. However, a perfectly balanced mode of growth in **all** the parts of the face and cranium **never** occurs in real life. Because regional imbalances always occur during the actual developmental processes, **changes** in facial shape and form always take place as the face grows into adulthood. That is, imbalances in the developmental process lead to corresponding imbalances in structure. Most of these "imbalances" are perfectly normal and are a regular part of the developmental and maturation process. They are unavoidable because of the complex design of the craniofacial composite in which many different parts develop at different times, in different directions at different velocities and perform many diverse functions. Making everything actually fit **requires** certain normal "imbalances." These factors are why the face of a child undergoes sequential alterations in profile and in facial proportions as developmental differentiation progresses.

The reason the facial growth descriptions that follow are presented first as a "balanced" series is twofold. First, they will show just what constitutes the concept of "growth balance" itself and how to understand what this actually means. Second, in order to be able to recognize and explain facial **imbalances**, normal and abnormal, one must know what constitutes deviations from the balanced mode of development, that is, exactly **where** disproportions develop to cause a given facial pattern, and **how much** is involved in terms of dimensional and angular departures from balanced growth. Only by understanding the balanced process can one accurately identify, measure and, importantly, account for the imbalanced changes. The face of each of us is the aggregate sum of all the many balanced and imbalanced craniofacial parts combined into a composite whole. Regional imbalances often tend to compensate for one another to provide functional equilibrium (growth works toward composite balance: Chapter 1). The process of **compensation** is a feature of the developmental process; it provides for a certain latitude of imbalance in some areas in order to offset the effects of disproportions in other regions.

The regional descriptions of the growth process outlined below are not randomly presented. Rather, a system is used that, in fact, is the same developmental plan utilized in the growth process itself. This is the **counterpart principle** of craniofacial growth. It states, simply, that the growth of any given facial or cranial part relates specifically to **other** structural and geometric "counterparts" in the face and cranium. For example, the maxillary arch is a counterpart of the mandibular arch. The anterior cranial fossae and the palate are counterparts, as are the palate and maxillary apical base. The middle endocranial fossa, mandibular ramus (it bridges the pharyngeal space established by the middle cranial fossa), and zygomatic arch (which bridges both the cranial fossa and the ramus) are all respective counterparts. These are **regional** relationships throughout the whole face and cranium. If each regional part and its particular counterpart enlarge to the same extent, balanced growth between them is the result. This is the key to what determines the presence or lack of balance in any region. Imbalances are produced by differences in respective amounts or directions of growth between parts and counterparts. Many part-counterpart combinations exist throughout the skull, and these provide a meaningful and effective way to evaluate the growth of the face and the morphologic relationships among all its structural components.

The "test" for a part-counterpart relationship in the face and cranium is not difficult. The question is simply asked: "If a given increment is added to a specific bone, or soft tissue part, **where** must an equivalent increment to be added to **other** bones or parts if the same form and balance are to be retained?" The answer to this question then identifies which other specific bones or parts of bones or soft tissue parts are involved as counterparts. This counterpart concept will be used repeatedly in this chapter as well as in following chapters dealing with facial variations and abnormalities. (See also page 159.)

Each regional growth change is presented as two separate processes. First, the changes produced by **deposition and resorption** (remodeling) are described and are shown by **fine arrows** in the illustrations. Second, the changes produced by **displacement** are described and are represented by **heavy arrows**. These two processes, it is understood, take place at the same time, but they must be described separately because their effects are quite different. Then the question asked is, "Where do counterpart changes also occur if the same pattern is to be maintained?" This identifies the **next** anatomic region, which is described in turn.

To illustrate the counterpart principle, an expandable photographic tripod is used here as an analogy (Fig. 3–1). The tripod has a series of tele-

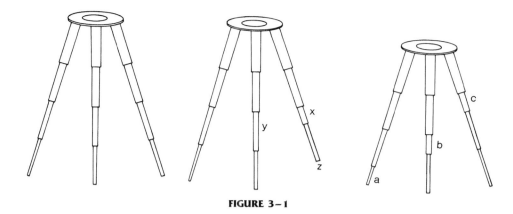

FIGURE 3–1

scoping segments in each leg; the length of each segment matches the length of its "counterpart" segments in the other two legs. If all the segments are extended to exactly the same length, the tripod retains geometric balance and overall symmetry. If, however, any one segment is not extended equal to the others, the leg as a whole is either shorter or longer, although the remainder of all the segments in that leg match their respective counterparts. One can thus identify **which** particular segment is different and determine the extent of imbalance. Segment x, for example, is short relative to y, thus causing a retrusion of z. In addition, the relative (not actual) length of a whole leg can also be altered by changing its **alignment**. A leg "rotated" into more vertical alignment, for example, increases the *expression* of that dimension without actually lengthening its real size.

Many other hypothetical combinations exist. For example, segments a, b, and c in Figure 3–1 are short with respect to their segment counterparts in the other legs. Overall symmetry is balanced, nonetheless, because of all these regional imbalances offset one another, and the total length of each leg is, therefore, the same.

Regional Change (Stage) 1

Note that two reference lines are used, a horizontal and a vertical,* so that directions and amounts of growth changes can be visualized (Fig. 3–2). The bony maxillary arch lengthens horizontally in a **posterior** direction (this always comes as a surprise to those new in the business). This is schematized by showing a posterior movement of the **pterygomaxillary fissure (PTM)**. Note its new location behind the vertical reference line (Fig. 3–3).

PTM is the routine radiographic landmark used to identify the **maxillary tuberosity**, and it appears on headfilms as an "inverted teardrop" produced by the gap between the pterygoid plates and the maxilla.

The overall length of the maxillary arch has increased by the same amount that **PTM** moves posteriorly. Bone has been deposited on the posterior-facing cortical surface of the maxillary tuberosity. Resorption occurs on the opposite side of the same cortical plate, which is the inside surface of the maxilla within the maxillary sinus.

---

*This vertical line is not arbitrary; it is the **PM** boundary, which is one of the most basic and important **natural** anatomic planes in the head (see Chapter 9). The horizontal line is the functional occlusal plane.

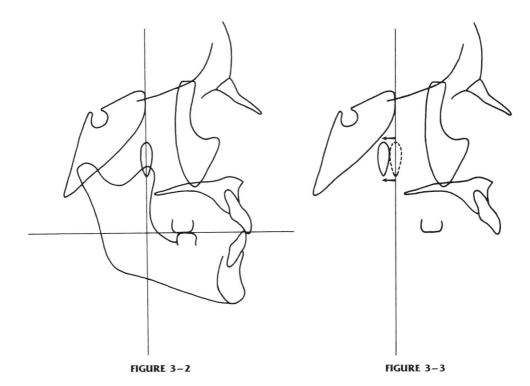

FIGURE 3–2   **FIGURE 3–3**

Regional Change (Stage) 2

The preceding stage is the first of the two-part growth process described for each region, that is, **remodeling** by deposition and resorption. The second part involves **displacement**, described in the present stage (Fig. 3–4). As the maxillary tuberosity grows and lengthens posteriorly, the whole maxilla is simultaneously **carried** anteriorly. The amount of this forward displacement exactly equals the amount of posterior lengthening. Note that **PTM** is "returned" to the vertical reference line. Of course, it never actually departed from this line because backward growth (Stage 1) and forward displacement (Stage 2) occur at the same time. This is a primary type of displacement because it occurs in conjunction with the bone's own enlargement; that is, as the bone is displaced, it undergoes remodeling growth that keeps pace with the amount of displacement. A protrusion of the forward part of the arch now occurs, not because of direct growth in the forward part itself, but rather because of growth in the **posterior** region of the maxilla as the whole bone is simultaneously displaced anteriorly. Note the Class II position of the molars. What is the source of the biomechanical force producing this maxillary movement? The answer, in brief, involves the developmental expansion of all the enclosing soft tissues which, attached to the maxilla by Sharpey's fibers, **carry** the maxillary complex anteriorly. (See also Figs. 1–6, 5–1, and 5–2.)

Regional Change (Stage) 3

The question is now asked: "When the elongation of the maxilla in Stage 1 is made, **where** must equivalent changes **also** be made if structural balance is maintained?" In other words, what are the **counterparts** to the bony maxillary arch? Several are involved, including the upper part

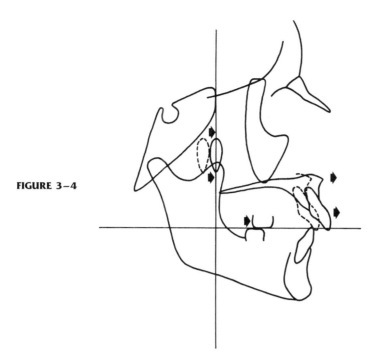

FIGURE 3–4

of the nasomaxillary complex, the anterior cranial fossa, the palate, and the corpus of the mandible. The mandible is described in this stage. The mandible is not to be regarded as a single functional element; it has two major parts, the **corpus** (body) and the **ramus**. These two parts must be considered separately because each has its own separate counterpart relationships with other, different regions in the craniofacial complex.

The bony mandibular arch relates specifically to the bony maxillary arch; that is, the body of the mandible is the structural counterpart to the body of the maxilla. The mandibular corpus now lengthens to match the elongation of the maxilla, and it does this by a remodeling conversion from the ramus (Fig. 3–5). The anterior part of the ramus remodels posteriorly, a relocation process that produces a corresponding elongation of the corpus. What **was** ramus has now been remodeled into a new addition for the corpus. The mandibular arch lengthens by an amount that equals the remodeling of the maxillary arch (Stage 1), and both elongate in a posterior direction. However, note that the two arches are still offset; the maxilla is in a protrusive position even though upper and lower arch lengths are the same, as seen in Figure 3–6. A Class II type of relationship still exists between the maxillary and mandibular molars. The proper Class I position is seen in Stage 1; the mandibular posterior tooth shown in the diagram should normally be about one-half cusp ahead of its maxillary antagonist, as seen in Figure 3–2.

Regional Change (Stage) 4

The second of the two growth processes (i.e., first, growth by deposition and resorption, and second, displacement) will now be described. Remember that these two changes actually occur **at the same time**. The whole mandible is **displaced** anteriorly, just as the maxilla also becomes carried anteriorly while it simultaneously grows posteriorly. To do this, the condyle and the posterior part of the ramus remodel posteriorly (Fig. 3–6). This returns the horizontal dimension of the ramus to the **same breadth** present in Stages 1 and 2 above; the amount of anterior ramus resorption is equaled by the amount of posterior ramus addition. This purpose is not to increase the width of the ramus itself, but to relocate it posteriorly for lengthening the **corpus**.

Regional Change (Stage) 5

The whole mandible, now, is displaced anteriorly by the same amount that the ramus has relocated posteriorly (Fig. 3–7). This is the primary type of displacement because it occurs in conjunction with the bone's own enlargement. As the bone becomes displaced, it simultaneously remodels (the stage just described) to keep pace with the amount of displacement. Note the following:

1. The corpus of the mandible elongates primarily in a **posterior** direction, just as the maxilla also lengthens posteriorly (Stage 1). It does this by remodeling from what **was** ramus into what then becomes a posterior addition to the mandibular arch. In this respect, mandibular arch elongation differs from maxillary arch elongation because the maxillary tuberosity is a free surface, unlike the posterior end of the mandibular corpus.

2. The whole ramus has moved posteriorly. However, the only actual change in horizontal dimension involves the mandibular corpus, which becomes longer. The horizontal dimension of the ramus remains constant during **this** particular remodeling stage (the widening of the ramus itself is part of another stage).

3. The anterior **displacement** of the whole mandible equals the amount of anterior maxillary displacement assuming everything is per-

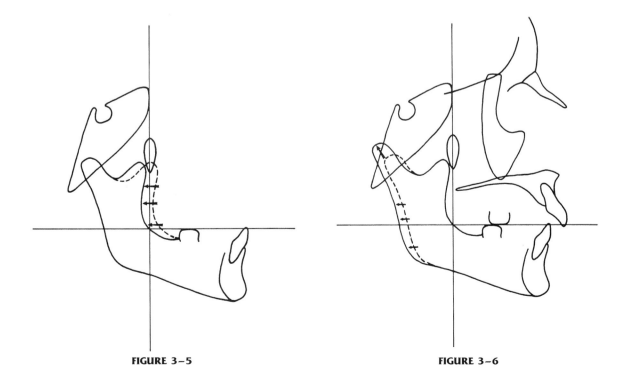

FIGURE 3–5   FIGURE 3–6

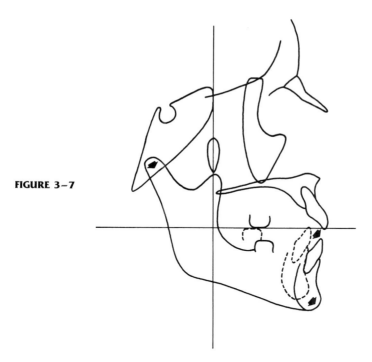

FIGURE 3–7

fectly balanced (which is unlikely; see Chapter 10.) This places the mandibular arch in proper position relative to the maxillary arch just above
it. The arch lengths and the positions of the maxilla and mandible are now
in balance, and a Class I position of the teeth has been "returned."

4.   Note, however, that the obliquely upward and backward direction of
ramus remodeling must also lengthen its **vertical** dimension in order to
provide for horizontal enlargement. This separates the occlusion (contacts
between the upper and lower teeth) because the mandibular arch is displaced inferiorly as well as anteriorly.

5.   In both the maxilla and mandible, the type of displacement is **primary** because it takes place in conjunction with each bone's own enlargement. The source of this displacement movement is comparable to that
just described for the maxilla.

6.   In summary thus far, the increment of backward growth at the maxillary tuberosity (Stage 1), the amount of forward displacement by the
whole maxilla (Stage 2), the extent of remodeling on the anterior part of
the ramus and the amount of corpus lengthening (Stage 3), the increment
of backward growth by the posterior part of the ramus (Stage 4), and the
amount of forward displacement of the whole mandible (Stage 5) are all
precisely equal in this "balanced" sequence of growth. What happens
when they are not all exactly equal (as usually happens), or when differentials in timing occur, or if developmental "rotations" occur to cause variations in alignment (which change the expression of actual dimensions)
is described later.

Regional Change (Stage) 6

While all of the growth and remodeling changes described in the preceding stages have been taking place, the dimensions of the temporal lobes
of the cerebrum and the middle cranial fossae have also been increasing

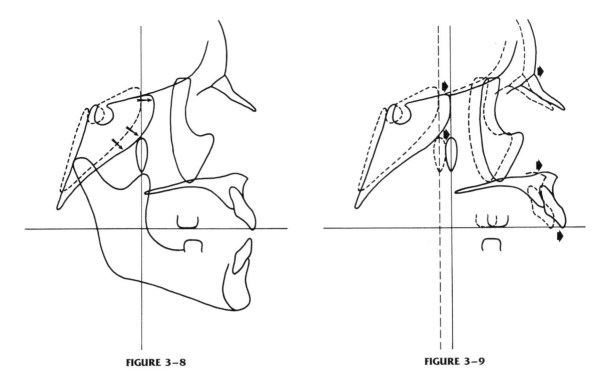

FIGURE 3-8   FIGURE 3-9

at the same time (Fig. 3–8). This is done by resorption on the endocranial side and deposition of bone on the ectocranial side of the cranial floor. The spheno-occipital synchondrosis (a major cartilaginous growth site in the cranium) provides endochondral bone growth in the midline part of the cranial floor.[†] The total growth expansion of the middle fossa would now project it anteriorly beyond the vertical reference line, except that this line itself is moved in the next stage.

Regional Change (Stage) 7

All cranial and facial parts lying anterior to the middle cranial fossa (in front of the vertical reference line) become **displaced** in a forward direction as a result (Fig. 3–9). The whole vertical reference line moves anteriorly to the same extent that the middle cranial fossa expands in a forward direction. This is because the line represents the anterior boundary between the enlarging middle cranial fossa and all of the cranial and facial parts in front of it. The maxillary tuberosity remains in a constant position on the vertical reference line as this interface line moves forward. The forehead, anterior cranial fossa, cheekbone, palate, and maxillary arch all undergo protrusive displacement in an anterior direction. This is a **secondary** type of displacement because the actual enlargement of these various parts is not directly involved. They are simply moved anteriorly because the middle cranial fossa behind them expands in this direction. The floor of the fossa, however, does not **push** the anterior cranial fossa and the nasomaxillary complex forward. Rather, they are **carried** forward as the frontal and temporal lobes of the cerebrum enlarge by respective

---

[†]Note the change in the position of the sella turcica. This is a highly variable structure, however, and other patterns of remodeling movements are also common. See Chapter 5.

growth increases. The nasomaxillary complex, suspended by sutures from the anterior cranial fossae and frontal lobes, is thus carried anteriorly as the combined frontal and temporal lobes progressively expand.

Regional Change (Stage) 8

The expansion of the middle cranial fossa, just described, also has a displacement effect on the mandible (Fig. 3–10). This too is a secondary type of displacement. The extent of the displacement effect, however, is much less than that for the maxilla. This, importantly, is because the greater part of middle cranial fossa growth occurs in **front** of the condyle and **between** the condyle and the maxillary tuberosity. The spheno-occipital synchondrosis also lies between the condyle and the anterior boundary of the middle cranial fossa. Thus, the extent of maxillary protrusive displacement far exceeds the amount of mandible protrusive displacement caused by middle fossa enlargement. The result is an offset horizontal placement between the upper and lower arches. The upper incisors show an "overjet," and the molars are in a Class II position, even though the mandibular and maxillary arch lengths themselves are matched in respective dimensions. **Sella-nasion** (again, a much used cephalometric plane) should not be used to represent the "upper face" or "anterior cranial base" in comparisons with the entire mandibular dimension, ramus and corpus, as is often done. The comparison is invalid because dissimilar effective spans (counterparts) are being compared and because sella-nasion itself does not represent any anatomically meaningful dimension, either for the cranial base or for the upper face.

Regional Change (Stage) 9

The question is now asked: "When this change in the middle cranial fossa takes place, **where** must an equivalent change **also** occur if balance

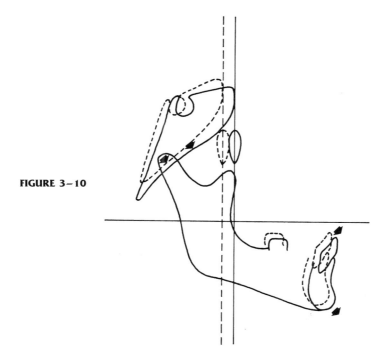

FIGURE 3–10

is to be sustained?" This identifies the "counterpart" of the middle fossa and shows where facial growth must take place to match it.

Just as the lengthening of the middle cranial fossa places the maxillary arch in a progressively more anterior position, the horizontal growth of the **ramus** places the mandibular arch in a like position. What the middle cranial fossa does for the maxillary body, in effect, the ramus does for the mandibular body. **The ramus is the specific structural counterpart of the middle cranial fossa.** Both are also counterparts of the **pharyngeal space.** The skeletal function of the ramus is to bridge the pharyngeal space and the span of the middle cranial fossa in order to place the mandibular arch in proper anatomic position with the maxilla. The anteroposterior breadth of the ramus is critical. If it is too narrow or too wide, the ramus places the lower arch too retrusively or too protrusively, respectively. This dimension and also the alignment must be just right. As will be described later, the horizontal dimension of the ramus can become altered during growth to provide intrinsic adjustments and compensations for morphogenic imbalances that may occur elsewhere in the craniofacial complex.

The horizontal extent of middle cranial fossa elongation is **matched** by the corresponding extent of horizontal increase by the ramus (Fig. 3–11). The horizontal (not oblique) dimension of the ramus now equals the horizontal (not oblique) dimension of the middle cranial fossa. The effective span of the latter, as it relates to the ramus, is the straight line distance from the cranial floor-condyle articulation to the vertical reference line. Recall that the ramus was previously involved in remodeling changes associated with corpus elongation (Stage 4), but the actual breadth of the ramus was not increased during that particular stage. The present stage represents that increase and is considered separately here. Both stages proceed simultaneously.

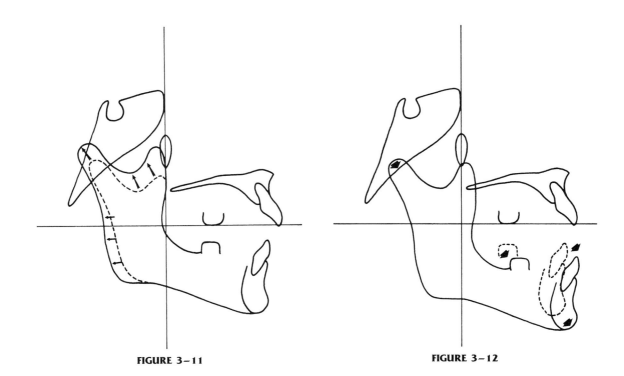

FIGURE 3–11   **FIGURE 3–12**

Regional Change (Stage) 10

The entire mandible is displaced anteriorly at the same time that it remodels posteriorly (Fig. 3–12). The amount of the anterior displacement equals (1) the extent of posterior ramus and condylar growth (Stage 9); (2) the amount of middle cranial fossa enlargement anterior to the mandibular condyle (Stage 6); (3) the extent of anterior movement of the vertical reference line; and (4) the extent of resultant anterior maxillary displacement (Stage 7).

The oblique manner of condylar growth necessarily produces an upward and backward projection of the condyle with a corresponding downward as well as forward direction of mandibular displacement. The ramus thus becomes vertically as well as horizontally enlarged. This results in a **further** descent of the mandibular arch and separation of the occlusion (it was also previously lowered during Stages 5 and 8). The total extent of this vertical growth (Fig. 3–12) must **match** the total vertical lengthening of the nasomaxillary complex (Fig. 3–15) and the upward eruption and drift of the mandibular dentoalveolar arch (Fig. 3–18) if the same facial balance is to be achieved.

Note that the protrusion of the maxilla during Stage 7 has now been matched by an equivalent amount of mandibular protrusion. The molars have once again been "returned" to Class I positions, and the upper incisor has no overjet. Note also that the anterior border of the ramus lies ahead of the vertical reference line. The "real" junction between the ramus and corpus, however, is the lingual tuberosity housing the last molar, not the "anterior border." The lingual tuberosity lies on the vertical reference line behind the anterior border, which overlaps this tuberosity (not shown in the figure because it cannot be seen in a lateral headfilm; observe on a dry mandible). This protruding overlap is an evolutionary result of the distinctive upright remodeling rotation of the ramus among higher primates relating to the more vertically elongate rotation of the midface (see Chapter 9) and the extension of a flange of the anterior border to accommodate the temporalis muscle.

Regional Change (Stage) 11

The **floor** of the anterior cranial fossa and the forehead grow by deposition on the ectocranial side with resorption from the endocranial side (Fig. 3–13). The nasal bones are displaced anteriorly. The posterior-anterior length of the anterior cranial fossa is now in balance with the extent of horizontal lengthening by its structural counterpart, the maxillary arch (Stage 1). Because these two regions have undergone equivalent growth increments, the profile retains its originally balanced form. (Actually, age differentials, both in time and amount together with male/female and headform differences, always occur, but our present purpose is to describe perfectly "balanced" growth.)

The enlarging brain displaces the bones of the **calvaria** (domed skull roof) outward. Each bone enlarges by sutural growth. As the brain expands, the sutures respond by depositing new bone at the contact edges of the frontal, parietal, occipital, and temporal. This expands the perimeter of each. At the same time, bone is laid down on **both** the ectocranial and endocranial sides to increase the thickness.

The upper part of the face, which is the ethmomaxillary (nasal) region, also undergoes equivalent growth increments. This facial area increases horizontally to an extent that matches (if the same balance is retained) the expansion of the anterior cranial fossa above and the maxillary arch and palate below it. These areas are all counterparts to one another. The growth process involves direct bone deposition on the forward-facing cortical surfaces of the ethmoid, the frontal process of the maxillary, and the nasal bones. Most of the internal bony surfaces of the nasal chambers are resorptive. In addition, anterior displacement takes place in conjunction with growth at the various maxillary and ethmoidal sutures. The composite of these changes produces an enlargement of the nasal chambers in an anterior (and also lateral) direction.

Regional Change (Stage) 12

The **vertical** lengthening of the nasomaxillary complex, as with its horizontal elongation, is brought about by a composite of (1) growth by deposition and resorption, and (2) a primary displacement movement associated directly with its own enlargement. The latter is considered in a later stage. The combination of resorption on the superior (nasal) side of the palate and deposition on the inferior (oral) side produces a downward remodeling movement of the whole palate from *1* to *2* in Figure 3–14. This **relocates** it inferiorly, a process that provides for the vertical enlargement of the overlying nasal region. The extent of nasal expansion is considerable during the childhood period to keep pace with the enlargement of the whole body and lungs. (Note: The pattern and extent of downward palatal and maxillary arch remodeling often varies between the mesial and distal parts of the area, as described on page 35 in Chapter 2. This provides for a range of positional adjustments of the arch to compensate for developmental variations and displacement rotations.) See also page 52.

The anterior part of the bony maxillary arch has a periosteal surface that is **resorptive** (the face of the human, with reduced jaws, is the only species that has this). The reason is because this area grows **straight**

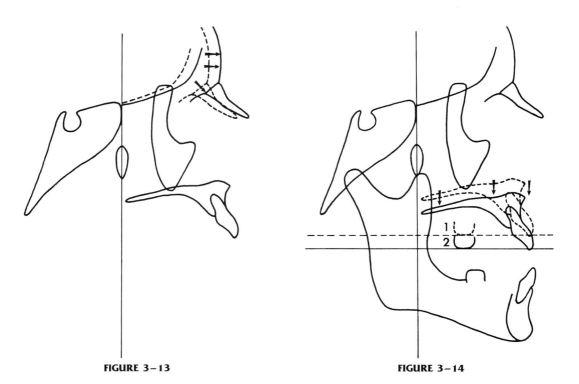

FIGURE 3–13 **FIGURE 3–14**

downward, as schematized in Figure 2–11. In other species (including primates), the premaxillary region remodels forward as well as downward to produce a much more elongate, protrusive muzzle.

As seen in Figure 2–11, the labial (external) side of the premaxillary region faces mostly upward and **away** from the downward direction of growth, and it is thus largely resorptive. The lingual side faces toward the downward growth directions and is depository. The growth pattern also provides for the remodeling of the alveolar bone as it adapts to the variable positions of the incisors (Fig. 3–15).

Regional Change (Stage) 13

Vertical growth by **displacement** is associated with bone deposition at the many and various **sutures** of the maxilla where it contacts the multiple, separate bones above and behind it. Bone is added at these sutures by amounts equalling whole maxillary displacement inferiorly (Fig. 3–16). The addition of new sutural bone does not "push" the maxilla downward, as presumed in years past. Rather, the maxilla is **carried** inferiorly by the physical growth forces of enclosing soft tissues (See Fig. 1–7). This is accompanied by bone deposition in the sutures responding to mutual growth signals relating to both displacement and remodeling. New bone is thus simultaneously laid down on the sutural edges keeping the bone-to-bone junction intact. The increment of bone growth in the suture exactly equals the amount of inferior displacement of the whole maxilla. This is primary displacement because it takes place in conjunction with the bone's own enlargement.

Of the total extent of downward movement by the palate and maxillary arch, that part from 2 to 3 is produced in association with sutural growth and primary **displacement** (Fig. 3–17). The part from 1 to 2, which can be about half of the total (depending on palatal remodeling rotations), is direct relocation by resorptive and depository remodeling. Similarly, the movement of the teeth from 2 to 3 is by the downward displacement of the whole maxilla, carrying the entire dentition passively with it. The movement from 1 to 2 is produced by each tooth's **own** movement as bone is added and resorbed on appropriate lining surfaces in each socket. This

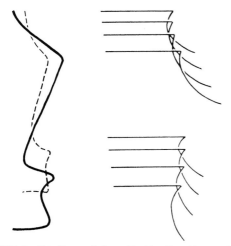

FIGURE 3–15. (From Enlow, D. H.: *The Human Face.* New York. Harper & Row, 1968, p. 244, with permission.)

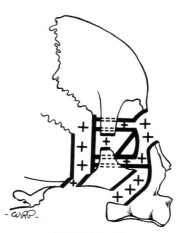

FIGURE 3–16

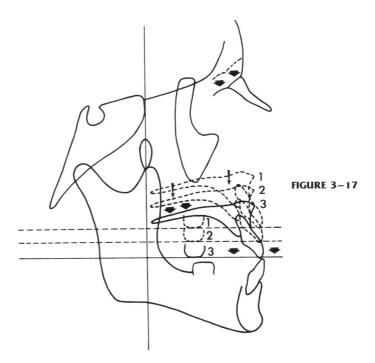

FIGURE 3-17

is the **vertical drift** of the tooth, a process that is accompanied by the **same** deposition and resorption of alveolar bone that works with the familiar "mesial drift" of the dentition (see Chapter 5). Vertical drift takes place **in addition to** eruption, which is a separate growth movement. The vertical drift process is important to the clinician because it provides a great deal of growth movement to "work with" during treatment.

"**Vertical drift**" is a most significant concept that somehow has been bypassed in the dental curriculum and literature. For the postdoctoral student, this concept deserves day-one attention because of its significance. Historically, vertical tooth movement has been called simply "eruption," **which it is not and which misses the point entirely**.

Tooth movement from *2* to *3* can also be clinically influenced. This involves the use of special appliances intended to either augment or retard the displacement movement of the entire nasomaxillary complex or to alter their directions. This in turn causes remodeling changes in the size or shape of the whole maxilla or of other separate bones (in contrast to remodeling of the alveolar bone supporting the teeth). Refer to the "Two Basic Clinical Targets" section in Chapter 1.

Another significant concept relates to the reason why the palate and maxillary arch are subject to both remodeling and displacement (*1* to *2* and *2* to *3*). Figures 2–11 and 3–14 illustrate the palate and maxillary arch moving inferiorly in an idealized manner, with the anterior and posterior regions remodeling downward to the same extent. Mesiodistal variations, however, are common. In displacement movements, a clockwise or counterclockwise **rotation** of the whole palate and arch often occurs. In conjunction with this, the remodeling movement (*1* to *2*) can compensate by producing an opposite direction of rotation, thereby leveling and fine-tuning the palate into definitive adult position. This, indeed, represents a primary function of the remodeling phase of the composite downward growth process. That is, selective remodeling in the anterior versus posterior parts can serve to adjust and counteract rotations produced during primary nasomaxillary displacement as well as secondary displacement rotations caused by growth of the middle and anterior cranial fossae.

Awareness of the distinction between the two categories of movements *1 to 2* and *2 to 3* should **also** be highlighted in any orthodontic or surgical training program. The clinician addresses one or the other in every patient, or some combination of both. Either the magnitude or the direction can be influenced by substituting "clinical control" for nature's own intrinsic control. The underlying biologic process actually producing the movements is the same, however, whether intrinsic or clinical. If the potential for growth movement does not already exist, as in an adult, this movement must be clinically induced in addition to providing direction. Also, a different "stability" situation then exists, since no subsequent childhood facial growth is involved that can either lead to a new, composite equilibrium or, conversely, that could disrupt it (relapse). See also Figure 1–1).

Keep in mind, also, this key point: the teeth themselves have very little capacity for remodeling. They can, essentially, only be moved by the displacement process, either in conjunction with remodeling of an individual alveolar socket or displacement of the entire arch as a unit. It is the **bone** that must undergo any remodeling required. (See "Anterior Crowding" in Chapter 10 and also refer to pages 16 and 112).

Regional Change (Stage) 14

In three previous stages (5, 8, and 10), it was seen that the mandibular corpus becomes lowered by the vertical enlargement of both the ramus and the middle cranial fossa. Their combined vertical dimensions represent the growth counterpart of the vertical dimensions of the nasomaxillary complex and the dentition. In other words, the amount of vertical separation between the upper and lower arches caused by the vertical growth of both the middle cranial fossa and the ramus must balance an equivalent amount of lengthening in the nasomaxillary complex and the dentoalveolar region of the mandible.

The maxillary arch has grown downward to Level 3 in Stage 13. Now, the mandibular teeth and alveolar bone drift **upward** to attain full occlusion (Fig. 3–18). This is produced by a superior **drift** of each mandibular tooth, together with a corresponding remodeling increase in the height of the alveolar bone. The extent of this upward growth movement plus that of the downward growth movement by the maxillary arch equals the combined extent of vertical remodeling by the ramus and middle cranial fossa **if** the pattern of the face is not changed. Note this factor: The extent of downward drift of the maxillary teeth can exceed the extent of upward drift by the mandibular teeth. Much less growth is thus available to "work with" in major orthodontic movements of the mandibular, as compared with the maxillary, teeth. However, there is a significant extent of vertical drift by the mandibular anterior teeth if a curve of Spee exists (See page 186).

Working with Growth and the Extraction Nonextraction Decision

Much has been written about the clinician's ability to treat malocclusions without the removal of permanent teeth. A major factor that has been largely overlooked in this debate is the potential for therapeutic modification of the vertical remodeling process. As stated, vertical remodeling occurs in response to and coincident with vertical displacement of the mandibular corpus and nasomaxillary complex. The remodeling that occurs around the individual sockets of maxillary and mandibular teeth can be modified by orthodontic forces. Indeed, it is this modification that allows the clinician to develop arch length by redirecting the alveolar remodeling process toward areas of natural deposition. In the maxilla the area of the tuberosity and in the mandible the posterior portion of the corpus are areas that can be used to biologically augment arch length. Interestingly, it is in the case of deep bite malocclusion that differential vertical alveolar remodeling can most easily be harnessed by the clinician. The reason deep bite malocclusions are more easily treated in this manner is that most orthodontic treatment mechanics tend to "extrude" (vertical drift) posterior teeth. As posterior teeth are moved, vertical overbite is reduced. This treatment response is desirable in the deep bite case, but would be disastrous in the open bite patient. The relationship between vertical remodeling and deep bite may be one reason for the observed clinical relationship between deep bite and nonextraction treatment. Variable extents of vertical drift of the mandibular teeth, from distal to mesial, occur during normal facial development, just as for the maxillary teeth (described earlier). This functions to adjust the occlusal plane to compensate for various displacement rotations. When the orthodontist "extrudes" a tooth, it is the equivalent of the vertical drifting movement of the tooth together with remodeling of its companion alveolar socket, and the essential purpose is the same.

Regional Change (Stage) 15

While the upward movements of the mandibular teeth and remodeling of the alveolar sockets are taking place, remodeling changes also occur in the incisor alveolar region, the chin, and the corpus of the mandible (Fig. 3–19). The lower incisors undergo a lingual tipping (a "retroclination"), so that the uppers overlap the lowers for proper **overbite**. This involves a

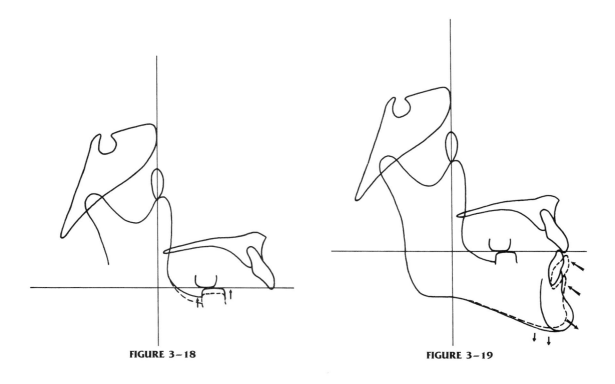

FIGURE 3–18   FIGURE 3–19

posterior rotational movement of the mandibular incisors as they simultaneously drift superiorly. The movement of the teeth is accompanied by **resorption** on the outside (labial) surface of the alveolar region just above the chin, and deposition on the lingual side. The alveolar bone thus moves backward as the incisors undergo lingual drift. This does not occur to the same extent in individuals having an "end-to-end" incisor relationship or an anterior crossbite.

Bone is progressively added to the external surface of the **chin** itself, as well as along the underside and other external surfaces of the corpus. This is slow accretion that proceeds gradually throughout childhood. At birth, the mental protuberance is small and inconspicuous. Many anxious parents naturally worry about the chinless appearance of their little child. However, the whole mandible usually tends to lag in differential growth timing and will later catch up to the maxilla in the normal face. This is because of the difference in the timing of growth expansion between the frontal cerebral lobes and anterior cranial fossae versus that of the temporal lobes and middle cranial fossae (Stages 10 and 11). The chin takes on more noticeable form year by year. The combination of new bone growth on the chin itself and the posterior direction of bone remodeling in the alveolar region just above it gradually causes the chin to become more prominent. The whole mandible, meanwhile, is also becoming displaced anteriorly in conjunction with continued remodeling additions at the condyle and ramus producing overall mandibular lengthening.

Regional Change (Stage) 16

The forward part of the zygoma and the malar region of the maxilla remodel in conjunction with the contiguous maxillary complex, and their respective modes of growth are similar. Just as the maxilla lengthens horizontally by posterior remodeling growth, the malar area also remodels posteriorly by continued deposition of new bone on its posterior side and resorption from its anterior side (Fig. 3–20). The front surface of the whole cheekbone area is thus actually resorptive. This remodeling process keeps this area's position in proper relationship to the lengthening maxillary arch as a whole. They **both** relocate backward, thereby maintaining the proper anatomic positions between them. The amount of deposition on the posterior side, however, exceeds resorption on the anterior surface, so that the whole malar protuberance becomes larger. Another way of understanding the rationale for the growth of the zygomatic process of the maxilla is to compare it with the coronoid process of the mandible. Just as the coronoid process relocates backward by anterior resorption and posterior deposition to keep pace with the overall posterior elongation of the whole bone, the zygomatic process similarly remodels posteriorly by anterior resorption and posterior deposition. (Refer to page 94.)

Note that the vertical length of the lateral orbital rim increases by sutural deposits at the frontozygomatic suture. The zygomatic arch also enlarges considerably by bone deposition along its inferior edge. The arch remodels laterally (not seen, of course, in lateral headfilms) by bone deposition on the lateral surface, together with resorption from the medial side within the temporal fossa.

Regional Change (Stage) 17

Just as the whole maxillary complex is displaced anteriorly and inferiorly as it simultaneously enlarges in overall size, the malar area is moved anteriorly and inferiorly by primary **displacement** as it enlarges

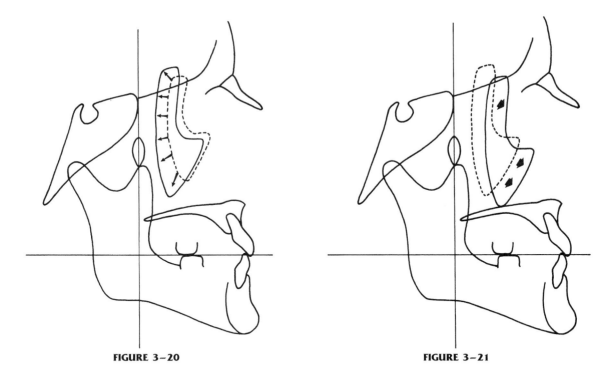

FIGURE 3–20   **FIGURE 3–21**

(Fig. 3–21). The cheekbone thereby proportionately matches the maxilla in (1) the directions and amount of horizontal and vertical remodeling relocation and (2) the directions and amount of primary displacement.

This completes the introductory survey of the regional growth changes taking place in the basicranium and face. The final result is a craniofacial composite that has essentially the same form and pattern present when the first stage was begun. Only the overall size has been altered. All the growth changes among the specific parts and counterparts have been purposefully balanced to give an understanding of the meaning of "balanced growth" and to provide a basis for analyzing **imbalanced** growth changes in a later chapter.

In Figure 2–24, the first and last stages are superimposed with sella as a registration point. When the sequence of changes described in Stages 1 through 17 are considered, it is apparent that the face does not simply grow directly from one profile to the other. Rather, all the regional changes just outlined are involved, including the complex array of many additional details as explained in following chapters. The overlay seen here is the traditional way of representing the results of the overall process of facial enlargement. This overlay does **not**, however, represent the actual growth processes themselves—that is, the changes produced (1) by remodeling resorption and deposition; (2) relocation; (3) by primary and (4) secondary displacement. Historically, this basic and important fact was not generally appreciated. The overlay shows the cumulative summation of all four processes and demonstrates the **locations** of all the regional parts, before and after, when registered on a plane such as sella-nasion.

4

Growth of the Mandible

Because the maxillary complex can respond to treatment procedures in ways that are similar to the mandible, but also in ways that are different, an evaluation of the **differences and the similarities** of the morphology, functions, and development of the mandible **compared** to the nasomaxillary complex is important. A listing is presented below. This is not merely academic, since virtually every factor herein is directly pertinent to basic treatment rationale. (Note, in seminar meetings with postdoctoral residents, a goodly number of significant additions were made to this preliminary list. Try your hand.)

1.   The mandible has a **ramus** jutting from the distal end of its arch (the lingual tuberosity), whereas the maxillary tuberosity has a free posterior surface (in childhood) with the pterygoid plates directly, but separately, behind.

2.   The mandible has movable articulation with the basicranium; the maxilla has fixed sutures with the cranial floor and also among its own multiple, separate bony elements.

3.   The temporomandibular joint is lined with cartilage, a pressure-tolerant articular tissue. The maxillary sutures are composed of collagenous connective tissue, which is tension adapted, but pressure sensitive at low threshold.

4.   The mandible has a condyle that involves endochondral ossification. The maxilla is entirely intramembranous.

5.   The mandible has masticatory (and other) muscles attached. The maxilla is not functionally mobile, and the maxilla itself is a paired bone with a midline suture.

6.   The mandible is a single bone (in primates). The nasomaxillary complex is an elaborate grouping of many separate bones and mostly without direct muscle attachments.

7.   The human mandible has a chin; the maxilla has a nasal spine attached to a septal cartilage with a septopremaxillary ligament. The mandible lacks a midline, vertical cartilage attached to the basicranium.

8.   Both are of "first pharyngeal arch" embryonic origin, and both are innervated by the fifth cranial nerve, but by different divisions.

9.   The maxilla incorporates orbital and nasal components not directly represented in the mandible, with diverse functions, structure, and development all involved. This is a *major* factor relating to clinical considerations. The vertical span of the mandibular ramus, however, is the vertical architectonic "counterpart" of these developing maxillary components.

10. The mandible has a coronoid process; the maxilla has a zygomatic process.

11. The maxilla has a maxillary tuberosity, the mandible has a lingual tuberosity, each a counterpart to the other.

12. The maxillary teeth drift inferiorly; the mandibular dentition drifts superiorly.

13. Both the maxilla and mandible remodel in a predominately posterior manner, and both become similarly displaced in an anteroinferior mode.

14. The maxillary dental apical base is linked directly to the perimeter of the hard palate. The mandible lacks an attached palate-equivalent altogether.

15. The vertical drifting process in both the maxilla and mandible have **considerable** adjustive capacity and potential for compensations relating to morphogenic variations elsewhere in the craniofacial composite.

16. The positioning of the mandibular corpus and dental arch is a function of remodeling adjustments in alignment, vertical height, and anteroposterior breadth of the **ramus**. The placement of the maxilla is primarily by the **basicranium**, but adjustive capacity occurs in sutural growth potential, both intrinsically and clinically.

17. Because the temporomandibular joint is located toward the rear of the middle cranial fossa, the secondary displacement effect caused by temporal lobe and middle cranial fossa expansion has a much lesser effect on the mandible than the maxilla (see page 47).

MANDIBULAR REMODELING

As introduced in Chapter 1, the mandible does **not** simply "grow" as pictured in Figure 2–17A. It "remodels" (B) and is simultaneously "displaced" as "forward and downward" movement proceeds from the temporomandibular interface (lower right).

The Ramus

In freshman gross anatomy lectures, the significance of the **ramus** of the mandible is mostly that it provides an attachment base for masticatory muscles, which, of course, is a basic function. What usually isn't mentioned, however, is the key role of the ramus in placing the corpus and dental arch into ever-changing fit with the growing maxilla and the face's limitless structural variations. This is provided by critical remodeling and adjustments in ramus alignment, vertical length, and anteroposterior breadth. A best fit with the maxillary arch and middle cranial fossa is thereby provided. Indeed, the **special developmental significance of the ramus is a highlight of craniofacial growth**. Of course, it is not the bony ramus itself that does the job, but rather its osteogenic, chondrogenic, and fibrogenic connective tissues receiving local input control signals that produce the adjustive shape and size of the ramus through time.

Contrary to old time theory, mandibular growth is not a product of, or singularly controlled by, a "master center." **Every** area and surface throughout the entire mandible participates directly in its remodeling process. Some parts, of course, represent more active growth sites than others; it would not be possible for a bone having such a complex architectonic configuration to be otherwise. Keep in mind, as emphasized in Chapter 1, that each local area has regionally local conditions, functions, and relationships. The growth signals generated locally are largely responsible for progressive maturation of each local region in concert with corresponding, but different, growth activities in all the other regions.

The mandibular remodeling description begins below with one of the most important structural parts, the ramus. It is important because (1) it **positions** the lower arch in occlusion with the upper, and (2) it is continuously **adaptive** to the multitude of changing craniofacial conditions.

As briefly described in Chapter 3, the principal vectors of mandibular "growth" are posterior and superior. The ramus is thereby **remodeled** in a generally posterosuperior manner while the mandible as a whole becomes **displaced** anteriorly and inferiorly, as schematized in two dimensions in Figures 2–17B; 2–17, *right*; 4–1; and 1–5. This allows posterior lengthening of the corpus and dental arch.

The posterior development of the mandibular bony arch simultaneously proceeds into the region that was previously occupied by the ramus. This requires a **remodeling conversion** from what used to be ramus into what then becomes mandibular corpus. That is, the whole ramus becomes relocated posteriorly by resorptive and depository remodeling, and the former anterior part of the ramus is structurally altered into an addition to the corpus, which thereby becomes lengthened by this remodeling process.

The remodeling movement of the ramus in a backward direction has usually been pictured as essentially a two-dimensional process (Fig. 2–3).

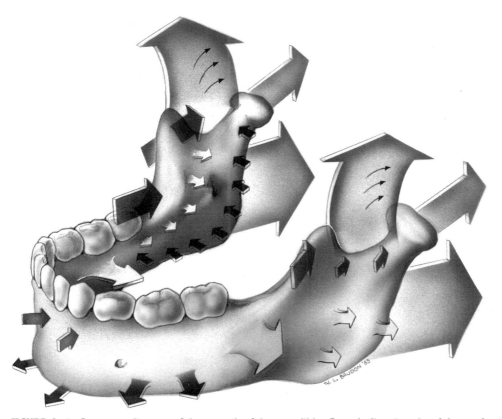

FIGURE 4–1. Summary diagram of the growth of the mandible. Growth directions involving periosteal resorption are indicated by arrows pointing into the bone surface, and growth directions involving periosteal deposition are represented by arrows pointing out of the bone surface. (From Enlow, D. H. and D. B. Harris: A study of the postnatal growth of the human mandible. Am. J. Orthod., 50:25, 1964, with permission.)

This is not merely an incomplete explanation; it is inaccurate as well. The problem is that some of the key anatomic parts that participate in the relocation and remodeling process of the ramus and corpus cannot be seen or represented in conventional two-dimensional headfilms and tracings. Among these is the **lingual tuberosity.**

The Lingual Tuberosity

This is an important structure because it is the direct anatomic equivalent of the maxillary tuberosity (Fig. 4–2). Just as the maxillary tuberosity is a major site of growth for the upper bony arch, so is the lingual tuberosity a major site of growth for the mandible. Yet, this structure is not even included in the basic vocabulary of cephalometrics. The reason, simply, is that it is not recognizable in the headfilm. This presents a severe handicap because the lingual tuberosity is not only a major growth and remodeling site but it also the effective boundary between the two basic parts of the mandible: the ramus and the corpus. The inaccessibility of the lingual tuberosity for routine cephalometric study is a great loss. Nonetheless, the changes this important structure undergoes during growth **must** be understood, all the more so since it cannot be visualized, at least directly, in headfilms.

The lingual tuberosity grows posteriorly by deposits on its posterior-facing surface, just as the maxillary tuberosity undergoes comparable growth additions. Ideally, the maxillary tuberosity closely overlies the lingual tuberosity (i.e., both are aligned on **PM**, a vertical reference line). Moreover, the lingual and maxillary tuberosities ideally have proportionate rates and amounts of respective remodeling. Variations are explained in Chapter 10.

Note that the lingual tuberosity protrudes noticeably in a lingual (medial) direction, and that it lies well toward the midline from the ramus. The prominence of the tuberosity is augmented by the presence of a large resorptive field just below it. This resorptive field produces a sizable de-

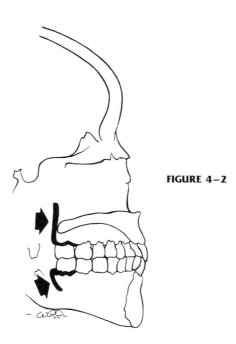

FIGURE 4–2

pression, the **lingual fossa**. The combination of periosteal resorption in the fossa and deposition on the medial-facing surface of the tuberosity itself greatly accentuates the contours of both regions (Figs. 4–3 and 4–4A).

The tuberosity remodels (relocates) in an almost directly posterior direction, with only a relatively slight lateral shift. The latter is because bicondylar width does not increase nearly as much as mandibular length beyond the early childhood period, since most of the bilateral growth of

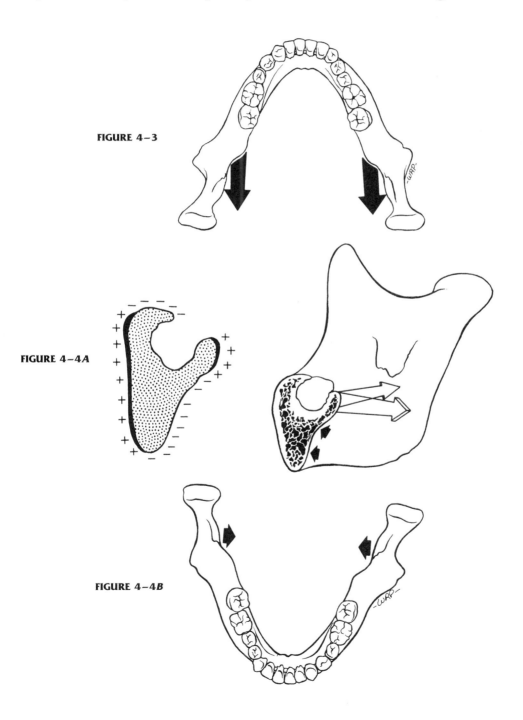

FIGURE 4–3

FIGURE 4–4A

FIGURE 4–4B

the basicranium has occurred by about the second and third years. Even so, the human basicranium is notably wide (and thus also the bicondylar dimension), and this calls for a key remodeling movement to accommodate the more narrow arch (described next).

The posterior growth of the tuberosity is accomplished by continued new deposits of bone on its posterior-facing exposure. As this takes place, that part of the **ramus** just behind the tuberosity remodels **medially** (Fig. 4–4*B*). This area of the ramus is coming into line with the axis of the arch in order to join it and thus become a part of the corpus, thereby lengthening it. As pointed out above, the whole ramus lies well lateral to the dental arch.

The Ramus-to-Corpus Remodeling Conversion

Keep in mind that the whole ramus is also becoming relocated in a posterior direction at the same time. What has happened, in summary, is that bony **arch length** has been increased and the corpus has been lengthened by (1) deposits on the posterior surface of the lingual tuberosity and the contiguous lingual side of the ramus and (2) a resultant lingual shift of the anterior part of the ramus to become added to the corpus.

The presence of resorption on the anterior border of the ramus is often described as "making room for the last molar." It is doing much more than this! The resorptive nature of this region is directly involved in the whole process of progressive relocation of the entire ramus in a posterior direction; this movement continues from the tiny mandible of the fetus to the attainment of full adult mandibular size. The overall extent of ramus movement amounts to several centimeters, not merely the width of the molar.

Another key point is that the traditional description of posterior ramus movement implies a **straight line** backward growth process in a two-dimensional plane, as represented by *a* and *b* in Figure 4–5. This is not the case at all. Such a picture of ramus growth shows, simply, resorption on the anterior edge and deposition on the posterior edge. Development actually takes place as indicated by *c*. (Refer to the "V" principle.) In *d*, the growth direction thus follows the *x* arrows, rather than the straight-line axis shown by the *y* arrows. As pointed out above, because the bicondylar dimension is established much earlier in childhood, bilateral growth separation between the right and left condyles is minimal beyond the early childhood years.

Remodeling activity does not occur **only** on the anterior and posterior margins of the ramus. The various parts of the ramus are oriented so that the span **between** also necessarily comes into play. The **coronoid process** has a propeller-like twist, so that its lingual side faces three general directions all at once: posteriorly, superiorly, and medially. When bone is added onto the lingual side of the coronoid process, its growth thereby proceeds **superiorly**, and this part of the ramus thereby becomes increased in vertical dimension (Fig. 4–6). Notice that each coronoid process lengthens vertically, even though additions are made on the medial (lingual) surfaces of the right and left coronoid processes. This is an example of the enlarging V principle, with the V oriented vertically.

These **same** deposits of bone on the lingual side also bring about a **posterior** direction of growth movement, because this surface also faces posteriorly. A backward movement of the two coronoid processes is the result, even though deposits are added on the inside (lingual) surface. This is also an example of the expanding V principle, with the V oriented horizontally. Notice further that this enables the whole posterior part of the

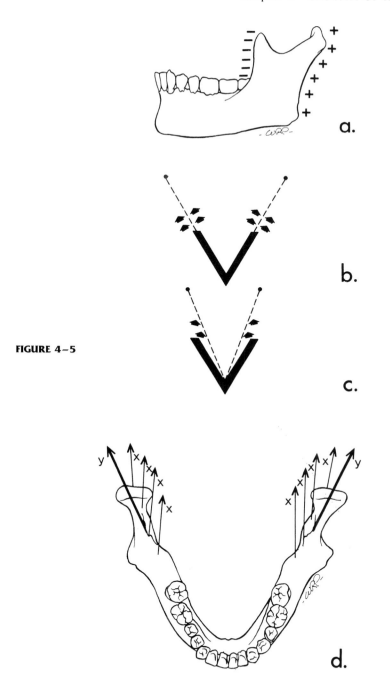

FIGURE 4-5

mandible to **widen** (although not very much except during the period of fetal and early childhood basicranial growth in width), even though deposition occurs on the inside of the V.

These **same** deposits of bone on the lingual side also function to carry the base of the coronoid process and the anterior part of the ramus in a **medial** direction in order to add this part to the lengthening corpus, which lies well medial to the coronoid process. This was underscored above, and, again, is an example of the V principle because a wider part undergoes

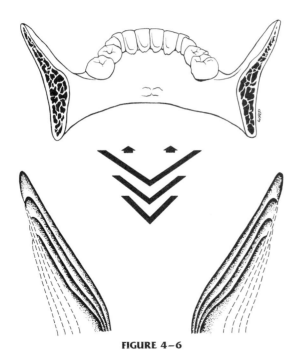

FIGURE 4-6

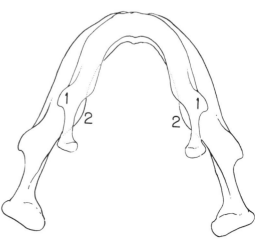

FIGURE 4-7. (Adapted from Enlow, D. H., and D. B. Harris: A study of the postnatal growth of the human mandible. Am. J. Orthod., 50:25, 1964, with permission.)

relocation into a more narrow part as the whole V moves toward its wide end. Thus, the area occupied by the anterior part of the early childhood ramus (Fig. 4–7) in *1* is **relocated** and its former location becomes remodeled into the posterior part of the corpus in *2*.

In all the above relationships, the **buccal** side of the coronoid process has a **resorptive** type of periosteal surface. This surface faces away from the combined superior, posterior, and medial directions of growth. The remainder of most of the superior part of the ramus, including the whole area just below the mandibular (sigmoid) notch and the **superior** (not lateral or medial) portion of the condylar neck, grows superiorly by deposition on the lingual side and resorption from the buccal side. The lower part of the ramus below the coronoid process also has a twisted contour. Its buccal side faces posteriorly toward the direction of backward growth and thus, has a depository type of surface (Fig. 4–8). The opposite lingual side, facing away from the direction of growth, is resorptive.

Keep in mind, in all such growth activities, that it is the enclosing distribution of osteogenic, fibrogenic, and chondrogenic connective tissues in respective local growth fields that actually conduct these remodeling activities. And, it is the signals from the composite of all related soft tissue parts and their growth and functioning that orchestrate the local remodeling patterns. (See Fig. 1–7.) The result is the complex configuration of the mandible that then carries out *its* diverse, regional functions, and grows and develops as it does so.

A single field of surface resorption is present on the inferior edge of the mandible at the ramus-corpus junction. This forms the **antegonial notch** by remodeling from the ramus just behind it as the ramus relocates posteriorly (Fig. 4–9). Other kinds of important mandibular rotations can also involve a sizable resorptive field on the ventral edge of the ramus, as illustrated by Figure 4–15.

The posterior margin of the ramus is a major remodeling site. The condyle generally has an obliquely upward and backward growth direction;

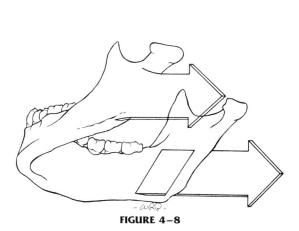

FIGURE 4–8

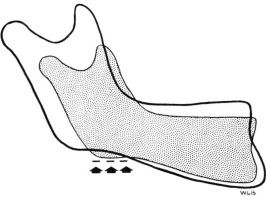

FIGURE 4–9. (Modified from Enlow, D. H.: *The Human Face.* New York, Harper & Row, 1968, p. 232, with permission.)

the trajectory of growth involved (i.e., how much upward and how much backward) is variable and depends on whether an individual is a "horizontal or vertical grower" with respect to the mandible. **Such variable directions are produced by selective cell divisions** in those parts around the periphery of the condyle pointing toward the growth direction, with retardation in other parts of the condyle. However, the growth of the rest of the ramus necessarily keeps pace (or actually determines) the amount of condylar proliferation (see Fig. 4–19). Although correlated, these two regional growth sites (posterosuperior part of ramus and condyle) are essentially separate and develop under different regional conditions, but interrelate in response to the common activating signals that both share. Together they represent the most active areas during mandibular growth in distance moved and amount of histogenic activity. Because of the relatively rapid rate of ramus growth, the bone tissue in the posterior part of the ramus is characteristically one of the more fast-growing types (see Chapter 16). Ramus development often involves a remodeling rotation of the whole ramus, and a resorptive field then occurs on the posterior margin below the condyle, as illustrated by Figures 4–13 and 4–15.

The gonial region is anatomically variable and, therefore, much variation is involved in its pattern of growth. Depending on the presence of inwardly or outwardly directed gonial flares, the buccal side can be either depository or resorptive, with the lingual side having the converse type of growth. However, many different histogenetic combinations can be encountered because of the variability of this region.

While the whole ramus grows posteriorly and superiorly, the mandibular foramen likewise relocates backward and upward by deposition on the anterior and resorption from the posterior part of its rim. The foramen, from childhood through old age, maintains a constant position about midway between the anterior and posterior borders of the ramus. Even when the ramus undergoes marked alterations associated with edentulism (during which it may become quite narrow), this foramen usually sustains a midway location.

The Mandibular Condyle

This is an anatomic part of special interest because it is a major site of growth, having considerable clinical significance. Historically, the condyle

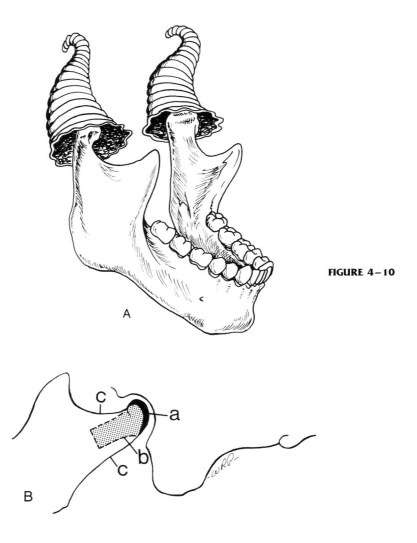

FIGURE 4–10

has been regarded as a kind of cornucopia from which the whole mandible itself pours forth (Fig. 4–10*A*). The condyle was believed (and is still regarded by some) to be the ultimate determinant that, essentially, establishes the mandibular rate of growth, the amount of growth, growth direction, overall mandibular size, and overall mandibular shape. Indeed, it was an attempt to explain what could not, in olden times, then be understood and explained. Present-day biologic theoreticians do not regard the condyle as a unique kind of structure actually functioning to "regulate" morphogenesis of the whole mandible, including its many regional parts. It is no longer believed to represent a pacesetting "master center" with all other regional growth fields subordinate to and dependent on it for direct control. Yet, the condyle is a major field of growth, nonetheless, and it is an important one. What, then, it must be asked, could be even more important than serving as a master center? That question is answered in the pages that follow. Indeed, there is a key function that **does**, in fact, transcend a mythical "master center" notion.

During mandibular development, the condyle functions as a **regional** field of growth that provides an adaptation for its own localized growth circumstances, just as all the other regional fields accommodate their own particular (but different) localized growth conditions. The growth of the mandible as a whole is the product of all the different **regional** forces and regional functional agents of growth control acting on it to produce the topographically complex shape of the mandible as a whole. Growth is the aggregate expression of the composite of all these localized factors. Every local growth site is independently self-contained, although all are bound as an interrelated mosaic proceeding as a "symphony of developmental movements."

The condylar growth mechanism itself is a clear-cut process. **Cartilage** is a special **non-vascular** tissue and is involved because variable levels of **compression** occur at its articular contact with the temporal bone of the basicranium. There are no capillaries in cartilage to press closed by a compressive surface force. In addition, importantly, the intercellular matrix of cartilage is markedly **hydrophilic** and, therefore, is turgid and unyielding to surface pressure. An **endochondral** growth mechanism is required for this part of the mandible because the condyle grows in a direction toward its articulation into the face of direct pressure. An intramembranous type of growth could not operate, because the periosteal mode of osteogenesis is not pressure adapted and has a low threshold for compressive forces. Endochondral growth occurs only at the articular contact part of the condyle, because this is where pressure exists at levels that would be beyond the tolerance of the bone's vascular soft tissue membrane. As seen in Figure 4–10B, the endochondral bone tissue (b) formed in association with the condylar cartilage (a) is laid down only in the medullary portion of the condyle. The enclosing bony cortices (c) are produced by periosteal-endosteal osteogenic activity; these vascular membranes are not subject to the compressive forces of articulation, but, rather, are essentially tension related because of muscle and connective tissue attachments. The real functional significance of the condylar cartilage thus involves an avascular and matrix-firm adaptation for regional pressure and movable articulation. This regional, **endochondral** bone-forming mechanism develops as a specific response to this particular **local** circumstance. The cartilage itself does **not** contain genetic programming that directly determines and governs the course of growth in all the other areas of the mandible, as presumed by obsolete theory. The pressure-tolerant condylar cartilage, however, provides another exceedingly basic and significant growth function, as described later.

The condylar cartilage is a **secondary** type of cartilage, which means that it does not develop by differentiation from the established **primary** cartilages of the fetal skull (i.e., the cartilages of the pharyngeal arches, such as Meckel's cartilage, and the definitive cartilages of the basicranium). Phylogenetically, the original ancestral reptilian endochondral bone (the articular) that provided for mandibular articulation became converted to an ear ossicle (the malleus) in mammals. Then, in mammalian evolution, a "secondary" cartilage was subsequently developed on the ancestral mandible (the intramembranous dentary bone) to provide for lower jaw articulation with the basicranium. It is believed that the unique connective tissue covering (capsule) of the "new mammalian" condylar cartilage was actually an original periosteum. Its undifferentiated connective tissue stem cells, however, metaplastically developed into chondroblasts, rather than osteoblasts, because of the compressive forces acting on this membrane. An adventitious type of "secondary" cartilage thereby developed, rather than bone, because of the changed functional and developmental conditions imposed upon this part of the mandible. It is thus not an "endochondral" bone in the sense that phylogenetically, the bones of the basicranium are endochondral in type. The mammalian mandible is essentially a membrane bone in which one part (i.e., what has become the new condyle) has developed in response to a phylogenetically altered developmental situation. This involved the ectopic presence of pressure that, in turn, caused localized ischemia and anoxia, factors known to induce chondrogenesis from the pool of undifferentiated connective tissue cells, rather than osteogenesis.

The condylar cartilage is thus phylogenetically and ontogenetically unique and differs in histologic organization from most other growth cartilages involved in endochondral bone formation. It is not structurally comparable to a long bone's cartilaginous epiphyseal plate. Further, it is now generally recognized that the secondary cartilage of the condyle is not the genetic pacemaker for the growth of the mandible. Its real contribution is to provide **regional adaptive growth** (i.e., growth that is secondarily responsive to a variety of circumstantial conditions) thus giving yet another meaning for the term "secondary." This maintains the condylar region in proper anatomic relationship with the temporal bone as the whole mandible is simultaneously being carried downward and forward. Thus, the condyle is not a "primary" center of growth, but rather (1) secondary in evolution; (2) secondary in embryonic origin; and (3) secondary in adaptive responses to changing developmental conditions.* It is now believed that the condyle does **not** establish the rate or the amount of overall mandibular growth. The condyle does, however, have a special multidirectional capacity for growth and remodeling in selective response to varied mandibular displacement movements and **rotations** (described below). The special structure of the condyle provides for this, unlike the committed unidirectional linear growth of long bone epiphyseal plates produced by the characteristic linearly oriented direction of chondroblast proliferation.

In summary, the condyle, rather than acting as a "master growth center," actually performs in a much more functional role. It (1) provides a pressure-tolerant articular contact, and (2) it makes possible a multidimensional growth capacity in response to ever-changing, developmental conditions and variations.

A unique **capsular layer** of poorly vascularized connective tissue covers the articular surface of the condyle (a in Fig. 4–11). This membrane is highly cellular early in development, but becomes densely fibrous with age and function. Just deep to it is a special layer of prechondroblast cells (b). This is the predominant site for cellular proliferation, and it is responsible for the tissue-feeding process providing an ongoing flow of new developing cartilage (layer c) for endochondral replacement by bone as the deeper layers advance.

The proliferative process produces the "upward and backward" growth movement of the condyle (Fig. 4–11). The condylar cartilage **moves** by prechondroblast cell divisions with an equal amount of cartilage removal at the cartilage-bone interface. The removal phase involves replacement with endochondral bone. A trail of continually forming endochondral bone thus follows the moving cartilage, as schematized by layer d.

The prechondroblast cells are closely packed, and very little intercellular matrix is present. This is due to their rapid proliferative activity. A relatively thin transitional zone or immature zone then occurs deep to the proliferative layer as new cells feed into it, with a somewhat increased amount of matrix. This layer does not appear to contribute materially to the cell division process. The deeper cells then become transformed into

---

*Another common definition is that secondary growth cartilages are those, simply, that have a type of structure that puts them in a separate category from the typical epiphyseal growth plates of long bones. Articular cartilages are another example of the secondary type. As shown by Moss, the condylar cartilage is comparable, both in structure and growth behavior, to an articular, rather than an epiphyseal plate, cartilage. It is not directly "articular," however, because of its special fibrous covering.

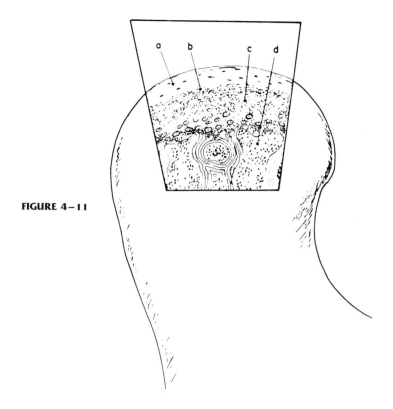

FIGURE 4–11

the next layer as it "moves up" behind the moving layers ahead of it and is composed of densely packed chondroblasts that are undergoing hypertrophy (*c*). The matrix is also noticeably scant.

The small amount of matrix in the deepest part of the hypertrophied zone becomes calcified, and a zone of resorption and bone deposition follows (*d*). Unlike the arrangement in typical *primary* growth cartilage (i.e., epiphyseal plates of long bones and synchondroses), these various zones **do not have linear columns of daughter cells. This is a notable histologic difference between primary and secondary types of growth cartilage**. The nonlinear arrangement of the daughter cells in the condylar cartilage thus does not reflect the direction in which the condyle is growing. It also means, importantly, that the cap of condylar cartilage has **multidirectional proliferative capacity**. This is one of the most significant developmental features of the condyle. Depending on *where* in the condylar cartilage that mitotic divisions occur, **that** part of the condyle (and ramus) thereby proliferates more vertically or more posteriorly, or virtually any point between, as determined by input signals. These input signals are related to both the demands of dynamic and static articulation of the teeth as well as the architectonic pattern of "fitting" among the multitude of craniofacial parts.

While all this is going on, the periosteum and endosteum are active in producing the **cortical** bone that encloses the **medullary core** of endochondral bone tissue. The overlying cap of pressure-tolerant cartilage has taken the brunt of the compressive forces acting on the condyle. The cortical ring of intramembranous bone continues down onto the condylar neck.

The lingual and buccal sides of the neck characteristically have **resorptive** surfaces (Fig. 2–2). This is because the condyle is quite broad and the neck is narrow. The neck is progressively relocated into areas previously held by the much wider condyle, and it is sequentially derived from the condyle as the condyle **moves** in a superoposterior course. What used to be condyle in turn becomes the neck as one is remodeled from the other (Fig. 4–12). This is done by periosteal resorption combined with endosteal deposition. Explained another way, the **endosteal** surface of the neck actually faces the growth direction; the periosteal side points away from the course of growth. This is another example of the V principle, with the V-shaped cone of the condylar neck growing toward its wide end. (See Figs. 2–2 and 2–9.)

All the while, as condylar and ramus development proceeds, the mandible, as a whole, is becoming displaced anteroinferiorly (Fig. 2–17). What is the physical force that produces the forward and downward primary **displacement** of the mandible? For many years it was presumed that growth of the **condylar cartilage**, because it is known that cartilage is a special pressure-adapted type of tissue, creates a "thrust" of the mandible against its articular-bearing surface in the glenoid fossa. The proliferation of the cartilage **toward** its contact thereby was presumed to **push** the whole mandible away from it.

Some students of facial biology still accept this explanation. However, most contemporary investigators and biologic researchers have concluded that this is either an incomplete or an off-target answer. The biologic reasons follow. See also Figure 1–7 and pages 6 and 85.

The Condylar Question

A great puzzle was created when it was pointed out that functional mandibles totally lacking condyles exist in nature. Yet their morphology is more or less normal in all other respects; only the condyle and part of the condylar neck are congenitally missing. Moreover, these **bilaterally** condyle-lacking mandibles occupy an essentially normal anatomic **position**; the bony arch is properly placed for occlusion, and the mandible functions (albeit with distress) in masticatory movements even though it lacks an articulation. These revealing observations suggested two conclusions. First, the condyles may not play the kingpin role of a "master center" pace-setting the growth processes in the other parts of the mandible. Second, the whole mandible can become **displaced** anteriorly and inferiorly into its functional position without a "push" against the basicranium. Many experimental studies have subsequently been carried out with similar results, although investigators are still arguing about the proper way to interpret their meaning.

These observations led to a consideration of the fabled "functional matrix" by students of facial biology. The idea is essentially that the mandible is **carried** forward and downward, just as the maxilla is presumably carried anteroinferiorly in conjunction with the growth expansion of the soft tissue matrix associated with it. It is a passive type of carrying in which condylar remodeling acts with displacement as co-participants but not as the driving force. They proceed together in mutual response to common activating signals. Thus, as the mandible is displaced away from its basicranial articular contact, the condyle and whole ramus **secondarily** (but virtually simultaneously) remodels toward it (see Fig. 1–5), thereby closing the potential space without an actual gap being created (unless the condyle does not develop at all, as mentioned above). There are still, however, actual but variable levels of pressure being exerted on the articular surface of the condyle because it is a movable joint; it is presumably a **relief** of the **amount** of pressure that relates to condylar growth. The enlarging soft tissue mass draws the mandible protrusively to cause this.

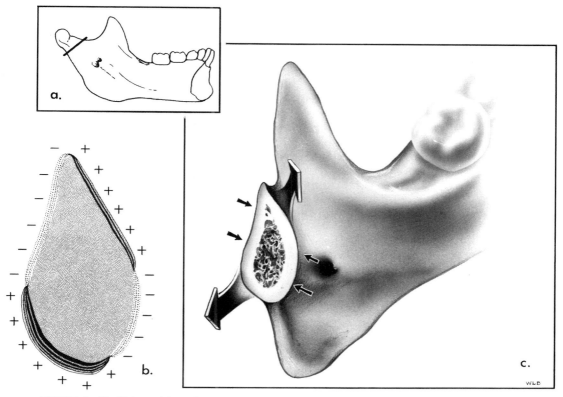

FIGURE 4–12. (Adapted from Enlow, D. H., and D. B. Harris: A study of the postnatal growth of the human mandible. Am. J. Orthod., 50:25, 1974, with permission.)

The clinical implications are apparent. Just how involved is the condyle as an underlying and causative factor in facial abnormalities? What happens to the mandible if the condyle is injured during the childhood period? To the orthodontist, a key question is whether the condyle itself is the **direct** and **primary** target of any given clinical procedure, or whether it **follows** in response to clinical signals acting on soft tissues (e.g., the masticatory musculature), which in turn activate the composite of osteogenic and chondrogenic connective tissues of the ramus and its condyle as a **whole**. How can overall mandibular length be clinically increased or decreased for Class II and III individuals by physiologic or mechanical intervention in this composite growth mechanism?

The current thinking is that the condylar cartilage **does** have some measure of intrinsic, genetic programming. This, however, appears to be restricted to a capacity for continued cellular proliferation. That is, the cartilage cells are coded and geared to divide and continue to divide, but extracondylar factors are needed to sustain this activity. The **rate** and **directions** of condylar growth are presumably subject to the influence of extracondylar agents, including intrinsic and extrinsic biomechanical forces and physiologic inductors. It is believed that increased amounts of pressure on the cartilage serve to inhibit the rate of cell division and proliferation. Decreased amounts of pressure appear to stimulate and accelerate growth. Presumably, forces applied to the mandible in such a way that they increase the level of pressure on the condyle would result in a shorter mandible **if** this were done during the period of active condylar growth. Similarly, a **release** of some of the compressive force acting on the condylar cartilage would produce a larger mandible if done during the active growth period. These conclusions are based largely on animal experiments and are not, at least at present, usable for everyday clinical practice. Moreover, recent research studies show that the nature of the condylar stimulus is more complex than simple forces acting directly on the condyle; rather, nerve-muscle-connective tissue pathways are involved, and changes utilize a **composite** of such tissue responses and chain feedbacks with the condyle as well as the other parts of the mandible that also participate. Sensory nerve input from the periodontal membranes and from the soft tissue matrix throughout the face pick up stimuli that are passed on via motor nerves to muscles that, in turn, alter the displacement and the positioning of the mandible, which then affects the course of growth and remodeling by the condyle and all other areas of the growing mandible. The key point is that **regional** areas within the condyle itself can be activated or inhibited by resultant, localized forces to grow regionally either more or less. This alters the **amount** of ramus growth in different **directions**, thereby continually adjusting both the alignment and the shape of the ramus to accommodate its multiple and changing anatomic and functional relationships.

This whole discussion of the condylar role, however, bypasses a most fundamental consideration. Is it the condyle itself or, more basically, the **whole ramus** with its condyle that is the real issue. This is evaluated later.

The Adaptive Role of the Condyle

The random arrangement of the condylar prechondroblasts, described earlier, is in contrast to the linear columns of daughter cells associated with the essentially unidirectional growth of long bones. This is a histogenetic adaptation of the condylar cartilage that provides opportunity for selected, multidirectional growth potential. Consider the virtually limitless range of anatomic variations that occur in the structural patterns of the nasomaxillary complex and basicranium. There are dolichocephalic and brachycephalic types of headforms, vertically long and short nasomaxillary regions, wide and narrow palates and upper arches, widely separated versus closely placed glenoid fossae, steep versus shallow cranial floor flexures, broad versus narrow pharyngeal regions, large versus small tooth sizes, male versus female patterns, and so on. If the growth, shape, and dimensions of the mandible were actually "preprogrammed" within the genes of condylar chondroblasts (according to old theory), and if the condyle were indeed to function as an ultimate "growth control center," without taking into account structural and developmental vagaries in the rest of the craniofacial complex, there is **no way** that a fitting of the mandible to the basicranium on one end and to the maxilla on the other could be achieved. If the condyle functioned as a self-contained, independent structure with its growth coded in an isolated cartilage unresponsive to variations and continual changes in the growth and morphology of contiguous regions, these many developmental and functional relationships simply could not be workable. However, it is the **adaptive responsive** nature of the condylar growth process that allows for a latitude of morphologic and morphogenic adjustments and a working (if not perfect) functional relationship among all of them. What could be more exalted in status than serving as a "master center of growth"? **The answer is the condyle's adaptive capacity.** A remarkable histogenic function.

The New Image of the Condyle and "Condylar Growth"

One specific point, however, needs to be clearly understood. Historically, it has been the **condyle** that has been given all the glory, whether as the primary **determinant** of mandibular growth or, as we now see it, as the **respondent** structure that makes possible adaptive, truly interrelated growth. The problem, however, is that we still use and endure the anachronistic, held-over term "condylar growth." This old term, unfortunately, implies an incomplete and inaccurate understanding of the whole picture. True enough, the condyle, of course, plays a significant role. It is directly involved as a unique, regional growth site; it provides an indispensable latitude for adaptive growth; it provides movable articulation; it is pressure tolerant and provides a means for bone growth (endochondral) in a situation in which ordinary periosteal (intramembranous) growth would not be possible; and it can also, all too frequently, become involved in TMJ (temporomandibular joint) pathology and distress. With regard to the growth and adaptive requirements for the mandible, **it is not just the condyle**, however, that participates as the key component. The **whole ramus** is directly involved. This is an all important point. The ramus bridges the pharyngeal compartment and places the mandibular arch in occlusal position with the maxillary arch. The horizontal breadth of the ramus determines the anteroposterior position of the lower arch, and the height of the ramus accommodates the vertical dimension and growth of both the nasal and masticatory components of the midface. The dimensions and morphology of the ramus are directly involved in the attachments of the masticatory muscles, and the ramus must accommodate their growth and size. It is the growth and development of the **whole** ramus, not merely the condyle, that accomplishes these multiple and basic ends. As already seen, the growth and remodeling of the ramus are complex maneuvers and involve many regional growth sites, only one of which is the condyle. The term "condylar growth" is misleading and conveys a biologic misconception. More properly, the terms needs to be "**ramus** and condylar growth." In a real sense, the condyle **follows** the growth of the whole ramus and does not lead it. This is important, because studies have shown, and continue to show, that the entire ramus and the muscles attached to it, not just the condyle, are a principal clinical target for many orthodontic procedures. Compare Figure 2–6 (an incomplete picture conveyed by the old term "condylar growth") with Figure 4–1 (whole ramus growth). Significantly, the "adaptive capacity" of the condyle discussed in the preceding paragraph **also** involves the entire ramus. The ramus, importantly, is also an important anatomic part directly involved in growth **compensations**, as described later.

The mandible has often been regarded as less responsive to orthopedic forces than the maxilla because the condyle itself is capped by the more pressure-tolerant cartilage, and also because its growth pre-program (old theory) has been presumed to resist extrinsic (clinical) forces. However, because the whole ramus is directly involved as well, consider that such clinical forces must overwhelm not just "the condyle" but also the massive masticatory musculature, a significant restraining factor. Furthermore, clinically induced changes in condylar cartilage growth may be negated by equal and opposite growth changes in the ramus. It follows then that mandibular orthopedics must modify growth signals targeted at both the ramus and condyle to be maximally effective.

The Ramus and Middle Cranial Fossa Relationship

This is a kinship that, at first thought, could seem unlikely considering their distant functions. However, the relationship becomes real during development and is indeed a significant consideration.

As the horizontal enlargement of the middle cranial fossa and brain growth advance the nasomaxillary complex by forward displacement, the horizontal span of the pharynx correspondingly increases (Fig. 3–9). The skeletal dimension of the pharynx is established by the size of the middle cranial fossa because the floor of this basicranial fossa is the roof of the pharyngeal compartment. The ramus must necessarily increase to an equivalent extent. The effective anteroposteral dimensions of the ramus and middle cranial fossa (not their respective oblique dimensions) are direct counterparts to each other. One structural function of the ramus, in spanning the pharynx, is to provide developmental potential for adaptations required to place the corpus in a continuously functional position because of variations elsewhere in the face and neurocranium. If such adjustments are fully or even only partially successful, a better occlusal fit is achieved. This is done by the same remodeling process that simultaneously relocates the ramus posteriorly as it becomes displaced anteroinferiorly.

Ramus Uprighting

The ramus normally becomes more vertically aligned during its development. As long as the ramus is actively growing in a posterior direction, this is accomplished by greater amounts of bone additions on the inferior part of the posterior border than on the superior part (Fig. 4–13). A correspondingly greater amount of matching resorption on the anterior border takes place inferiorly than superiorly. A "remodeling" rotation of ramus alignment thus occurs. Condylar growth becomes directed in a more vertical course along with the rest of the ramus. See page 34.

The reason the ramus becomes progressively more upright as childhood development proceeds is that it must lengthen vertically to a much greater extent than it broadens horizontally, and this creates a developmental problem for the "genic" tissues involved (Fig. 4–14). In this schematic diagram, the pharynx (and middle cranial fossa) enlarges horizontally from a to a'. The ramus enlarges, correspondingly, from b to b' to match

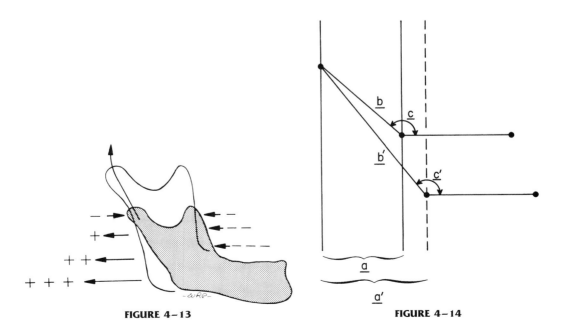

FIGURE 4–13   FIGURE 4–14

it. It also **lengthens vertically,** however. Angle c is thereby reduced to c' in order to accommodate the vertical **nasomaxillary growth** also taking place at the same time. The "gonial angle" thus must undergo change (close) in order to **prevent** change in the occlusal relationship between the maxillary and mandibular arches.

However, vertical lengthening of the ramus continues to take place **after** horizontal ramus growth slows or ceases (when the horizontal growth of the middle cranial fossa begins to slow and cease). This is to match the continued vertical growth of the midface. To achieve this, condylar growth may become more vertically directed, and a different pattern of ramus remodeling can also become operative (Fig. 4–15). The direction of deposition and resorption reverses. A **forward** growth direction can then occur in some individuals on the **anterior** border in the upper part of the coronoid process. Resorption takes place on the upper part of the posterior border. A posterior direction of remodeling takes place in the lower part of the posterior border. The result is a more upright alignment and a longer vertical dimension of the ramus without a material increase in breadth. This remodeling change, when it occurs, appears to be more marked when the backward relocation of the ramus, to provide for corpus lengthening, has decreased. There are probably other relationships involved as well, including different facial and headform types, although the biologic basis is presently not fully understood. (See Hans, et al., 1995.)

The ramus thus undergoes a remodeling alteration in which its angle becomes changed in order to **retain** constant positional relationships between the upper and lower arches. Otherwise, development among all the diverse parts involved at different times, by different amounts, and in different directions would result in a marked misfit between the upper and lower jaws. This is another example of a developmental "compensation" (intrinsic adjustment) at work.

If mandible a in Figure 4–16 is superimposed over b in the anatomically functional position, it can be seen that all the complex remodeling changes outlined above serve simply to alter the ramus angle without increasing its breadth. This also accommodates the growing muscle sling and muscular adaptations associated with mandibular rotations. In addition, increased space for third molar eruption is provided.

The composite of vertical growth changes of the mandibular dentoalveolar arch, the ramus, and the middle cranial fossae must **match** the

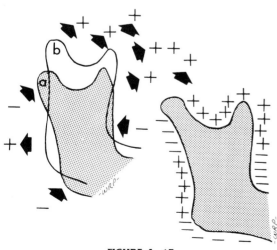

FIGURE 4–15

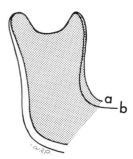

FIGURE 4–16

composite of vertical nasomaxillary growth changes to achieve continuing facial balance. Any differential will lead to a displacement type of mandibular rotation, either downward and backward or forward and upward. Normal variations of facial type and headform pattern are a common basis for such mandibular rotations.

During the descent of the maxillary arch and the vertical drift of the mandibular teeth, the anterior mandibular teeth simultaneously drift **lingually** and superiorly (Fig. 4–17). This produces a greater or lesser amount of anterior **overjet** and **overbite**. The remodeling process that brings this about (Fig. 4–18) involves periosteal resorption on the labial bony cortex (*a*), deposition on the alveolar surface of the labial cortex (*b*), resorption on the alveolar surface of the lingual cortex (*c*), and deposition on the lingual side of the lingual cortex (*d*).

At the same time, bone is progressively added onto the external surface of the mandibular basal bone area, including the mental protuberance (chin). The reversal between these two growth fields usually occurs at the point where the concave surface contour becomes convex. The result of this two-way growth process is a progressively enlarging mental protuberance. Man is one of only two species having a **"chin"** (the elephant is the other, although the analogy is loose). Whatever its mechanical adaptations, the human chin is a phylogenetic result of downward-backward whole-face rotation into a vertical position, decreased prognathism (as described in Chapter 9), the marked extent of vertical facial growth, and the development of an overbite (in comparison to an end-to-end type of occlusion).

The Human Chin

In Chapter 9, the evolutionary factors of upright (bipedal) body posture and the greatly enlarged human brain, as they relate to a marked downward and backward rotational placement of the nasomaxillary complex, are described. For the mandible and its development, that situation has led to a serious evolutionary problem. This midfacial rotation has caught the human mandible in a closing vice, with the maxilla on the one side and the airway and other cervical and pharyngeal parts on the other. The result has placed these vital parts in real jeopardy. However, there have been three evolutionary adjustments, each based on contrasting headform and facial types. First, in many long-midface individuals, the "fitting" of the lower jaw has led to a characteristic overbite and overjet bimaxillary feature, thus relieving the closing vise. Second, in many short-face types, a tendency toward an anterior cross bite or bimaxillary protrusion has

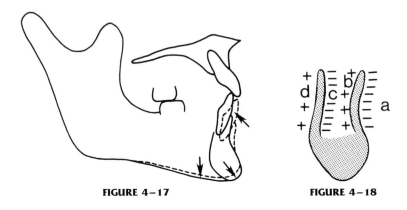

FIGURE 4–17   FIGURE 4–18

achieved an alternate adaptation to the problem. A third way is by anterior crowding, which shortens the mandible. All three are "malocclusions" in the clinical context, but nonetheless have served as phylogenetic answers (biologic compensations) to this evolutionary problem.

There is considerable variation in the placement of the reversal line between the resorptive alveolar and the depository parts of the chin; it may be fairly high or low. Variations also occur in the relative amounts of resorption and deposition. There are, correspondingly, marked variations in the shape and the size of the chin among different individuals. It is one of the most variable (but slow-growing) areas in the entire mandible as seen among the different basic facial types and patterns.

The Ramus-Corpus Combine

Most of the outer surfaces of the mandibular corpus receive progressive deposits of bone on both its buccal and lingual sides, with resorption occurring from the endosteal surfaces. (Resorptive periosteal areas occur, however, on the labial side of the incisor region and below the lingual tuberosity, as previously described.) The above changes enlarge the breadth of the corpus; the buccal side remodels, to a slightly greater extent than the lingual side because bony arch width increases slightly during postnatal mandibular development, but not as much as the bony maxillary arch increases in width. The ventral border of the corpus is also depository; this is a prolonged growth process, however, and progresses in concert with long-term masticatory development and dental arch maturation.

The amount of upward alveolar growth greatly exceeds the extent of downward enlargement by the "basal bone." (Note: Basal bone is a term sometimes used to denote that part of the corpus not involved in "alveolar" movements of the teeth. This area has a higher threshold of resistance to extrinsic forces than alveolar bone, which is extremely labile. There is no distinct structural line, however, separating basal from alveolar bone tissue. This is more of a physiologic than an anatomic difference.)

Whenever a change in the angle between the ramus and corpus develops, multiple sites of remodeling are involved. The adaptive trajectory of condylar growth is usually a factor (Fig. 4–19), as shown by *a, b,* and *c.* **Variable growth directions are produced by selective proliferation of prechondroblasts in some parts around the periphery of the condyle, with retardation of cell divisions in other parts.** Thus, "condylar growth" is an active **respondent** in developmental function that can adapt to the widely variable conditions imposed on it.

If **backward** (but not yet upward) condylar *and* ramus growth has slowed or largely ceased (Fig. 4–13), remodeling can produce angular changes of the ramus relative to the corpus by direct remodeling. Such remodeling processes can either close or open the "gonial angle." In fact, some clinical intervention strategies (most notably the vertical chin cup) attempt to alter gonial angle by **ramus** (not just "condylar") remodeling to achieve the desired clinical result.

Note these two fundamental points: It is the **entire ramus** that is involved, not just "condylar growth." Also, any change in the ramus-corpus ("gonial") angle is largely produced by **ramus** remodeling, not the corpus, and **is determined by the remodeling direction of the ramus with its condyle** (Fig. 4–20). This is a most important point because the **whole** ramus (not just the condyle) is a primary clinical target. It is remodeling combinations such as those shown in Figure 4–13) that are primarily responsible for ramus and corpus alignment positions relative to each other. Direct upward remodeling of the corpus, involving resorption on its infe-

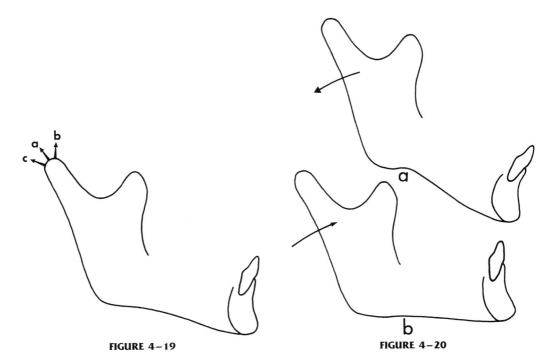

FIGURE 4-19   **FIGURE 4-20**

rior surface, does not ordinarily occur. A marked superior extent of alveolar bone growth and the drifting of anterior mandibular teeth, however,
is common (see curve of Spee). The size of the antegonial notch is determined largely by the nature of the ramus-corpus angle and also by the
extent of bone deposition on the underside (inferior margin) just posterior
or anterior to the notch. The notch itself is also increased in size owning
to its resorptive periosteal surface. A mandible characteristically has a less
prominent antegonial notch (Fig. 4–20*b*) if the angle between the ramus
and corpus becomes closed, and a much more prominent antegonial notch
(a) if it becomes opened. The antegonial notch itself is surface resorptive
because it is relocated posteriorly, as the corpus lengthens, into the former
gonial region of the ramus (Fig. 4–9).

A significant point is that clinical manipulation of the ramus is effective
only so long as it is actively engaged in mandibular growth. Thereafter,
how to unlock its responsive remodeling capacity is poorly understood,
since a developmental "balance" (Chapter 1) has long since been achieved
with the vertical, anteroposterior and bilateral relationships with the basicranium, airway, nasomaxillary complex, dentition, tongue, and the masticatory and hyoid musculature.

5

The Nasomaxillary Complex

Just as the mandible **remodels** in a predominately posterosuperior manner as it simultaneously becomes **displaced** in an opposite anteroinferior direction, the nasomaxillary composite also "grows " in a generally comparable way. Because of the notable differences between mandibular and nasomaxillary circumstances, however, the midface necessarily involves additional and significant developmental operations.

The Maxillary Tuberosity and Arch Lengthening

The horizontal lengthening of the bony maxillary arch is produced by remodeling at the maxillary tuberosity. The area shown in Figure 5–1A is the specific growth field that carries this out. It is a **depository** field in which the backward-facing periosteal surface of the tuberosity receives continued deposits of new bone as long as growth in this part of the face continues. The arch also widens, and the lateral surface is, similarly, depository. The endosteal side of the cortex within the interior of the tuberosity (the maxillary sinus) is resorptive. The cortex thus moves (relocates) progressively posteriorly and also, to a lesser extent, in a lateral direction. The maxillary sinus increases in size as a result. In the newborn, this sinus is quite small but becomes greatly expanded as growth continues and eventually occupies the greater part of the large suborbital compartment. (See page 154 for the interesting evolutionary significance of this region.)

Because distal movement of the maxillary first molar is often part of an orthodontic treatment plan, the maxillary tuberosity is important in clinical orthodontics. Every mechanical option designed to move the maxillary first molar distally exploits the growth potential of the tuberosity. It is **this** depository field that allows the clinician to "expand the arch" by moving teeth into an area of bone deposition. Orthodontists often extract teeth to adjust arch length. This decision is based primarily on the **lower** arch discrepancy because of the potential to expand the upper arch both laterally and distally. A second reason is that, in a Class II molar relationship, such distal molar movement aids the clinician in achieving the treatment goal of a Class I molar relationship.

The maxillary tuberosity is a major "site" of maxillary growth. It does not, however, provide for the growth of the whole maxilla, but relates only to that area associated with the posterior part of the lengthening arch.

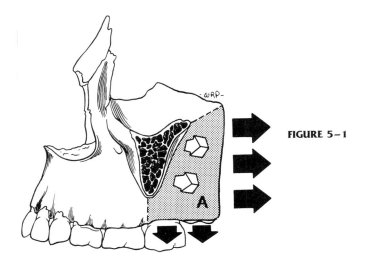

FIGURE 5–1

Many other basic and important sites of growth also exist throughout the various parts of this architecturally and functionally complex bone (Figs. 5–2 and 5–3). Remember, also, that the position of the maxillary tuberosity is actually established by the posterior boundary of the anterior cranial fossa, and any clinically induced deviation could result in a developmental rebound. (See the **PM Plane** in other chapters.)

The whole maxilla undergoes a simultaneous process of **primary displacement** in an anterior and inferior direction as it grows and lengthens posteriorly (Fig. 5–4). In Figure 5–5, extensive remodeling occurs throughout the nasomaxillary complex (*B* and *C*) as the entire region undergoes inferior (and anterior) displacement (*D*). The nature of the force that produces this anterior movement has, historically, been a subject of great controversy. One early theory (long since abandoned) suggested that additions of new bone on the posterior surface of the elongating maxillary tuberosity "push" the maxilla against the adjacent muscle-supported pterygoid plates. This presumably would cause a resultant shove of the entire maxilla anteriorly because of its own posterior bone growth activity. The idea was aborted, however, when it was realized that a bone's osteogenic membrane is pressure sensitive, and that the bone growth process does not have the physiologic capacity to actually push the whole bone away from the other bones by itself. The reason, simply, is that a surface force exerting pressure causes compression that would press closed the sensitive capillary plexus within the vascular osteogenic connective tissue. This renders it inoperable and leads to necrosis.

Another theory held that bone growth within the various maxillary *sutures* produces a pushing-apart of the bones, with a resultant thrust of the whole maxilla anteriorly (and inferiorly as well). Although this old explanation is still sometimes heard, it has been soundly rejected for the reason just mentioned: bone tissue is not capable of growth in a field that requires the levels of compression needed to produce a "pushing" type of displacement. The sutural connective tissue is not adapted to a pressure-related growth process (in contrast to cartilaginous types of bone-to-bone articular contacts, which are much more compression tolerant). The suture is essentially a **tension-adapted** tissue. This is a basic difference. Its collagenous fiber construction is a functional design for traction accommodation across the connective tissue bridge between separate bones. The presence of any unusual pressure on a suture triggers bone resorption, not depo-

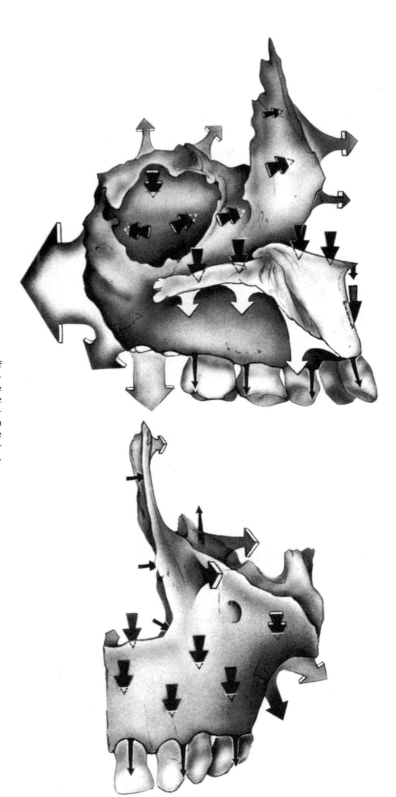

FIGURE 5–2. Summary diagram of maxillary remodeling. Growth directions involving surface resorption are represented by arrows entering the bone surface. Directions of growth involving surface deposition are shown by arrows emerging from the bone surface. (From Enlow, D. H.: *The Human Face.* New York, Harper & Row, 1968. p. 164, with permission.)

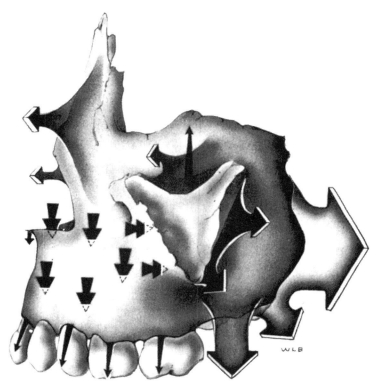

FIGURE 5–3. (From Enlow, D. H.: *The Human Face.* New York, Harper & Row, 1968, p. 164, with permission.)

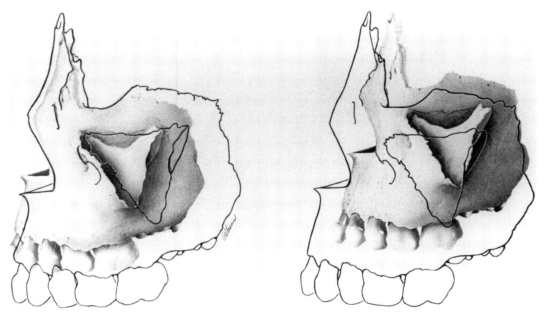

FIGURE 5–4. (From Moyers, R. E., and D. Enlow: In: *Handbook of Orthodontics*, 4th Ed. Chicago, Mosby-Yearbook, Inc., 1988, with permission.)

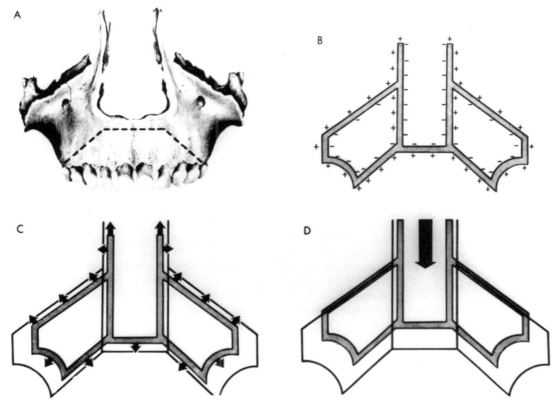

FIGURE 5–5. (From Moyers, R. E., and D. Enlow: In.: *Handbook of Orthodontics*, 4th Ed. Chicago, Mosby-Yearbook, Inc., 1988, with permission.)

sition, to relieve the pressure. This decreases the pressure by removing some of the bone.

It is believed that the stimulus for sutural bone growth (remodeling) relates to the tension produced by the **displacement** of that bone. The deposition of the new bone is in tandem to the displacement, rather than the force that causes it. (See later in this chapter and also Chapter 16 for further discussion of the sutural growth process.) Thus, as the entire maxilla is **carried** forward and downward by displacement, the osteogenic sutural membranes form new bone tissue that enlarges the overall size of the whole bone and sustains constant bone-to-bone sutural contact.

The Biomechanical Force Underlying Maxillary Displacement

An early explanation for maxillary displacement is the now famous "*nasal septum*" theory (Fig. 5–6). This was developed largely by Scott, and the premise for the idea was quite reasonable. It developed from the criticisms of the "sutural theory" described above. The hypothesis was soon adopted by many investigators around the world and became more or less the standard explanation for a number of years, replacing the sutural theory. **Cartilage** is specifically adapted to certain pressure-related growth sites, as mentioned before, because it is a special tissue uniquely structured to provide the capacity for growth in a field of compression. (See Chapter 16.) Cartilage is present in the epiphyseal plates of long bones,

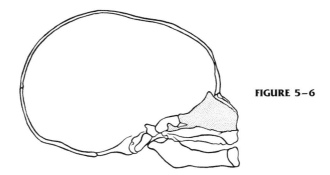

FIGURE 5–6

in the synchondroses of the cranial base, and in the mandibular condyle, where it relates in each case to linear growth by endochondral proliferation. Whereas the cartilaginous nasal septum itself contributes only a small amount of actual endochondral growth, the basis for the "septal" theory is that the pressure-accommodating **expansion** of the cartilage in the nasal septum provides a source for the physical force that displaces (pushes) the whole maxilla anteriorly and inferiorly. This sets up fields of tension in all the maxillary sutures. The bones then secondarily, but virtually simultaneously, enlarge at their sutures in response to the tension created by the displacement process. (See also page 205.)

As with any important explanatory theory, the nasal septum concept subsequently received a great deal of laboratory study to test validity. Ingenious experiments led to inconclusive results subject to multiple and uncertain interpretations, however. The concensus today is that the septum functions essentially to support the roof of the nasal chamber, but does not actively participate in the displacement movements of the palate itself.

There are two basic reasons why this problem hobbled on unresolved, and why such divergent opinions were inevitable. The first is that the source of maxillary displacement is multifactorial in nature. If the nasal septum itself is indeed involved, many other factors contribute as well, and it is impossible to separate respective effects in controlled laboratory experiments. The second reason is that experimental studies usually involve surgical removal of parts (such as the septum) to presumably test the nature of their functional roles in growth. Such studies simply cannot account for the multiple variables introduced by the experimental procedure itself, such as the destruction of tissues, blood vessels, and nerves playing a role in the growth process. Critics of these studies point out that the experimental removal of a given part does not necessarily demonstrate what the role of that part actually is when present *in situ*. It merely shows how the growth process functions in the absence of that part, rather than in its presence. A basic point is usually not acknowledged: if one experimentally changes some structure, as by surgical deletion, and this, in turn, affects the growth process, one simply cannot thereby conclude that this structure, thus, "controls the growth process."

Another important biologic consideration is the concept of *"multiple assurance"* (Latham and Scott, 1970). The processes and mechanisms that function to carry out growth are virtually always multifactorial. Should any one determinant of the growth process become inoperative (as by pathology or by experimental deletion of an anatomic part), other morphologic components in some instances have the capacity to "compensate." That is, they provide an alternative means to achieve more or less the same developmental and functional end result, although perhaps with

some degree of anatomic distortion. This concept has far-reaching implications, necessitating caution in the interpretation and evaluation of facial
growth experiments utilizing laboratory animals.

As with the cartilaginous mandibular condyle, there can be no actual
genetic determinates within the septal cartilage itself (a blueprint for the
maxilla).

A notable advance was made with the development of the **functional
matrix** concept, largely by Moss. It deals with the determinants of bone
and cartilage growth in general. The functional matrix concept states, in
brief, that any given bone grows in response to functional relationships
established by the sum of all the soft tissues operating in association with
that bone. This means that the bone itself and its osteogenic membranes
do not genetically regulate the rate and directions of their own growth;
the functional soft tissue matrix, rather, is the "epigenic" governing determinant of the skeletal growth process. The course and extent of bone
growth are secondarily dependent upon the growth and the functioning of
pacemaking soft tissues. Of course, the bone and any cartilage present are
also involved in the operation of the functional matrix, because they participate in giving essential feedback information to the governing soft tissues (muscles, etc., see Fig. 1−7). This causes the osteogenic and chondrogenic tissues to inhibit or accelerate the rate and amount of subsequent
bone remodeling activity, depending on the status of functional and mechanical equilibrium between the bone and its soft tissue matrix. A basic
concept is that genetic as well as functional determinants of the growth
process reside wholly in the related soft tissues, giving control signals to
the "genic" tissues, and not in the hard part of the bone itself.

The functional matrix concept is basic to an understanding of the fundamental nature of a bone's role in the overall process of growth control.
This concept, historically, has had great impact in the field of facial biology.

The functional matrix concept also comes into play as a source for the
mechanical force that carries out the process of displacement. According
to this now popular explanation, the facial bones grow in a subordinate
growth control relationship with all the surrounding, pace-making soft
tissues. As those tissues continue to grow, the bones become passively (i.e.,
not of their own doing) **carried** along (displaced) with the soft tissues
attached to the bones by the Sharpey fibers. Thus, for the nasomaxillary
complex, the growth expansion of the facial muscles, the subcutaneous and
submucosal connective tissues, the oral and nasal epithelia lining the
spaces, the vessels and nerves, and so on, all combine to move the facial
bones passively along with them as they grow. This continuously places
each bone and all of its parts in correct anatomic positions to carry out its
functions, **because the functional factors are the very agents that
cause the bone to develop into its definitive shape and size and to
occupy the location it does**.

The functional matrix concept, as a generalized picture, is established
and valid. It is basic in helping to understand the complex interrelationships that operate during facial growth. It is to be realized, however, that
this principle is not intended to explain **how** the growth control mechanism actually functions. This concept describes essentially **what** happens
during growth; it does not presume to account for the regulatory processes
at the cellular and molecular levels that carry it out. This is a basic point.

The term "functional" matrix, however, can be misleading in the sense
that it unintentionally implies that function, as in the forces of muscle
contractile function, is the only or primary determinant. Just as basic to
the big picture of "growth" is the expansive biomechanical **force of
growth itself**. A significant force is exerted by the process of growth ex-

pansion that has a major traction effect on attachment fibers to bone, thereby moving the bones in displacement. (See Fig. 1−7). The forces of (1) function and (2) growth itself are equally basic, and **both** must be taken fully into account; either without the other is incomplete.

NASOMAXILLARY REMODELING

An important concept, clinically as well as biologically, is that *all* inside and outside parts, regions, and surfaces participate directly in growth (Figs. 5−2 and 5−3). The old idea of centralized and self-contained "growth centers" (such as presumed growth-controlling sutures) is contrary to the actual biology involved and prevents any realistic grasp of the developmental interplay that occurs. There are, of course, differentials in the timing and magnitude among all the localized regions, but they all nonetheless take active part in response to the activating signals that trigger their local "genic" tissues. Furthermore, because of the developmental and functional interrelations among them, what occurs in any one region is not developmentally isolated from the others. This has profound clinical implications in terms of responses to treatment procedures presumably targeting on some particular area. See also page 89.

The Lacrimal Suture: A Key Growth Mediator

This is a significant but unsung growth site that provides a developmental function so important and so basic and so interesting that it merits special consideration. What it does as a growth function has gone unrecognized, yet its unique role in facial development has made possible a headform design that **works**. Without it, human (and mammalian) craniofacial development could not have evolved and could not have resulted in a functional assembly of parts. It is simply that important and fundamental.

The **lacrimal** bone is a diminutive flake of a bony island with its entire perimeter bounded by sutural connective tissue contacts separating it from the many other surrounding bones. As all these other separate bones enlarge or become displaced in many directions and at different rates and different times, the **sutural system** of the lacrimal bone provides for the "slippage" of the multiple bones along sutural interfaces with the pivotal lacrimal as they all enlarge differentially. This is made possible by collagenous linkage adjustments within the sutural connective tissue (see page 272). The lacrimal **sutures** make it possible, for example, for the maxilla to "slide" downward along its orbital contacts. This allows the whole maxilla to become displaced inferiorly, a key midfacial growth event, even though all the **other** bones of the orbit and nasal region develop quite differently and at different times, amounts, and directions. Without this adjustive developmental "perilacrimal sutural system," a developmental **gridlock** would occur among the multiple developing parts. The lacrimal bone and its suture is a developmental hub providing key traffic controls.

The lacrimal bone itself undergoes a remodeling rotation (Fig. 5−7), because the more medial **superior** part remains with the lesser-expanding nasal bridge, while the more lateral **inferior** part moves markedly outward to keep pace with the great expansion of the ethmoidal sinuses. This remodeling change is illustrated by *a*; the primary rotational displacement that accompanies it is shown by *b*. (See page 217 for additional information on lacrimal and orbital development and the biologic rationale involved.) Refer also to page 92.

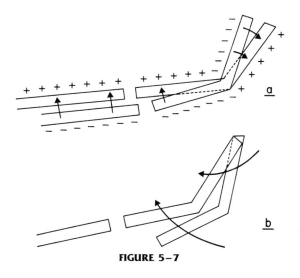

FIGURE 5-7

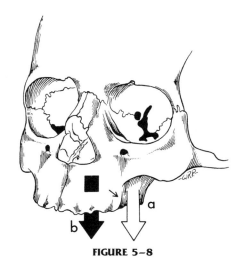

FIGURE 5-8

The Maxillary Tuberosity and the Key Ridge

In the growth of the bony maxillary arch, area A in Figure 5–1 is moving in three directions by bone deposition on the external surface: it lengthens **posteriorly** by deposition on the posterior-facing maxillary tuberosity; it grows **laterally** by deposits on the buccal surface (this widens the posterior part of the arch); and it grows **downward** by deposition of bone along the alveolar ridges and also on the lateral side, because this outer surface slopes (in the child) so that it faces slightly downward. The endosteal surface is resorptive, and this contributes to maxillary sinus enlargement.

In Figure 5–8, note that a major change in surface contour occurs along the vertical crest just below the malar protuberance (small arrow). This crest is called the "key ridge." A **reversal** occurs here. Although a range of variation occurs in the exact placement of the reversal line, anterior to it most of the external surface of the maxillary arch (the protruding "muzzle" in front of the cheekbone) is **resorptive**. This is because that part of the bony arch in area b is **concave**, and the labial (outside) surface faces upward, rather than downward. The resorptive nature of this surface provides an inferior direction of arch remodeling in conjunction with the downward growth of the palate. This is in contrast to area a, which grows downward by periosteal **disposition**. See page 79 for descriptions of this region as it participates in the posterior (distal) remodeling of the tuberosity and malar region.

In Figure 5–9, surface a is resorptive; b is depository. A reversal occurs at "A point" (indicated by arrow, a much-used cephalometric landmark). Periosteal surface c is resorptive, d is depository, e is resorptive, and f is depository.

The Vertical Drift of Teeth: An Important Clinical Consideration

A basically important term and the concept underlying it is highlighted here. It is important because of the significant growth and clinically involved growth movement it represents. This term is "vertical drift." Every student of dentistry is familiar with the well-known process of "mesial drift." However, the accompanying and equally important (perhaps clinically even more so) process of **vertical drift** has not yet become a part of

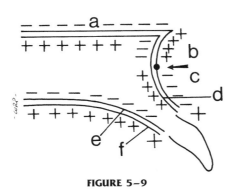

FIGURE 5–9

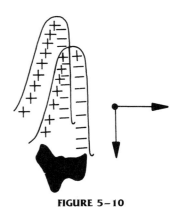

FIGURE 5–10

everyday working vocabulary. This is a great loss. Everything "vertical" has been labeled simply "eruption or extrusion/intrusion" when applied clinically. This is missing a very important clinical point. The developmental **vertical** movements of teeth in normal growth are marked in extent and play a key role in maxillary and mandibular morphogenesis. All orthodontic teachers emphasize that "working with growth" is a primary objective. Yet, "vertical drift," a significant intrinsic growth factor, lies virtually untouched in clinical theory. This makes no sense at all.

As a tooth drifts mesially (or distally, depending on species and which tooth), note that the same process of alveolar remodeling (resorption and deposition) relates to a vertical movement of the tooth as well. Any tipping, rotations, or buccolingual tooth movements are also simultaneously carried out by the same versatile remodeling process. As a tooth bud develops and its root elongates, the growing tooth undergoes **eruption**, bringing its crown into definitive occlusal position above the bone and gingiva. Now, the vertical drift of a tooth **thereafter** (which is considerable) is **in addition to** eruption, and use of the term eruption for this vertical drifting is quite inappropriate (although always still used by nearly everyone). As the maxilla and mandible enlarge and develop, the dentition drifts both vertically and horizontally to keep pace in respective anatomic positions. The process of drift moves the whole tooth **and** its socket; that is, the tooth does not drift vertically out of its alveolar housing as it does in eruption (or as implicit in the term "extrusion"). Rather, in vertical drift, the socket and its resident tooth drift **together** as a unit (Fig. 5–10). Actually, unerupted tooth buds also undergo drifting in order to sustain their anatomic positions. The periodontal connective tissue also moves together with drifting teeth, but it does not merely "shift" along with its tooth. Rather, it undergoes extensive **remodeling** within itself to relocate (see page 114). It is this important periodontal connective tissue membrane that (1) provides the intramembranous (hence periodontal "membrane" rather than "ligament") bone remodeling that changes the location of the alveolar socket and (2) moves the tooth itself. The horizontal and, especially, the vertical distances moved by the socket, its tooth, and the periodontal membrane can be substantial. By harnessing the vertical drift movement, the orthodontist can more readily guide teeth into calculated positions, thereby taking advantage of the growth process ("working with growth"). In cases where only the upper and lower anterior teeth are bonded along with the first molars, the clinician will use the vertical drift of the teeth without braces as a guide. In these partially banded cases, the clinician is attempting to selectively modify vertical drift in one area and allowing normal drift to occur in others. This concept may be useful to understand treatment response in partially banded cases.

When the teeth are "full banded" by the orthodontist, the objective, even though the whole dental arch can be wired, is control of each individual tooth's drifting movement. The specific target is regulation of each individual periodontal membrane, to bring about the remodeling ("relocation") of each individual alveolar socket as the connective tissue simultaneously moves the tooth as directed by the clinically controlled "signals." In these instances, the clinician does not have any vertical drift reference to help gauge treatment response. This can be problematic if the clinically induced "signals" lead to biologically unstable tooth movements. The biologic target of full banded tooth movements is to be distinguished from other biologic targets utilized to control the "displacement" movements of the entire maxilla, as described later.

The Nasal Airway

The lining surfaces of the bony walls and floor of the nasal chambers are predominantly resorptive except for the nasal side of the olfactory fossae (See Fig. 1–9.) This produces a lateral and anterior expansion of the nasal chambers and a downward relocation of the palate; the oral side of the bony palate is depository. The small, paired olfactory fossae have a resorptive endocranial surface that lowers them in conjunction with the downward cortical remodeling of the entire anterior cranial floor.

The ethmoidal conchae generally have depository surfaces on their lateral and inferior sides and resorptive surfaces on the superior and medial-facing sides of their thin bony plates. This moves them downward and laterally as the whole nasal region expands in like directions. (The developmentally separate inferior concha, however, can show remodeling variations because it is carried inferiorly, to a greater extent than the others, by maxillary displacement.) The lining cortical surfaces of the maxillary sinuses are all resorptive, except the medial nasal wall, which is depository because it remodels laterally to accommodate nasal expansion (Fig. 5–5).

A basic and important concept of the facial growth process is underscored in Figure 1–9: it is the **entire** facial complex that participates in the growth process. **All** parts and bony surfaces are directly involved, not merely certain special sites and "centers." All are necessarily interrelated, and the developmental positioning, shaping, and sizing of any one part affects all the others. (See the "keystone" analogy, page 12.)

The bony portion of the internasal septum (the vomer and the perpendicular plate of the ethmoid) lengthens vertically at its various sutural junctions (and to a much lesser extent by endochondral growth where the cartilaginous part contacts the perpendicular plate of the ethmoid). The bony septum also warps in relation to variable amounts and directions of **septal deviation**. The remodeling patterns involved are individually variable, and the thin plate of bone typically shows alternate fields of deposition and resorption on the right and left sides, producing a buckling to one side or the other.

Note that the breadth of the nasal bridge in the region just below the frontonasal sutures does not markedly increase from early childhood to adulthood (Fig. 5–11). More inferiorly in the interorbital area, however, the medial wall of each orbit (lateral walls of the nasal chambers between the orbits) expands and balloons out considerably in a lateral direction in conjunction with the considerable extent of lateral enlargement of the nasal chambers. The ethmoidal sinuses are thereby enlarged greatly.

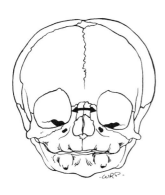

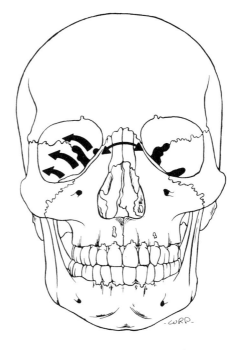

FIGURE 5–11

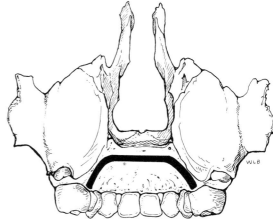

FIGURE 5–12. (From Enlow, D. H., and S. Bang: Growth and remodeling of the human maxilla. Am. J. Orthod., 51:446, 1965, with permission.)

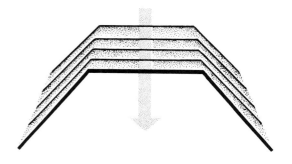

Palatal Remodeling

Even though the external (labial) side of the whole anterior part of the maxillary arch (the protruding "muzzle") is resorptive, with bone being added onto the **inside** of the arch, the arch nonetheless increases in width, and the palate becomes wider (Fig. 5–12). This is another example of the V principle. In addition, growth along the midpalatal suture is known to participate to a greater or lesser extent in the progressive widening of the palate and alveolar arch (not shown in this schematic diagram). The extent can vary between the anterior and posterior regions. (See also pages 35, 52, and 184 for other palatal growth adjustments.)

As the palate grows inferiorly by the remodeling process, a nearly complete exchange of old for new hard and soft tissue occurs. At each succeeding descending level, the palate becomes, literally, a different palate. It occupies a different position and is composed of different bone, connective tissue, epithelia, blood vessels, nerve extensions, and so on. When one visualizes the palate of a newborn and a young child, it should be realized that the palate in that same person at an older age is not the same palate at all.

The rotations, tipping, and inferior drift of the individual maxillary teeth, in combination with the characteristic external bony resorptive surface of the whole forward part of the maxilla, sometimes result in a localized rupture and protrusion of a tooth root tip through the bony cortex. Such penetration results in a normal defect (i.e., a tiny surface hole in the bone) called a fenestra.

Rapid or slow palatal expansion has become a very common clinical technique. Historically, the process of expanding the maxilla by "splitting" the midpalatal suture has been thought of as "biologic" procedure. Such is not the case. Natural increases in palatal width are the result of vertical drift of the posterior teeth with expansion laterally occurring according to the V principle of growth. Therapeutically induced expansion of the midpalatal sutures is an entirely different process. In rapid palatal expansion the maxillae are first displaced laterally. Remodeling of the displaced maxillae follows the clinically induced displacement. Understanding that this process is **not** the same as the natural biology of increasing maxillary arch width has two important clinical consequences. First, it **is** possible to expand the maxilla into an unstable (imbalanced) position and, if the clinician retains the maxillary shelves with a tooth-born device, fenestration of the molar and bicuspid roots is an almost certain consequence. Remember that the lateral aspect of much of the maxilla is resorptive, **not** depository. Moving teeth into areas of natural resorption is problematic at best and disastrous at worst. The second important clinical point is that, because the midpalatal suture probably plays only a small role (if any) in the displacement of the maxillary shelf laterally, it should be clinically possible to increase maxillary arch width even after fusion of the midpalatal suture. Such increases in arch width would necessarily result from remodeling of the alveolar process laterally and inferiorly. Stability of such nonsutural expansion should be subject to the same rules of biologic balance that apply to expansion achieved by the separation of the suture.

How palatal remodeling participates in adjustments for maxillary rotations was explained in Chapters 2 and 3.

Downward Maxillary Displacement

The **primary displacement** of the whole ethmomaxillary complex in an inferior direction (Fig. 5–5) is accompanied by simultaneous remodeling (resorption and deposition) in all areas, inside and out, throughout the entire nasomaxillary region.

New bone is added at the frontomaxillary, zygotemporal, zygosphenoidal, zygomaxillary, ethmomaxillary, ethmofrontal, nasomaxillary, nasofrontal, frontolacrimal, palatine, and vomerine sutures. These multiple sutural deposits accompany displacement and are not the pacemaker for it. The process of displacement produces the "space" within which remodeling enlargement occurs. Sutural bone growth does not **push** the nasomaxillary complex down and away from the cranial floor. The displacement of the bones is produced by the expanding soft tissues (Fig. 1−7). As the bones of the ethmomaxillary region (Fig. 1−6) are displaced downward (*a*), sutural bone growth (*b*) takes place at the same time in response to it, thus enlarging the bones as the soft tissues continue to develop. This places all the bones in new positions in conjunction with the generalized expansion of the soft tissue matrix and maintains continuous sutural contact as the bones become "separated." See also page 51.

The balance between the greater or lesser amounts of displacement and remodeling growth in the posterior and anterior parts of the maxilla is a response to the clockwise or counterclockwise rotatory displacements caused by the downward and forward growth of the middle cranial fossa. The nasomaxillary complex must correspondingly undergo a compensatory ***remodeling rotation*** in order to sustain its proper position relative to the vertical reference (PM) line and to the neutral orbital axis (see also descriptions for Figs. 2−11 and 3−14).

Maxillary Sutures

Most sutures in the facial complex do not simply grow in directions perpendicular to the plane of the suture itself. This was pointed out in a previous stage with respect to the lacrimal sutures. Because of the multidirectional mode of primary displacement and the differential extents of growth among the various bones, a slide or slippage of bones **along** the plane of the interface can be involved. As the whole maxillary complex is displaced downward and forward, or as it remodels by deposition and resorption, it undergoes a frontal **slide** at sutural junctions with the lacrimal, zygomatic, nasal, and ethmoidal bones. This is schematized by a slip of *b* over the sutural front of *a* as shown in Figure 5−13. The process requires adjustment remodeling and relinkages of the collagenous fiber connections within the sutural connective tissue across the suture (see Chapter 16).

It is apparent that the downward **and** forward directions of movement occur at the same time, and that they are produced by the same actual displacement process. Moreover, the sutures do not represent special "centers" of growth (and old but now obsolete theory). Historically, sutural

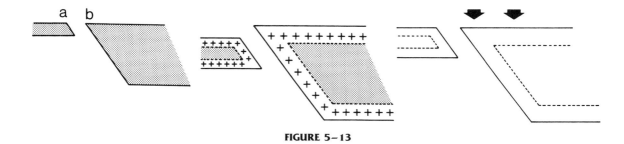

FIGURE 5−13

articulations were spotlighted but were given developmental functions that were biologically unreal, even though making good sense at the time. A suture is just another regional site of growth adapted to its own localized, specialized circumstances, just as all the other parts of the bone have their own regional growth processes. It is not possible for a bone to grow **just** at its sutures, as was sometimes implied in years past. Nor is it possible for a bone to have "generalized surface growth" without sutural involvement (in areas where sutures are present, of course; nonsuture regions may enlarge by direct remodeling). Another old but invalid idea is that "the suture growth system closes down at a given age, but the bone continues to enlarge simply by generalized **surface** deposition." To dispel this notion, bone additions on surface x in Figure 5–14 enlarge the surface area of the bone, but additions must **also** be made by deposits at sutural surface y in order to maintain morphologic form. It is apparent that it would not be possible for the bone to enlarge in surface area without corresponding additions at the sutural contacts.

The downward movement of the teeth from *1* to *2* in Figure 3–17 is accomplished by a **vertical drift** of each tooth in its own alveolar socket as the socket itself **also** drifts (remodels) inferiorly with it in lock-step by deposition and resorption. The movement of the dentition from *2* to *3*, however, is a passive **carrying** of the maxillary dental arch as a whole, the palate and bony arch, all associated soft tissues, and all of the alveolar sockets as the **entire** maxilla is **displaced** downward as a unit. The *1* to *2* and *2* to *3* movements are shown separately, but, of course, actually proceed simultaneously. Recognition and understanding of the biologic difference between them are of basic importance because each represents a separate biologic target for different clinical procedures.

Some orthodontic procedures are designed to alter the vector (magnitude and course) of the displacement movement (e.g., to accelerate or restrain it or to change direction). The specific target is thus the growth activity of the various maxillary sutures and other regional growth sites associated with the displacement process. A good example of an orthopedic force system designed to modify displacement at the sutures is the use of maxillary orthopedic traction, using a face mask attached to a rapid palatal expander. The expander is used to separate the maxillary sutures by lateral movement of the maxillae. Subsequent to this lateral movement, anterior traction is applied to literally pull the maxilla forward and transiently disarticulate the bone at its sutural margins. This is in contrast to orthodontic procedures in which the periodontal connective tissue and drift movements of individual teeth (*1* to *2*) are the direct clinical target. In the mandible, similarly, the displacement movement is one target for treatment (as by a restraining chin cup), and horizontal and vertical drift movements of teeth, separately, are another. The former utilizes (it is hoped) regulation of ramus (and with it, condylar) growth, and the latter involves control of growth movements related to the periodontal "genic" tissues. In both the maxilla and the mandible, **both** types of movements occur most actively during childhood growth, of course. Utilization for clinical purposes can be less effective in adult patients if considerable move-

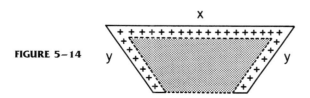

FIGURE 5–14

ment is needed, since extant growth movements are not available to "work with." Clinically activated displacement and remodeling movements are thus needed. Also, importantly, any significant extent of clinically induced movement after growth is complete could invite "rebound," because the state of functional equilibrium can be disturbed. Some clinicians hold that so long as growth continues, opportunity for achieving better stability is possible because the growth process itself can help lead to a state of physiologic balance. Others hold that the converse is true. This, however, is a complex, multifactorial biologic problem (see Figure 1–1).

The remodeling and displacement changes of both the ramus and the middle cranial fossa produce a lowering of the mandibular arch. This accommodates the vertical expansion of the nasomaxillary complex. To bring the upper and lower teeth into full occlusion, the mandibular teeth must drift (not simply erupt) vertically (Fig. 3–18). The extent can vary considerably among different individuals having different facial types, and it can also vary markedly between the anterior and posterior parts of the arch. The latter is involved in occlusal plane rotations (see Figure 10–31). Significantly, the amount of upward mandibular tooth drift can be much less than the downward drift and displacement of the maxillary teeth, depending on headform type and location within the arch. This is one of several reasons that orthodontic procedures, at least at present, often attack the maxillary dentition, even though a given malocclusion can be based on positioning of the mandible. That is, an "imbalance" is clinically produced in the maxilla to offset the effect of an existing skeletal situation in the mandible (or basicranium), because it is the maxilla that can most readily be altered and controlled. Because imbalances may still exist, however, long-term stability can be involved, and retention is a problem.

The Cheekbone and Zygomatic Arch

The growth changes of the malar complex are similar to those of the maxilla itself. This is true for the remodeling process as well as the displacement process (Figs. 5–15 to 5–17).

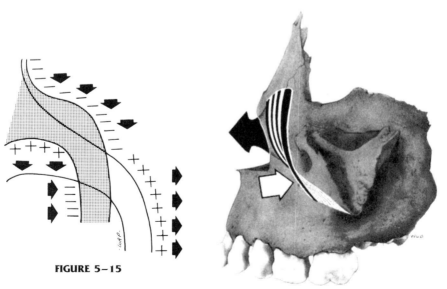

FIGURE 5–15.

FIGURE 5–16. (From Enlow, D. H., and S. Bang: Growth and remodeling of the human maxilla. Am. J. Orthod. 51:446, 1965, with permission.)

The posterior side of the malar protuberance within the temporal fossa is depository. Together with a resorptive anterior surface, the cheekbone relocates **posteriorly** as it enlarges. It would seem untenable that the whole front surface of the cheek area can actually be **resorptive**, considering that the face "grows forward and downward." However, as the maxillary arch remodels posteriorly, the malar region must also move backward at the same time to keep a constant relationship with it. The extent of malar relocation is somewhat less in order to maintain **relative** position along the increasing length of the maxillary arch. The zygomatic process of the maxilla thus behaves in a manner similar to that of the coronoid process of the ramus. Both move posteriorly as the maxillary and mandibular arches develop posteriorly to complement each other.

Some published implant-growth studies have not detected this posterior remodeling (relocation) movement of the malar region and anterior part of the zygoma. The reasons are twofold. First, implant insertion can be too close to the reversal lines between resorptive-to-depository remodeling fields (see Fig. 1–3), or too medial, and would thus not show the relocation movement because the remodeling extents here are not great enough to detect in serial headfilms. **Second, importantly, posterior relocation of the malar area slows and ceases after dental arch length is achieved during childhood development, and implant studies subsequent to this will not demonstrate the prior active posterior relocation of the malar protuberance, but which is no longer active.** Histologic sections, however, clearly demonstrate the active resorptive nature previously present. This factor was not taken into account in previous implant studies. (See also Kurihara and Enlow, 1980a, in which resorptive surfaces are documented in histologic sections and the timetable involved.)

The inferior edge of the zygoma is heavily depository. The anterior part of the zygomatic arch and malar region thereby become greatly enlarged vertically as the face develops in depth.

The zygomatic arch moves **laterally** by resorption on the medial side within the temporal fossa and by deposition on the lateral side (Fig. 5–

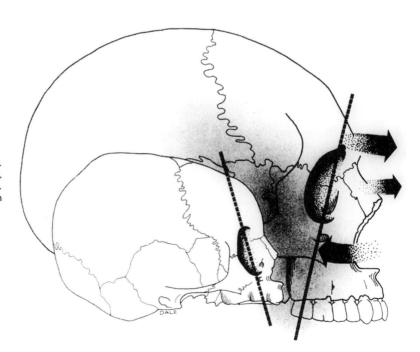

FIGURE 5–17. (From Enlow, D. H., and J. Dale: In: *Oral Histology,* 4th Ed. Ed. by R. Ten Cate, St. Louis, C. V. Mosby, 1994, with permission.)

15). This enlarges the temporal fossa and keeps the cheekbone proportionately broad in relation to face and jaw size and the masticatory musculature. It also moves the arches bilaterally, thus increasing the space between for overall head and brain enlargement. The anterior rim of the temporal fossa moves posteriorly by the V principle.

As the **malar** region grows and becomes relocated posteriorly, the contiguous **nasal** region is enlarging in an opposite, anterior direction (Fig. 5–16). This draws out and greatly expands the contour between them, resulting in a progressively more protrusive-appearing nose and an anteroposteriorly much deeper face (see Fig. 5–17). This is a major topographic maturational change in the childhood-to-adult face. Note how the facial contours become opened, the protrusions more prominent, and the depths all increased.

The zygoma and cheekbone complex becomes **displaced** anteriorly and inferiorly in the same directions and amount as the primary displacement of the maxilla. The malar protuberance is a part of the maxillary bone and is carried with it. The separate zygomatic bone is displaced inferiorly in association with bone growth at the frontozygomatic suture and anteriorly in relation to growth at the zygotemporal suture. The growth changes of the malar process are similar to those of the mandibular coronoid process, its counterpart. Both remodel backward, along with the backward elongation of each whole bone, by anterior resorption and posterior deposition (Fig. 5–18). Both become displaced anteriorly and inferiorly along with each whole bone.

Orbital Growth

The remodeling changes of the **orbit** are complex. This is because many separate bones comprise its enclosing walls, including the maxilla, ethmoid, lacrimal, frontal, zygomatic, and the greater and lesser wings of the sphenoid. Many different rates, timing, directions, and amounts of (1) remodeling growth and (2) displacement occur among these multiple bony elements and their parts, thereby adding substantially to the developmental complexities.

The elaborate remodeling activities in the medial wall of the orbit, including the lacrimal and ethmoid bones, were mentioned above. In other parts of the orbit, most of the lining roof and the floor are depository. The

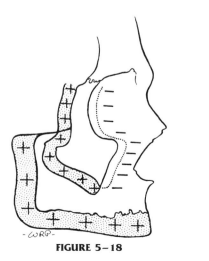

FIGURE 5–18

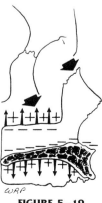

FIGURE 5–19

orbital roof is also the ectocranial side of the floor of the anterior cranial fossa. As the frontal lobe of the cerebrum expands forward and downward (until about 5 to 7 years of age), the orbital roof remodels anteriorly and inferiorly by resorption on the endocranial side and deposition on the orbital side. It might seem that a depository type of orbital roof and orbital floor would decrease the size of the cavity. However, two changes come into play that actually increase it, although the amount is relatively small in the older child. First, the orbit grows by the V principle (Fig. 6–13). The cone-shaped orbital cavity **moves** (relocation by remodeling) in a direction toward its wide opening; deposits on the inside thus enlarge, rather than reduce, the volume. Second, the factor of enlarging **displacement** is directly involved. In association with sutural bone growth at the many sutures within and outside the orbit, the orbital floor is displaced and enlarges in a progressive downward and forward direction along with the rest of the nasomaxillary complex.

An interesting developmental situation is seen involving the nasal and orbital parts of the **same** bone (the maxilla). The floor of the nasal cavity in the adult is positioned **much lower** than the floor of the orbital cavity (Fig. 2–12). Compare this with the situation in the child, in which they are at about the same level. As described earlier, about half the process of palatal descent is produced by downward **displacement** of the whole maxilla accompanied by maxillary sutural growth. The greater part of the orbital floor is a component of the maxillary bone. Because both the orbital and nasal floors are regional portions of the **same** bone, the same displacement process that carries the palate downward **also** carries the floor of the orbit inferiorly at the same time. The extent of this downward palatal and nasal/oral displacement, however, greatly exceeds the much smaller amount required for orbital enlargement; that is, a lesser increase is needed for the much earlier growing eyeball and other orbital soft tissues than for the marked expansion carried out by the longer-growing nasal chambers. The floor of the orbit offsets this by **remodeling upward** as the whole maxilla **displaces inferiorly**. Deposition takes place on the intraorbital (superior) side of the orbital floor and resorption on the maxillary (inferior) sinus side (Fig. 5–19). This sustains the orbital floor in proper position with respect to the eyeball above it. The nasal floor, in contrast, approximately doubles the amount of displacement movement by **additional** downward cortical remodeling. Thus, the orbital and nasal floors are necessarily displaced in the same direction because they are parts of the same bone, but they undergo remodeling relocation movements in opposing directions.

The floor of the orbit also remodels laterally. It slopes in a lateral manner, and deposits on the surface of the floor thus relocate it in this same direction (as shown in Fig. 5–11). The lateral wall of the orbital **rim** remodels by resorption on the medial side and by deposition on the lateral side. This intraorbital field of resorption continues directly onto the anterolateral surface of the orbital roof beneath the overhanging supraorbital ridge. This is the only part of the orbital roof and lateral wall that is resorptive, and it provides for the lateral expansion of the domed roof. The cutaneous side of the supraorbital ridge is depository, and this combination causes the superior orbital rim to become protrusive. An upper orbital rim that extends forward beyond the lower rim is a characteristic of the adult face, particularly in the male because of the larger nose associated with larger lungs. (See Chapter 6 and refer to Figure 6–12 for an account of forehead and frontal sinus development in relation to nasal protrusive growth.)

The growing child's facial topographic profile undergoes a characteristic clockwise rotation (facing right). Several developmental relationships underlie this maturational change. **The two-way combination of (1) forward remodeling of the nasal region and superior orbital rim together with (2) backward remodeling growth of the inferior orbital rim and the malar area, and (3) the essentially straight downward remodeling of the premaxillary region, all combine to produce a developmental rotation in the alignment of the whole of these middle and upper facial regions** (Fig. 5–17; see Figs. 5–16 and 5–18). Keep in mind that all parts, regardless of regional remodeling directions, become **displaced** in an anteroinferior direction (Fig. 3–16).

The lateral orbital rim undergoes remodeling growth in an obliquely posterior and a lateral direction at the same time. The lateral growth change increases the side-to-side dimension of each orbit and also contributes to the lateral movement of the whole orbit added to the small increase in the interorbital (nasal) dimension. The backward growth change of the lateral orbital rim keeps it in proper location with respect to the posterior direction of remodeling by the zygoma. **The forward remodeling of the superior orbital ridge and the whole anterior part of the nasal region, combined with the backward remodeling of the lateral rim and cheekbone, cause the orbital rim in the adult human face to slant obliquely forward, in contrast to all other mammalian faces. This reflects the forward remodeling rotation of the entire upper part of the human face and the backward rotation of the lower part**. Additional discussion is provided in Chapter 9.

The resorptive nature of the cheekbone surface area, combined with the depository nature of the whole external nasal region of the maxilla, **greatly expands the surface contour between them and markedly deepens the topography of the face**. This changes the relatively flat early childhood face into the much bolder adult topography. The medial rim of the orbit is only slightly in front of the lateral rim in the young child. In the adult, the medial rim has grown forward with the anterior-growing nasal wall, and the lateral rim has remodeled backward with the cheekbone. The medial and lateral rims are thus drawn apart in divergent posterior-anterior directions as the face deepens. Note the greatly increased depth of the contour of the lateral orbital rim and the midface as a whole resulting from these topographic changes.

Note this Feature of Facial Growth

In many of the growth and remodeling processes described throughout this chapter, one major difference exists between the female and the male. In the female, skeletal changes in the developing face slow markedly shortly after puberty. In the male, however, topographic and dimensional changes continue through the late adolescent period. The distinct facial similarities that exist between the sexes during earlier childhood, therefore, become substantially altered and divergent in the teenage years. This includes the preteenage composite of a more upright and bulbous forehead with lesser eyebrow ridges, the smaller and less protrusive nose, a lower nasal bridge, a more rounded nasal tip, flatter face, a wider appearing face with more prominent-appearing cheekbones, and a vertically shorter midface, all features of the prepubertal facial complex characterizing both sexes.

6

The Neurocranium

The housing for the brain impacts directly on many aspects of the developing facial complex (the latter known also as the viscerocranium or the splanchnocranium). The basicranium is involved in this fundamental and important relationship because the ectocranial side of the cranial floor is the interface with the face suspended beneath it. The perimeter, alignment, and configuration of the basicranium prescribes a "template" that establishes the growth fields within which both the mandible and naso-maxillary complex develop. The calvaria is largely removed from direct growth effects on the face.

The skull roof is described first, the basicranium second. There are basic growth differences between them and the developmental conditions relating to each.

The Calvaria

First, the proper singular spelling is calvar*ia*, not calvar*ium*, even though the latter seems to make sense given the related term "cranium," which is correct. The proper plurals are calvariae and crania, respectively. This common error is so pervasive, even by some anatomists, that one medical dictionary now even includes the incorrect form as a second spelling. Proper use, however, is a badge of scholarship.

The lining bony surface of the whole cranial **floor** is predominantly resorptive (darkly shaded, Fig. 6–1). This is in contrast to the endocranial surface of the **calvaria**, which is predominantly depository (lightly shaded; note the **circumcranial reversal line** indicated by the arrow). The reason for this major difference is that the inside (meningeal surface) of the skull roof is not compartmentalized into a series of confined pockets. The cranial floor, in contrast, has the **endocranial fossae** and other depressions, such as the sella turcica and the olfactory fossae. Why this calls for a difference in the mode of growth is explained below.

As the brain expands (*a* in Fig. 6–2), the separate bones of the calvaria are correspondingly displaced in outward directions (*b*). This is a passive movement on the part of the bones themselves in conjunction with the brain's expansion. Brain enlargement does not directly "push" the bones outward; rather, each separate bone is enmeshed within a connective tissue stroma attached to it. This stroma, in turn, is continuous with the meninges endocranially and the integument outside. As these enclosing

99

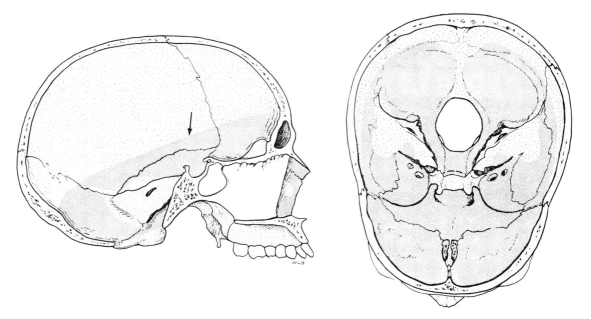

FIGURE 6–1. (From Enlow, D. H.: *The Human Face.* New York, Harper & Row, 1968, p. 197, with permission.)

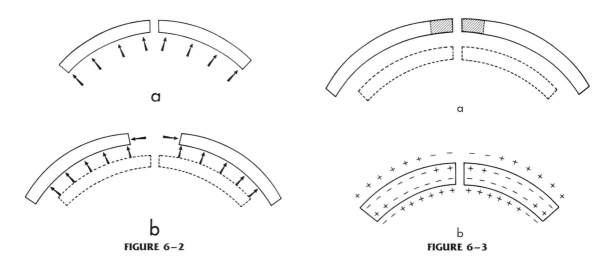

a

b

FIGURE 6–2

a

b

FIGURE 6–3

connective tissue membranes anchored to the bones enlarge with the growing brain, the bones are carried outward (displaced) by them, thereby "separating" all of the bones at their sutural articulations. In Figure 6–3, the primary displacement causes tension in the sutural membranes, which, according to present theory, respond immediately by depositing new bone on the sutural edges (*a*). Each separate bone (the frontal, parietal, and so forth) thereby enlarges in circumference. At the same time, the whole bone receives a small amount of new deposition on the flat surfaces of **both** the ectocranial and endocranial sides (*b*). The endosteal surfaces lining the inner and outer cortical tables are resorptive. This increases overall thickness and expands the medullary space between the inner and outer tables. The deposition of bone on the ectocranial surface, however, is **not** the growth change that causes the entire bone to move (displace) outward. Note that the endocranial surface, which is in contact with the dura that functions as a periosteum, is **not** a resorptive surface. This is an error in the older literature, still sometimes encountered.

The arc of curvature of the whole bone decreases, and the bone becomes flatter (Fig. 6–4). Although **remodeling** is not extensive in any of these "flat" bones because of their relatively simple contours, reversals can occur in areas mostly adjacent to the sutures. Here, either outside or inside surface resorption can take place (Fig. 6–3b), depending on the local nature of the changing contour.

The Basicranium

It has often been presumed that the face is more or less independent of the basicranium, and that facial growth processes and the topographic features of the face are unrelated to the size, shape, and growth of the floor of the cranium. This is not the case at all. What happens in the floor of the cranium very much affects the structure, dimensions, angles, and placement of the various facial parts. The reason is that the cranial floor is the **template** from which the face develops. How differences in the architecture of the basicranium as a whole affect facial pattern is explained in other chapters.

The neural side of the cranial floor requires an entirely different mode of development compared to the calvaria because of its topographic com-

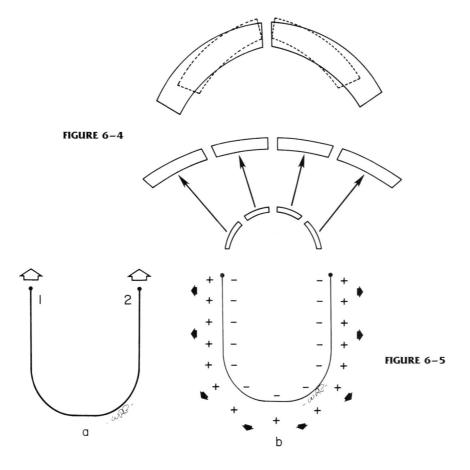

FIGURE 6–4

FIGURE 6–5

plexity and the tight curvatures of its fossae. The endocranial surface of the basicranium, in contrast to the roof, is characteristically **resorptive** in most areas (see Fig. 6–1). The reason for this is that the alignments of the sutures do not have the capacity to provide for the multiple directions of enlargement and the complex magnitude of remodeling required. The relatively simple system of sutures inherited from our mammalian ancestors cannot fully accommodate the markedly deepened endocranial fossae of the massively enlarged human brain and basicranium. Additional, widespread remodeling of the cranial floor is necessarily involved. For example, Figure 6–5a schematically represents an enlarged human basicranial fossa with sutures located at 1 and 2. These produce unidirectional sutural growth as indicated by the arrows. However, the two sutures present cannot produce the growth for the **other** directions also needed to accommodate brain expansion, as shown in Figure 6–5b. Fossa enlargement is accomplished by direct remodeling, involving deposition on the outside with resorption from the inside. This is the key remodeling process that provides for the direct expansion of the various endocranial fossae in **conjunction** with sutural (and also synchondrosis) growth. Thus, the pattern of sutures present (as inherited from the flat basicranium of our early ancestors) cannot provide for this more elaborate remodeling design.

The various endocranial compartments are separated from one another by elevated bony partitions. The middle and posterior fossae are divided by the petrous elevation; the olfactory fossae are separated by the crista galli; the right and left middle cranial fossae are separated by the longitudinal midline sphenoidal elevation just below the sella turcica; and the right and left anterior and posterior cranial fossae are divided by a longitudinal midline bony ridge. All these elevated partitions, unlike most of the remainder of the cranial floor, are **depository** in nature (Figs. 6–1 and 6–6a). The developmental basis for the depository nature of these partitions is schematized in Figure 6–6b. The reason, simply, is that, as the fossae expand outward by resorption, the partitions between them must enlarge inward, in proportion, by deposition.*

The **midventral segment** of the cranial floor grows much more slowly than the floor of the laterally located fossae. This accommodates the slower development of the medulla, pons, hypothalamus, optic chiasma, and so forth, in contrast to the massive, rapid expansion of the hemispheres. Because the floor of the neurocranium enlarges by remodeling in addition to sutural and synchondrosis growth, these differential extents and rates of expansion can be carried out. A markedly decreasing and tapering gradient of sutural growth occurs as the ventral midline is approached, but direct remodeling also occurs to provide for the varying extents of expansion required among the different midline parts themselves and between

---

*The activity of the bone lining the **sella turcica**, however, is quite variable and can be either depository or resorptive in different areas. Several reasons contribute to this, including the varying degrees of cranial base flexure and the variable amounts of downward and forward displacement of the midventral segments of the whole basicranium by the different shapes and proportionate sizes of the cerebral lobes. The sella turcica, however, must remain in contact with the hypophysis and also adjust to the variable size of the growing gland itself. If the pituitary fossa is carried downward by whole basicranial displacement disproportionately to the hypophysis itself, the floor of the sella will correspondingly rise by surface deposition to maintain contact with the pituitary, or the floor may be partly or entirely resorptive in other individuals to adjust to the balance between cranial base displacement and hypophyseal contact. A common combination is a resorptive posterior lining wall of the hypophyseal fossa and a depository surface on the sphenoidal part of the clivus. This causes a backward flare of the dorsum sellae to accommodate a pituitary gland that is being displaced to a lesser extent than the sphenoidal body below it. The jugum sphenoidal, like the floor of the sella turcica, shows variations for the same reasons. Its dorsal surface may be resorptive in some individuals, but depository in others.

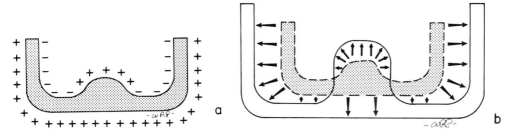

FIGURE 6–6

the midline parts and the much faster growing lateral regions (see Fig. 6–10*b*).

The following point is developmentally significant. Unlike the skull roof, the floor of the neurocranium provides for the passage of cranial nerves and the major cerebral blood vessels. Because the expansion of the hemispheres would cause marked displacement movements of the bones in the cranial floor if only sutural growth mechanism were operative (as in the skull roof), the process of **remodeling** growth in the basicranium provides for the changing stability of these nerve and vascular passageways. That is, they do not become disproportionately separated because of the massive expansion of the hemispheres of the brain, as would happen if the basicranium enlarged primarily at the sutures. The foramen enclosing each cranial nerve and major blood vessel also undergoes its own drift process (+ and −) to constantly maintain proper position. The foramen moves by deposition and resorption, keeping pace with the corresponding movement of the nerve or vessel it houses as the brain expands carrying the nerves with it. This relocation movement is differential in magnitude and direction related to the remodeling movements of the lateral walls of the fossa, thus requiring sensitive differences in respective regional remodeling.

The differential remodeling process maintains the proportionate placement of the spinal cord, even though the floor of the posterior cranial fossa, which rims the cord, expands to a considerably greater extent than the circumference of the foramen magnum (Fig. 6–7). Note the much larger growth increments of the hemispheres and the squama of the occipital bone, in contrast to the much smaller growth increments of the spinal cord and foramen magnum. Differential remodeling, not merely sutural growth, again provides for this. Recall, as emphasized in Chapter 1, that bone and soft tissue remodeling proceeds in whatever mode is required by the **regional** conditions that produce **local** developmental control signals in response to those architectonic circumstances.

The midline part of the basicranium is characterized by the presence of **synchondroses**. They are a retention left from the primary cartilages of the chondrocranium after the endochondral ossification centers appear during fetal development. A number of synchondroses are operative during the fetal and early postnatal periods. During the childhood period of development, however, it is the spheno-occipital synchondrosis that is the principal "growth cartilage" of the basicranium. As with all growth cartilages associated directly with bone development, the spheno-occipital synchondrosis provides a pressure-adapted bone growth mechanism. This is in contrast to the tension-adapted sutural growth process of the calvaria, lateral neurocranial walls, and the endocranial fossae. Compression is involved in the cranial floor, unlike the calvaria, presumably because it supports the mass of the brain and the face, which bear on the fulcrum-like

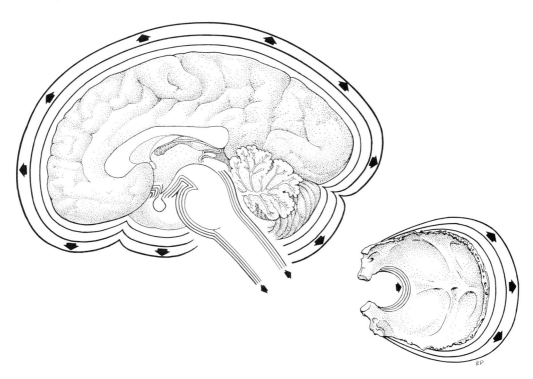

FIGURE 6–7. (Modified from Enlow, D. H.: *The Human Face.* New York, Harper & Row, 1968, p. 202, with permission.)

synchondrosis in the midline part of the cranial floor, and also presumably because it is more subject to cervical and masticatory muscle forces. Beyond these presumed pressure-adapted conditions, what other possible factors may be involved are not presently understood. The spheno-occipital synchondrosis is retained throughout the childhood growth period as long as the brain and basicranium continue to develop and expand. It ceases growth activity at about 12 to 15 years of age, and the sphenoid and occipital segments then begin to become fused in this midline area through about 20 years of age.

The presence of the spheno-occipital synchondrosis provides for the elongation of the **midline** portion of the cranial floor by its pressure-adapted mechanism of endochondral ossification. The floor of the cranium also has sutures in the lateral areas, but (1) the force of the compression produced by the growing neural mass is accommodated by the synchondrosis, not the sutures, and (2) the expansion of the laterally located **hemispheres** produces tension in these lateral sutural areas, unlike the more slowly growing midline part of the brain and basicranium not related directly to the hemispheres. Sutures are connective tissue membranes that provide tension-adapted sites of intramembranous bone growth, as described in Chapter 16.

Historically, the spheno-occipital synchondrosis has been regarded as **the** growth "center" and pacemaker that programs the development of the basicranium. This overly simplistic notion, however, as with the mandibular condyle, is a conceptual anachronism. The development of the basicranium is **quite** multifactorial and not merely the product of localized, midline cartilages that do not relate to the many regional growth circumstances throughout all parts of the basicranium as a whole. Only a very small percentage of the actual bone of the cranial floor is formed endochondrally in conjunction with the synchondroses, a parallel truism previously noted for the mandibular condyle.

The structure of the synchondrosis is similar to the basic plan for all "primary" types of growth cartilages, in contrast to the secondary variety of cartilage, which is basically different (see Chapter 4). As in the epiphyseal cartilage plate of long bones, the synchondrosis has a series of "zones," including the familiar reserve, cell division, hypertrophic, and calcified zones (Fig. 6–8). Similar to an epiphyseal plate, but unlike the condylar cartilage, the chondroblasts in the cell division zone are aligned in distinctive columns that point along the line of growth. Unlike the epiphyseal plate, the synchondrosis has **two** major (bipolar) directions of linear growth. Structurally, the synchondrosis is essentially two epiphyseal plates positioned back-to-back and separated by a common zone of reserve cartilage.

Endochondral bone growth by the spheno-occipital synchondrosis relates to primary **displacement** of the bones involved. The sphenoid and the occipital bones become **moved apart** by the primary displacement process (Fig. 6–9), and at the same time, new endochondral (medullary fine-cancellous) bone is laid down by the endosteum within each bone. Compact cortical (intramembranous) bone is formed around this core of endochondral bone tissue. Each whole bone (the sphenoid and the occipital) thereby becomes lengthened. Both bones also increase in girth by periosteal and endosteal remodeling. The interior of the sphenoid bone eventually becomes hollowed to form the sizable **sphenoidal sinus**. This sinus is just behind and in direct line with the bony nasal septum of the nasomaxillary complex. As the midface becomes progressively displaced forward and downward, the sphenoidal body must remodel to retain contact with it. The sphenoidal sinus is thereby formed and progressively enlarges. Sphenoidal sinus expansion does not "push" the maxilla, however. This sinus secondarily "grows" as the body of the sphenoid bone expands around it keeping constant junction with the moving nasomaxillary complex.

Two key questions exist with regard to the lengthening of the basicranium at a synchondrosis and the process of displacement that accompanies the elongation of each whole bone. First, do the synchondroses **cause** dis-

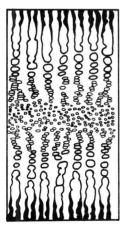

FIGURE 6–8

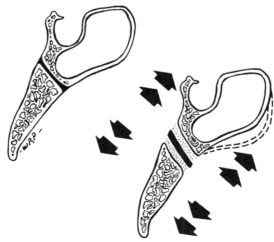

FIGURE 6–9

placement by the process of growth expansion, or is their endochondral growth a **response** to displacement caused by other forces (such as brain expansion)? Second, does the cartilage have an intrinsic genetic program that actually regulates the rate, amount, and direction of growth by the cranial base? Or, is the cartilage dependent on some **other** pacemaking factors for growth control and secondarily responsive to them?

Traditionally, the cranial cartilages (and the whole basicranium in general) have been regarded as essentially autonomous growth units that develop in conjunction with the brain, but somehow independent of it. This is difficult to understand. Basicranial growth has historically, also, been presumed to be controlled by some genetic code residing within the cartilage cells of the synchondrosis. In other words, the shape, size, and characteristics of the cranial floor have evolved in direct phylogenetic association with the brain it supports (i.e., a "phylogenetic type" of functional matrix), but the basicranium itself has presumably developed a genetic capacity for its own growth that is somehow self-contained and independent of the brain and which is capable of growth without the brain during ontogenetic growth (as can happen to some extent in agenesis of the brain). Better and more complete biologic insight is presently needed on the morphogenic relationships involved in basicranial development, but present presumptions seem uncertain and incomplete at best.

Experimental studies show that the independent proliferative capacity of a synchondrosis does not approach that of epiphyseal plates in long bones. This suggests that whatever capacity the basicranium (not calvaria) does have for continued growth, extrinsic control factors are also required. Just what these factors actually are and to what extent they are involved also is not fully understood, since the cranial floor **can** develop to a greater or lesser extent, even though the brain is malformed or absent. In contrast, the calvaria is largely dependent on its surrounding endocranial and ectocranial matrix for growth control.

As previously pointed out, the contribution of the synchondrosis relates to the midventral axis of the cranium and not the **entire** cranial floor. Note that the overall enlargement of the midline part of the basicranium is much less than the marked expansion of the more laterally located middle (and posterior) cranial fossae. This is because the lateral fossae house the various lobes of the huge hemispheres, which enlarge considerably more than the closer-to-midline medulla, pituitary gland, diencephalon, hypothalamus, optic chiasma, and so forth. Endocranial resorption occurs on the endocranial surface of the clivus and, laterally, the sizeable floor of the middle cranial fossa. For the clivus, this produces an oblique anteroinferior remodeling movement **in addition to** the linear growth by the synchondrosis.[†] For the middle and also posterior cranial fossae, it produces massive expansion in conjunction with the sutural growth also taking place. The clivus also lengthens by bone deposition on the ectocranial side of the occipital bone at the lip of the foramen magnum.

The expansion of the middle cranial fossa and its neural contents have a major **secondary** displacement effect on the anterior cranial floor, the underlying nasomaxillary complex suspended from the latter, and the mandible. Because the posterior boundary of the maxillary complex is developmentally positioned to exactly coincide with the boundary between the anterior and middle cranial fossae, a like amount of forward displace-

---

[†]The dorsum sellae, however, shows much variation in shape and size. In some individuals it flares markedly in an upward and backward direction, and the sphenoidal part of the clivus may be correspondingly depository, rather than resorptive.

ment of both the anterior cranial fossa and the nasomaxillary complex suspended beneath it occurs. The amount of horizontal displacement for the mandible, however, is much less because most of the enlargement of the middle cranial fossa takes place **anterior** to the mandibular condyles. Historically, these various facial effects have almost never been taken into account, yet they are of basic developmental significance.

The enlarging middle cranial fossa does not in itself **push** the mandible, anterior cranial fossa, and maxillary complex forward. Visualize the enlarging temporal and frontal lobes of the cerebrum as two expanding rubber balloons in contact. They are each displaced **away** from the other, although the net effect is a forward direction of movement from the foramen magnum. The temporal and frontal "balloons" have fibrous attachments to the middle and anterior cranial fossae, respectively. As **both** balloons expand, these two fossae are thus **pulled away** from each other, but both also being moved together in a protrusive direction. This sets up tension fields in the various frontal, temporal, sphenoidal, and ethmoidal sutures, and this presumably triggers sutural bone responses (in addition to direct basicranial remodeling expansion by resorption and deposition all over all other inside and outside surfaces). Both fossae are thus enlarged, and the nasomaxillary complex is carried along anteriorly with the floor of the anterior cranial fossa from which it is suspended. At about 5 or 6 years of age, frontal lobe growth and anterior cranial fossa expansion are largely complete. Thus, any further developmental protrusion of the forehead is a result of thickening of the frontal bone and enlargement of the frontal sinus within it (Fig. 6–12). The temporal lobe and middle fossa, however, continue to enlarge for several more years, and ongoing expansion of each temporal lobe continues to displace the frontal lobe forward, and this, in turn, causes tension in the osteogenic suture systems between these two areas. The anterior fossae and the maxillary complex are carried anteriorly by the frontal lobes, which is moved forward because of temporal lobe enlargement behind it. (Note: This "tension" trigger in response to **brain** and other soft tissue enlargements is the present-day theory. Time may or may not prove this to be fully correct, but the rationale is at least reasonable as we now see it.)

As schematized in Figure 6–10*a*, the composite picture shows that resorption occurs from the lining side of the forward wall of the middle cranial fossa (*1*), deposition on the orbital face of the sphenoid and in the sphenofrontal suture (*2*), and forward displacement of the anterior cranial fossae as the frontal lobes are displaced anteriorly (*3*). The petrous elevation (*4*) increases by deposition on the endocranial surface, and lengthening of the clivus occurs by growth at the spheno-occipital synchondrosis (*5*). The foramen magnum is progressively lowered by resorption on the endocranial surface and deposition on the ectocranial side. This also contributes to the lengthening of the clivus (*6*), and the perimeter of the foramen enlarges to match myelination and further enlargement of the spinal cord. Inferior to the circumcranial reversal line (see Fig. 6–1), the endocranial fossae enlarge by a combination of endocranial resorption and ectocranial deposition (*7*) that occurs in addition to growth at the basicranial sutures.

In Figure 6–10*b*, a decreasing gradient of sutural growth occurs approaching the midventral part of the basicranium is schematized (lightly shaded areas, *1*). The endocranial fossae enlarge by a corresponding gradient of direct cortical remodeling, as shown by the darkly shaded areas (*2*). The clivus lengthens by endochondral bone growth at the spheno-occipital synchondrosis (*3*) and also by direct downward remodeling of the basicranial floor around the rim of the foramen magnum. The sphenoid

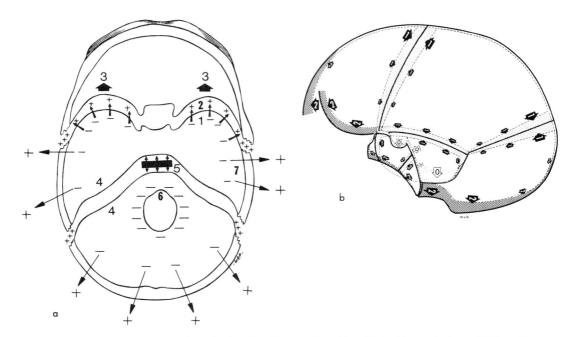

FIGURE 6–10. (b) From Enlow, D. H.: *The Human Face.* New York, Harper & Row, 1968, with permission.

and occipital complex remodels and rotates anteriorly and inferiorly by endocranial resorption (*0*) and ectocranial deposition.

The vertical enlargement of the middle cranial fossae has a major effect on the respective vertical placements of both the mandibular and maxillary arches. The effect is a progressive separation of the arches.

Each anterior cranial fossa enlarges in conjunction with the expansion of the frontal lobes. Wherever sutures are present, they contribute to the increase in the circumference of the bones involved. Thus, the sphenofrontal, frontotemporal, sphenoethmoidal, frontoethmoidal, and frontozygomatic sutures all participate in a closely coordinated, traction-adapted bone growth response to brain and other soft tissue enlargements. The bones all become **displaced** "away" from each other as a consequence. This is a primary type of displacement, because the enlargement of each bone is involved. Together with this, the bones also enlarge outward by ectocranial deposition and endocranial resorption, as described below. The aggregate of all these processes produces the composite growth changes seen in Figure 6–10*b*.

As previously pointed out, sutural growth alone cannot accomplish the extent of cranial fossa expansion required. In addition to bone additions at the various sutures, direct cortical remodeling also takes place extensively (Fig. 6–11). About midway up the forehead a reversal line encircles the inner side of the skull and separates the resorptive endocranial remodeling fields of the basicranium from the separate depository field of the roof (see arrow in Fig. 6–1).

As long as the frontal lobes of the cerebrum enlarge, the **inner** table of the forehead correspondingly remodels anteriorly (Fig. 6–11). When frontal lobe enlargement slows and largely ceases sometime before about the sixth year, the growth of the inner table stops with it. The outer table, however, continues to remodel anteriorly (Fig. 6–12). This progressively

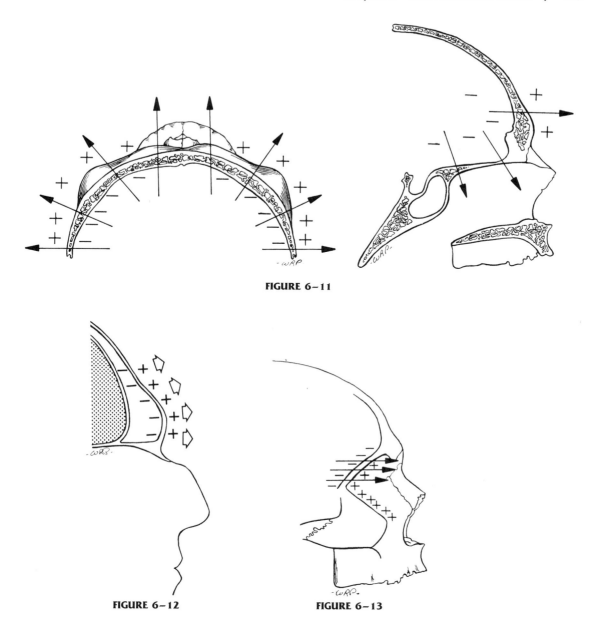

FIGURE 6–11

FIGURE 6–12   **FIGURE 6–13**

separates the two tables, and an enlarging frontal sinus develops by re-sorptive replacement of the cancellous medullary bone (diploë). The size of the sinus, however, and the amount of forehead slope vary considerably according to age, sex, and headform characteristics (see Chapter 8). The reason the frontal sinus develops is that the upper part of the nasomax-illary complex continues to remodel protrusively, and the outer table of the contiguous forehead necessarily must remodel with it.

Note that the floor of the anterior cranial fossa is also the roof of the underlying orbital cavity (Fig. 6–13). The endocranial side is resorptive, and the orbital side of this very thin bony plate is depository; it relocates by remodeling progressively downward and outward. While this serves to enlarge the bottom part of the cranial fossa, does it also then reduce the size of the orbital cavity? The answer is no, for two reasons. First, the orbits relocate anteriorly by the V principle, which itself serves to enlarge, not reduce, orbital size (Fig. 6–13). Second, the multiple parts of the whole orbit are also becoming **displaced** out and away from each other at the same time in association with bone deposition at the various orbital sutures, as described in the chapter dealing with the maxilla.

Facial Growth and Tooth Movement Basics

7

A developmental process previously highlighted in Chapter 1 is that "tooth movement" has functions beyond just placing the dentition into occlusion. It is, indeed, a key part of facial growth. Tooth movement (1) positions a tooth into changing functional locations, and (2) sustains progressively changing anatomic relationships as the entire craniofacial assembly around it continues to undergo massive development. Additionally, (3) the periodontal membrane (PDM) serves as a pressure-to-traction converting buffer to masticatory forces. These basic growth functions require an elaborate and intricate biologic system of closely orchestrated histologic actions involving multiple "genic" tissues. An intrinsic control process selectively activates and coordinates the complex histogenic interplay.

To "work with growth," clinical control signals are introduced to augment, modify, or replace the intrinsic, regionally distributed intercellular messengers already ongoing. The objective is to manipulate (1) the directions, and (2) the magnitude of the underlying biologic actions sensitive to these signals. The biologic process itself is the same; it is the signal input to the genic tissues that is altered by the clinical procedure. The result is to selectively accelerate or inhibit **regional** cellular responses, and to alter directions of movement. The clinician, thus, is a "growth programmer," analogous to a computer programmer, with signal input directing the outcome.

The **periodontal membrane*** is an osteogenic connective tissue comparable to the periosteal membrane and, because it is a "back-to-back,"

---

*Also commonly called the **periodontal ligament**. It is indeed a mature ligament in terms of its histologic structure in the more stable, adult form. However, the term "membrane" is much more appropriate for the childhood growth period. The periodontium has a connective tissue membrane that is quite active and dynamic, not one that merely physically supports a tooth (i.e., a ligament). It (1) contributes to the growth and development of the tooth; (2) is involved directly in the eruption of the tooth; (3) is involved directly in the drifting, tipping, and rotation movement of the tooth; (4) provides for the formation of the bone tissue lining the alveolar socket; (5) is an active and essential sensory receptor and vascular pathway; and (6) is involved directly in the extensive remodeling of the bone associated with the movements of the teeth. For these reasons, the term periodontal "membrane" is more closely associated with the truly dynamic functions of this connective tissue layer. "Ligament," on the other hand, connotes a more stable, inactive, nonchanging type of tissue that has a single function—fibrous attachment. Alveolar bone, of course, is of intra-**membranous** origin, being produced by the periodontal **membrane**.

double-sided histogenic membrane, it is also comparable to a sutural histogenic membrane. Phylogenetically, it is the adaptive answer to a basic functional problem. A vascular membrane, such as the periosteum, is known to be quite pressure sensitive, and resorptive necrosis results when a surface compressive force acts to close off its vascular supply (see page 266). Pressures produced by chewing teeth would seem to cause such destructive compression on a jaw bone's osteogenic membranes, and a neutralizing factor is thereby needed. Would cartilage, a tissue specially resistant to pressure, function satisfactorily as a neutralizing buffer between the tooth root and the bony alveolar surface? No, because cartilage is severely limited in its capacity for remodeling and could not accommodate the dynamic changes required for tooth development, eruption, and the drift needed as an integral part of the facial growth process.

The phylogenetic problem of pressure on the bone surface beneath a tooth has been overcome in a simple but effective way (Fig. 7–1). Pressure is converted directly into **tension** (which fibrous membranes are adapted and can handle) by the suspension of each tooth in a connective tissue **sling** of fibers within a socket.[†] By this means, the compressive force by a tooth being pushed into its socket is translated, not as pressure, but as direct tension on the alveolar bone. Thus, the sensitive, vascular periodontal membrane is not exposed to the killing effects of compression as the tooth is depressed into the socket or as it is tipped or rotated in one direction or another by masticatory forces. This relatively simple plan accomplishes several needed functions. It provides effective mechanical support for the tooth, gives resilient yet nonbrittle stability, provides a biologic system (connective tissue remodeling) for eruption, enables each individual tooth to acquire a functional occlusal position, provides for the growth and remodeling maintenance of the alveolar bone, provides a vascular and nerve supply as well as a pool of undifferentiated cells that are needed for continued development, and provides for the vertical and horizontal drifting of the tooth and the accompanying remodeling movements of the alveolar bone. These are all major requirements essential to the biology of tooth movement. All of these functions performed by the PDM are lacking in the rigid osseo-integrated implants being used to replace teeth prosthetically. The impact of this important difference between implants and natural tooth-membrane physiology is yet to be fully appreciated by the dental profession.

Teeth drift for two basic, functional reasons. One, as described in all basic oral histology texts, is to close-up the dental arch during growth and keep it closed as the contact edges along interproximal contacts of the teeth progressively wear. This braces the arch to better withstand masticatory forces. **The second reason, much less known but of great importance, is to anatomically place and progressively relocate the teeth as the whole mandible and maxilla grow and remodel.** Each tooth (and the unerupted tooth buds as well) must drift vertically, laterally, and either mesially or distally in order to sustain proper but changing anatomic position. The "molar" region at an early age level, for example, becomes the "premolar" region of the jaw at a later age as the corpus lengthens posteriorly. The maxillary teeth, another example, must drift (not merely "erupt") inferiorly for a considerable distance as the whole bony maxillary arch relocates downward to provide (1) enlargement of the overlying nasal chambers, and (2) adjustments for palatal displacement

---

[†]A violation of this biologic relationship is the basis for many of the problems encountered by the prosthodontist. Dentures are pressure-causing appliances fitted onto bone without a tension-converting sling of periodontal fibers. Uncontrolled resorption can be a consequence.

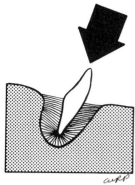

FIGURE 7–1

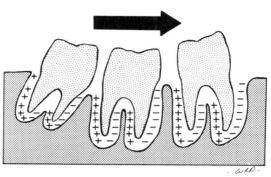

FIGURE 7–2

rotations to "level" the occlusal plane. Anterior versus posterior differences in the extents of this vertical dental drift, in conjunction with palatal remodeling, function to achieve constant and ongoing proper palate and dental arch alignment (see pages 184 and 187). Thus, the function of horizontal **and** vertical **drift** is far more significant than merely "closing up" the dentition. It is one of the basic developmental factors involved in facial growth. As pointed out in Chapter 1, importantly, it is the "growth" a clinician "works with" in tooth movements.

The customary diagram used to illustrate "mesial drift" shows deposition and resorption on the "tension" (depository) and "pressure" (resorptive) sides of the alveolar socket, respectively (Fig. 7–2). A posteroanterior section through the jaw showing several tooth roots gives the familiar histologic picture schematized here. However, only the **mesial** direction of drift movement is pointed out in most standard textbooks; the important **vertical** drift movements that **also** take place are never explained. This other movement is carried out by the **same** alveolar bone deposits and resorption usually associated only with mesial drift. Drift is a three-dimensional growth process, and the oversimplified, two-dimensional, diagrammatic picture illustrated here does not adequately represent it (see page 88). This is an exceedingly important point: it represents significant components of the "growth" that a clinician "works with." An alveolar socket can move by remodeling in virtually **any** direction, when accompanying its resident tooth's movement, by appropriate patterns of its periodontal remodeling fields.

The old "pressure and tension" concept of the mesial and distal sides of the alveolar socket, however, is an oversimplification, and it masks the actual biology involved. The collagenous fibers of the periodontium on the pressure side are actually under tension in nonclinical movements (see Fig. 7–8). Although heavy tooth-to-periodontal membrane-to-alveolar bone compression can be indeed involved in extreme **clinical** tooth movements (as by an orthodontist using heavy forces), such severe levels of sustained force are not involved in ordinary physiologic (growth) conditions. On the "tension" side, furthermore, the cells of the periodontal membrane are actually under compression between the taut collagenous fibers.

It has been a major point of controversy for many years whether the pressure presumed to trigger alveolar bone resorption acts first on the connective tissue membrane or directly on the bone, which, in turn, causes the membrane to respond (see below). One concept is that very minute **distortions** of alveolar bone caused by shifting of the tooth's root, or through other forces created by growth, serve to trigger alveolar remodeling. The **piezo effect** is held by many investigators to be the response to this stress trigger, and it is widely believed that this bioelectric stimulus serves as a "first messenger" that fires receptor sites on osteoblastic and osteoclastic cell surfaces within the periodontium. Some investigators have suggested that the viscous intercellular fluid matrix functions as the biomechanical intermediary. It presumably acts as a "hydraulic system" that can transmit variable amounts of pressure to the alveolar bone surface by vessel or matrix distention or compression.

If the extent of pressure exerted by a tooth on the periodontal membrane produced, for instance by heavy orthodontic forces, results in a severe compression of the membrane, a closing-off of the blood vessels and cellular necrosis follows. The growth capacity of the membrane is destroyed, and remodeling changes on the alveolar bone surface are precluded. This is presumed to trigger **undermining resorption.** In this process, the resorptive changes then proceed from the endosteal cancellous spaces **deep** to the alveolar bone surface, since the hyalinized connective tissue on the alveolar surface itself is histogenically inert owing to vascular occlusion.

As pointed out above, the periodontal membrane is an equivalent of both the periosteum and sutures. Its general structure is similar, and its own internal mode of growth is comparable. The notable difference, of course, is that one side attaches to a tooth, rather than to a muscle or another bone. The periodontal membrane is a reflection of the overlying periosteum into the alveolar socket, and these two histogenic, vascular membranes are directly continuous.

In its "stable," nonremodeling and histogenically inactive form, the periodontal membrane is then essentially a mature ligament composed of dense bundles of thick collagenous fibers with correspondingly few fibroblasts and little ground substance. During the active period of facial growth, dental development, and the establishment of occlusion, however, this membrane has a much more dynamic function, and its histologic structure is adapted to the complex developmental role in facial growth that it plays. During the growth period, the periodontal membrane is much more highly cellular, and much more than just ligament attachment fibers and a scattering of pyknotic fibroblasts are present. As comprising the histogenically active periosteal and sutural connective tissues, the periodontal membrane has three basic layers. The middle layer, called the "intermediate plexus," is composed of the same slender, precollagenous **linkage fibrils** that are present in the intermediate layers of the osteogenic periosteum and sutures. Linkage fibrils (layer B in Fig. 7–3) provide connections and sequential reconnections between the innermost and outermost dense, coarse fibrous layers (layers A and C). Their key function is for **adjustments** involved in tooth drift, eruption, rotations, and alveolar bone movements produced by remodeling. This layer may be poorly differentiated or absent in nonremodeling periods and in regional locations (and species) where tooth movements are relatively slow. Or, the distribution of the linkage fibrils may be more diffuse rather than forming a separate recognizable zone. During active tooth movements, nonetheless, they are necessarily **always** present, as histochemical tests clearly show, whether or not a separate, discrete zone is apparent (Kraw and Enlow, 1967). During tooth movement and companion alveolar remodeling relocations, the PDM is not simply "moved," *in toto,* to progressively new positions. Rather, it undergoes **its own remodeling**, just as the bone does, to provide the movement, and this requires considerable and on-going relinkages of the connecting fibers.

It has been proposed that the actual source of the propulsive mechanical force that brings about eruption, vertical and horizontal drift, and other

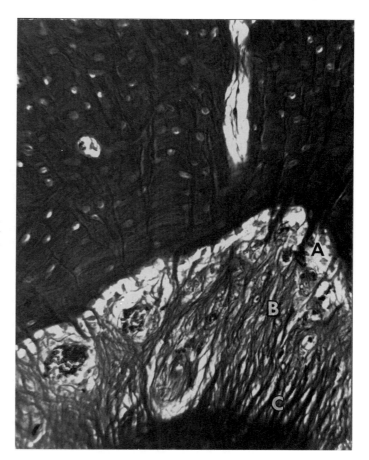

FIGURE 7–3. (From Kraw, A. G., and D. H. Enlow: Continuous attachment of the periodontal membrane. Am. J. Anat., 120:133, 1967, with permission.)

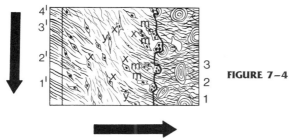

FIGURE 7–4

tooth movements is provided specifically by an abundant population of actively contractile fibroblasts ("myofibroblasts") on the **resorptive** sides of the socket (Azuma et al., 1975). The contraction of these special cells (m in Fig. 7–4) is believed to **pull** the collagenous framework within the periodontal membrane, and thereby the tooth, in the direction of the resorptive bone front. The contractile cells also presumably transport fibers into new linkage positions. These contractile fibroblasts are all interattached by desmosomes, and interconnected physiologically by a nexus between cells. The cells are anchored to fibers by hemidesmosomes. Simultaneously, special collagen-degrading and collagen-producing cells (x and y in Fig. 7–4) within the linkage zone provide the fiber remodeling and relinkages described below. This occurs in conjunction with ground substance degradation and synthesis, and the tooth is thus propelled in horizontal and vertical drift movements (arrows). Multinuclear osteoclasts resorb the bone in advance of tooth's movement. The same process also appears to provide for eruption and rotatory movements. The fibers at level *1*, formerly linked with *1'*, thus become relinked with fiber level *2'*, and so on, in the inferior direction of maxillary dental eruption. It is suggested, importantly, that these various cells are the specific targets of the clinical forces utilized by the orthodontist to move teeth. Some histogenic process such as this, or similar variation to it, must necessarily be operative.

As seen in Figures 7–5 to 7–7, on one side of the zone of linkage fibrils (*b*) is a layer of coarse collagenous fibers that attach to the alveolar bone (*a*), and on the other side a layer of coarse fibers attaching to the cementum of the tooth (*c*). The activity on the "tension side" is schematized in Figure 7–6. This old term is used because the pull of the tooth to the right presumably sets up tension on the bone surface by the periodontal fibers, and tension was presumed to be osteoblastic activating (see below). A new layer of bone is deposited on the alveolar surface. This embeds the periodontal fibers of layer *a* (Fig. 7–6). Note that the attachment fibers are not driven into the bone as with a nail; they become progressively enclosed and buried as new bone deposits form around them. It is apparent that the fibers of zone *a* would soon be used up and become completely enclosed. However, the **linkage** fibrils of the intermediate zone *b* (or its histologic equivalent) become remodeled into *a*, thereby lengthening *a* in advance of the drifting alveolar wall. The fibers of layer *a* are thus enclosed by new bone on one side while being lengthened by an equal amount on the other. The conversion from *b* to *a* is accomplished by a bundling together of the thin, precollagenous linkage fibrils into the thick, "mature" fibers of layer *a*. Ground substance is believed to be the binding agent, and the process is carried out by the abundant resident population of periodontal fibroblasts. Layer *b* retains its breadth by elongation of the precollagenous linkage fibrils. It is not presently known whether this lengthening process occurs within zone *b* or at the interface between *b* and *c*. New unit fibrils are also constantly added as the tooth grows and as the membrane drifts

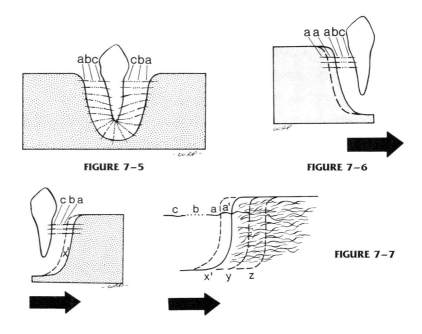

FIGURE 7–5

FIGURE 7–6

FIGURE 7–7

in conjunction with tooth drift. The fibers of layer c are carried in the direction of the tooth's movement. Throughout this membrane remodeling process, continuous attachment between tooth and alveolar bone is thereby maintained. Note that the periodontal membrane as a whole is not simply pushed or pulled along as the tooth moves. It **grows** from one location to the next.

Figure 7–7 shows the activity on the "pressure side" of the tooth root ("pressure," as mentioned above, because the tooth root, according to long-standing but inadequate theory, has been presumed to exert direct compression on the periodontal membrane and bony alveolar wall). It is the reverse of the remodeling sequence on the opposite ("tension") side. A layer of bone is **resorbed** (x') from the alveolar surface by an abundant sheet of osteoclasts. The resorptive side of the alveolar socket can easily be distinguished microscopically from the depository side by the characteristic chiseled, pitted, eroded appearance of the bone's surface. If the resorptive process was active at the time, numerous osteoclasts are seen in the erosion pits (Howship lacunae).

An effective means for periodontal attachment onto resorptive alveolar bone surfaces is operative and involves an adhesive mode of new fiber attachment onto the resorptive bone surface. (Kurihara and Enlow, 1980b and 1980c).

As the alveolar resorptive front (Fig. 7–7) proceeds from x' to y and on to z, the linkage fibrils (b), the attachment fibers on the bone side (a and a'), and those on the tooth side (c) **remodel** to sustain their proportionate lengths, with new fibers and relinkages sustaining continuous attachments as the tooth moves. The whole membrane thus grows in a direction toward the bone surface and away from the tooth as the tooth simultaneously moves in a like direction. The process is continuously repetitive. The tooth movement itself is presumably provided by myofibroblasts, as described above and schematized in Figure 7–4. Even though the bone on the resorptive side of the alveolar socket undergoes progressive removal, periodontal connection between bone and tooth nonetheless is still sustained. Periodontal membrane reattachment is rapidly achieved by deposition of a layer of adhesive ground substance (a component of proteoglycans) on the resorbed bone surface, followed by the formation of new precollagenous fibrils. This can be done almost immediately after the resorptive action of the osteoclasts. Indeed, the fibroblast-like cells that do this trail just behind the ameboid-moving osteoclasts and reestablish attachment as the osteoclast moves from its Howship lacuna. The new fibrils, embedded in the adhesive proteoglycans secretion on the bone surface, become "stuck" onto the bone. They link with older collagenous fibers deeper within the periodontal membrane, and transitory attachment between bone and membrane is thereby produced. As the resorptive front continues, such adhesive attachments undergo removal in turn, to be replaced by new ones. Should a reversal occur in which the bone surface becomes depository, rather than resorptive, calcification of the interface proteoglycans layer becomes a "reversal line." Such reversals may be more or less permanent, with substantial new deposits formed. Or they may occur, as frequently seen, as temporary, thin scales of bone ("spot" deposits) that serve to reinforce transient attachments (Fig. 7–8). In either case, the reversal shows clearly as a refractile line at the interface.

Wherever connective fiber-to-bone anchorage attachments are made on resorptive alveolar bone surfaces, the fibers of the periodontal membrane are **taut between bone and tooth**. Thus, even though the "resorptive" side of the socket is often referred to as the "pressure side," the fibers are actually under tension, as seen in Figure 7–8, top, side B.

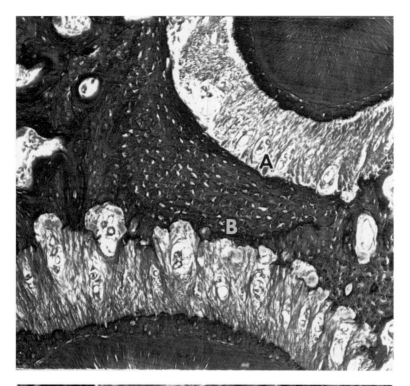

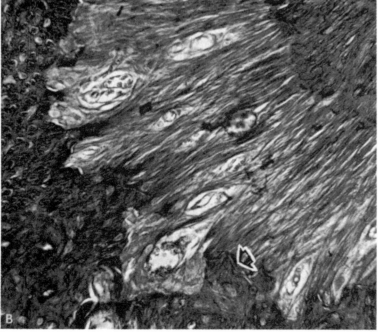

FIGURE 7–8 In the upper photomicrograph, alveolar surface *A* is depository and alveolar surface *B* is resorptive. The entire bony plate was produced by the periodontal membrane of the upper socket. Note that the fibers on the resorptive side (*B*) are taut and under tension, even though this has frequently been referred to as the "pressure" side. In the lower photomicrograph, a "spot deposit" of bone (arrow) has maintained fibrous attachment with the tooth. Note the **reversal line** separating this thin, transient scale of new bone from the resorptive surface just deep to it (From Kraw, A. G., and D. H. Enlow: Continuous attachment of the periodontal membrane. Am. J. Anat., 120:133, 1967, with permission.)

The periosteal and periodontal vascular, connective tissue membranes are constructed to function in a field of traction (as by the pull of a muscle or biting force on a tooth), not marked surface pressure. Covering membranes are quite sensitive to direct compression because any undue amount causes vascular interference and impedes osteoblastic formation of new bone. Osteoclasts can function to "relieve" the degree of pressure by removing bone. A commonly heard cliché is that "bone" is "pressure sensitive," and that high-level pressure induces resorption. Actually, it is the covering membrane and not the hard part of the bone itself that responds in such a manner. However, there are two general targets for biomechanical forces acting on bone: (1) the bone's membrane and, (2) the bone's calcified matrix. The nature of response is different for each. If surface pressure is exerted on the membrane, the resultant compressive effect is to restrict the vascular bed with an osteoclastic result (if the compression is not so great as to cause complete necroses and a close-out of function), and the tissue response is resorption in the specific, localized area so involved. **Tension** acting on the membrane, in contrast, is generally osteoblastic, and the response is new bone deposition. These responsive actions presumably continue until physiologic and biomechanical equilibrium is attained, whereupon the blastic and clastic activities are turned off.

The above biomechanical relationships deal with growth actions on a bone's **vascular membranes**. An additional **bone matrix** factor exists. Stresses on bone's intercellular matrix have been shown to have a different but also important mode of remodeling action, as shown schematically in Figure 7–9. The **piezo** (bioelectric) response to a physical force results in a histogenic bone response accompanying a bone's displacement. The action of a muscle or tooth, the bearing of weight, and the forces of growth itself cause minute distortions within a bone at the ultrastructural level (arrows). This leads to regional changes in configuration involving localized surface convexities and concavities. A concavity results in matrix com-

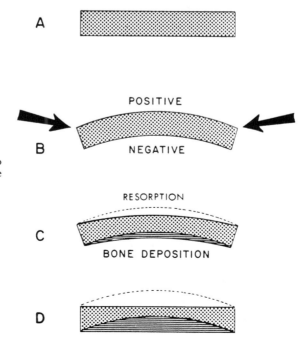

FIGURE 7–9. Piezo response to forces acting on the bone matrix. See text for description.

pression and a negative surface charge (*B*), and a convexity causes tension in the bone matrix and a resultant positive surface charge. This triggers bone deposition and resorption (*C*), respectively, by the piezo effect (page 208) acting on surface cell receptors of osteoblasts and osteoclasts. The bone thereby remodels until biomechanical and bioelectric neutrality (remodeling equilibrium) is attained (*D*), and the signals activating the whole process are turned off.

Note that the nature of this bioelectric response is **opposite** to that seen for forces acting on a bone's covering soft tissue. This is significant. Pressure on the (1) periosteum or periodontal membrane leads to resorption, and tension can trigger deposition. Pressure in the bone's matrix (2), conversely, leads to deposition with tension relating to resorption. The nature of the operations and balance between these seemingly opposite remodeling effects is interesting if not presently fully understood. This is a basic question that needs to be addressed, and it suggests a biologic interplay that is very significant.

As an exercise, see if an advanced student can account for orthodontic tooth movements on the basis of the membrane/bone matrix information provided in the preceding paragraph. A seeming obstacle, however, is that **all** of the alveolar surfaces are concave. One theoretical idea will be helpful in addressing that problem. If an existing concave surface becomes **more concave**, the effect is active compression and the action-response thereby depository. If an existing concave surface becomes **less** concave, however, the action results in less compression and in a "direction" toward tension; the response is thereby resorption. If a convex surface becomes either more or less convex, similarly, the results are believed to be resorption and deposition, respectively.

A reflective thought with regard to the biology of tooth movement: consider the **remarkable degree of precision** operative among the separate movements of a tooth, its alveolar bone, the periodontal connective tissue, and the remodeling of all the other surrounding hard and soft tissues affected by these movements. It is, in effect, a "symphony" of movements having **zero** latitude of misplay among them. Otherwise, everything would soon become developmentally mismatched, and the whole process would end quickly in gridlock. This wondrous growth system is a **precisely** coordinated, interactive composite of movements.

A tooth cannot move itself; it must be physically moved by the soft tissue surrounding its root. The directions, the amounts, and the timing of the tooth's movement must be **precisely** matched with no variance **at all** by the connective tissue remodeling of the periodontal membrane and alveolar bone remodeling movements. Attachments must be sustained all the while. If the tooth moves farther than, faster than, or at a time different from that of the resorptive bone side, for example, the periodontal space would become lost, and tooth-to-bone ankylosis would result. Similarly, the same matching growth actions on the depository alveolar bone surface must proceed in precise coordination between both and tooth for the same reason. Too much or too little, in any varying directions, one way or the other, or with off-timing, the periodontal space would either be lost or enlarged beyond functional tolerance. The PDM must remodel itself, sustain its breadth, provide relinkages, maintain attachments, and continue to relocate with the bone/tooth all the while. The whole process works because of the exceedingly finely tuned, exact operation of the signals activating the closely interrelated developmental responses involving all of these separate parts. This underscores concordance within a communal organization in which everything happens with mutual and reciprocal precision and harmony. Function continues uninterrupted throughout.

This remarkable developmental system operates under an intrinsic system of control and implementation responsive to functional conditions and complex developmental circumstances that spread throughout the craniofacial assembly during ordinary development. **Orthodontic** tooth movement harnesses and manipulates this control system through clinically induced signals that override and replace or modify the intrinsic signals. These signals can be produced by fixed and/or removable orthodontic appliances. The genic tissues respond to the signals without regard to their source. Therefore, clinical orthodontics should concentrate on identifying the type of signals generated by various appliances, rather than simply the mode of attachment. The common misconception that fixed appliances move teeth and removable appliances adjust bone is both inaccurate and incorrect. Importantly, the system of operation itself, however, is biologically the same and utilizes the same intrinsic histogenetic mechanisms. That is, in conclusion, the essential point. The future of orthodontics lies in the sophistication of "control input" regulating histogenic biologic systems.

8

Facial Form and Pattern

If a child's facial form and pattern are essentially balanced, "balanced growth" will then sustain it. Imbalanced growth, however, will alter the pattern into an imbalanced state. If a child's face is imbalanced, "balanced growth" will sustain the imbalance. An imbalanced child's face requires, in effect, imbalanced growth in order to achieve a structural craniofacial balance. Whichever, the infinite balance/imbalance mix and headform variations, population differences, and sex dimorphic variations result in a bewildering spectrum of facial "types." This chapter addresses basic developmental reasons. Other chapters evaluate anatomic patterns underlying categories of variations.

In your lifetime, you have seen the faces of thousands of people, and each face is recognizable to you as distinctively individual. No two are quite alike, even those of identical twins. Every person's face is a custom-made original; there has never been another face exactly the same before, and there never will be again. Yet consider how relatively few parts comprise a face: a lower jaw and chin, cheekbones, a mouth and upper jaw, a nose, and two orbits. Add a forehead and supraorbital ridges for the neurocranial parts relating to the face. How is it possible that so few components can underlie such great variation in facial form?

The answer is that we have the ability to perceive exceedingly subtle differences in the relative shape, spread, and proportions of both hard and soft tissue parts and minute variations in the topographic contours among all of them. Very slight alterations in the configuration of the nose, for example, make a substantial difference in the appearance and the character of one's face as a whole. (Fig. 8–1, shows a sketch from photographs of the same person before and after rhinoplasty; they look like two quite different individuals, although only a minor nasal contour has been altered.) Furthermore, there is the particular "set" to a person's mouth, the personal sparkle in the eyes, and the tone in the muscles of facial expression that are quite individualized. Often we ask, "Who does that person remind you of?" because there is some unique combination of nasal contour, lip configuration, jaw shape, and so on, that resembles some other face known to us.

Anthropologists can "reconstruct" the face from a dry skull by use of normative population data that provide integument thicknesses in the different areas of the face. However, the results can provide only a general approximation, because population "averages" can never match the delicate topographic features of a given individual in all, or even most, re-

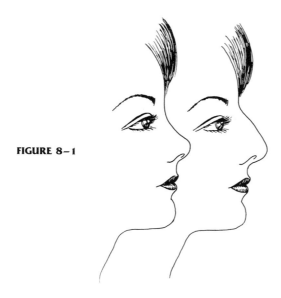

FIGURE 8–1

gards. Everybody is familiar with the method by which a police department artist attempts to draw a suspected felon's face from the recollections
of eyewitnesses. Sometimes the artist's "composite" picture can be close
enough to give a more or less recognizable likeness, but often it is vague
at best. It depends on how thoroughly a witness can recall and visualize
key facial features. Also, the effectiveness of the artist's rendering depends
on how accurately the witness can select the proper features from the
police department's "catalogue," picturing different noses, cheekbones,
hairlines, eyebrows, chins, and so on. As pointed out before, relatively
subtle differences in a given feature can produce a quite noticeably different overall facial "character."

In the next few pages, the biologic rationale underlying common variations in facial features is described. Three general considerations are
taken into account: (1) different facial types as they relate to variations in
the development of overall form and shape of the whole head, (2) male
and female developmental facial differences, and (3) child and adult facial
differences. As you study these variations, you will begin to realize that
most of the same characteristics relate to all three categories, essentially
for similar physiologic, developmental, and morphologic reasons.

HEADFORM

Two general extremes exist for the shape of the head: the long, narrow
(dolichocephalic) headform and the wide, short, globular (brachycephalic)
headform. The facial complex attaches to the basicranium, and the early
growing cranial floor is the template that establishes many of the dimensional, angular, and topographic characteristics of the face. The dolichocephalic headform, therefore, sets up a developing face that becomes correspondingly narrow, long, and protrusive. This facial type is termed
leptoprosopic. Conversely, the brachycephalic headform establishes a
face that is more broad, but somewhat less protrusive, and this is called
the **euryprosopic** facial type.

In Figure 8–2, observe what happens when a skull is dolicho- or brachycephalized. If faces are cast onto rubber balloons and the balloons then

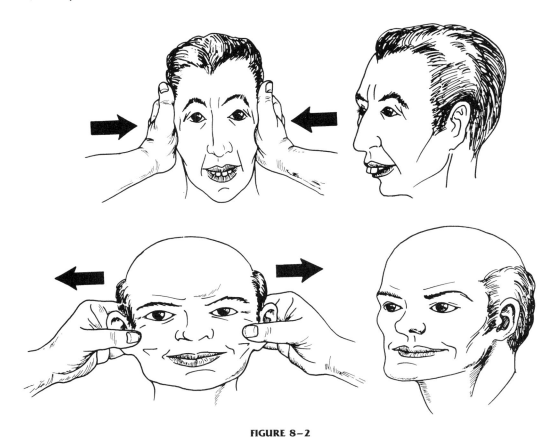

FIGURE 8-2

either squeezed or stretched, as shown, distinctively divergent facial patterns occur with regard to the forehead, the shape of the nose, the set of the eyes, the prominence of the cheekbones, the contour of the facial profile, the degree of flatness (depth) of the face, and the position of the mandible. Note that the dolichocephalic nose is vertically longer and much more protrusive (Fig. 8-3). The pug-like brachycephalic nose is vertically and protrusively shorter, and it has a more rounded tip. Even though quite different in configuration, this latter nasal design is such that approximately equivalent airway capacity exists nonetheless, because it is proportionately wider. The vertically shorter midfacial feature of the wide-face type (europrosopic), in turn, establishes a number of other facial features distinguishing it from the longer and more narrow midface of the leptoprosopic type (including differing basic malocclusion tendencies, as described in other chapters). Because the proboscis in the long and narrow facial form is also much more protrusive, the bridge and root of the nose tend to be much higher. In the dolichocephalic, also, the slope of the nasal profile tends to follow the same slope of the forehead, in contrast to the brachycephalic nose as it breaks from a more bulbous and upright forehead. Because the **upper** part of the dolichocephalic nose is also quite protrusive, the nose sometimes "bends" to produce an aquiline* ("Roman or Dick Tracy") type of convex nasal contour; and the end of the more pointed nose frequently tips down (the effect increases as age advances).

---

*Aquila** is the generic name for the eagle, with its characteristic beak.

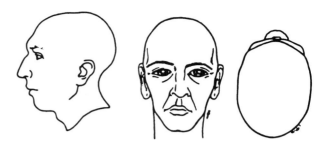

DOLICHOCEPHALIC

FIGURE 8–3. The dolichocephalic headform has a cranial index of .75 or less. The brachycephalic cranial index is .80 or greater. Between lies the mesocephalic (not shown). The dinaric cranial index is often hyperbrachycephalic (e.g., about .90 or greater). However, intermediate dinaric configurations with other headform types exist. In the lateral dinaric view, note the posterosuperior bossing. A variation is biparietal bossing (right). Note: The "cranial" index refers to a dry skull. The "cephalic" index includes covering soft tissue and has slightly different ratio values.

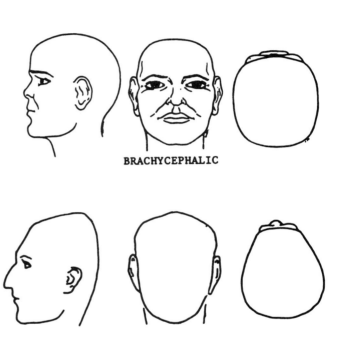

BRACHYCEPHALIC

DINARIC

The degree of the bending and downturning also increases with increasing height of the nose. Thus, aquiline convexity becomes much more marked in persons having vertically longer noses. In contrast, the more stubby brachycephalic nose tends to be straighter or often concave, and it frequently tips up, with the external nares usually showing in a face-on view. (Note: A "third" nasal configuration also exists among some long-nosed dolichocephalics and dinarics in which the **middle** part of the external nose is protrusive relative to an upper part that is much less so. In this type, the nose displays a graceful, recurved, S-shaped configuration.)

Because the nasal part of the narrow (leptoprosopic) type of face is more protrusive, the external bony table of the contiguous forehead is correspondingly more sloping, and the glabella and upper orbital rims tend to be much more prominent. The forehead of the wide (euryprosopic) facial type is more bulbous and upright, and the frontal sinus tends to be thinner because of the lesser degree of separation between the inner and outer tables of the forehead. The more protrusive nature of the nasal region and the supraorbital ridges in the dolichocephalic type of headform gives the cheekbones a much less prominent appearance, and the eyes appear more deep-set for the same reason. As seen from above (Fig. 8–3) as well as laterally, the dolichocephalic face (Fig. 8–6, left) is more angular and less flat. In the brachycephalic headform (right), the wider, flatter and less protrusive face gives the cheekbones a noticeably squared configuration and a more prominent-looking character. The brachycephalic eyeballs are characteristically more exophthalmic (proptotic) because of the shorter anterior cranial fossa (the floor of which serves as the roof for each orbit). The orbital cavities are thus more shallow causing the eyeballs to bulge in appearance. The broad brachycephalic face also appears quite shallow in comparison with the deeper and topographically more bold contours of the dolichocephalic face.

The vertically long nature of the dolichocephalic midface and the "open" (obtuse) form of its basicranial flexure (see Chapter 10) relate to a downward-backward rotational alignment of the mandible. This results in a tendency for a retrusively placed mandible and retrusive lower lip with a retrognathic (convex) facial profile (Fig. 8–4). The brachycephalic face, conversely, relates to a more "closed" basicranial flexure. As a result, the lower jaw tends to be variably more protrusive, with a greater tendency for a straighter or even concave facial profile and a more prominent-appearing chin (Fig. 8–5) The vertically shorter midface in this facial type tends to highlight a more prominent appearance of the mandible. The more upright (closed) nature of the brachycephalic basicranium produces a tendency for more erect head posture, in contrast to a tendency for a more slumped stance and head posture in many individuals with a dolichocephalic headform. The narrow but longer anterior cranial fossa in the dolichocephalic headform (Fig. 8–6) results in a correspondingly longer but narrower and deeper (high vaulted) maxillary arch and palate. The broad but anteroposteriorly shorter brachycephalic type of anterior cranial fossa sets up a wider but shorter and more shallow palate and maxillary arch. **The palate is a configurational projection of the anterior cranial fossa. The configuration of the apical base of the maxillary dental arch, in turn, is established by the perimeter of the palate.** These are basic developmental and anatomic relationships. As emphasized in earlier chapters, the development of any given region is **not** wholly "preprogrammed" within itself. Rather, factors external to the region can largely determine size and shape. A link thereby exists between brain and basicranium down to actual palatal and dental arch configuration. These same long-narrow and short-wide cranial and facial relationships are also routinely seen in other mammalian species (e.g., the Doberman pinscher or collie versus the bulldog or boxer).

Among most of the world's different human population groups, either the brachycephalic or the dolichocephalic type of headform tends to predominate. Keep in mind that very few population groups are truly genetically homogeneous, even though "assumed" otherwise. Genetic admixtures and diverse population blends are nearly always operative, whether European, Asiatic, New World, or anywhere. A distribution **range** from one extreme headform or facial type to the other thereby usually exists within a given population, even though one or the other particular side of the range is the more common. An intermediate headform type (mesocephalic) can occur, and the facial features tend to be correspondingly intermediate. In the northern and southern edges of continental Europe, as well as in most of England, Scotland, Scandinavia, northern Africa, and some Near and Middle Eastern countries (e.g., Iran, Afghanistan, India,

FIGURE 8–4. Mandibular retrusive/maxillary protrusive effects (+) are seen when there is (a) an anterior inclination of the middle cranial fossa; (b) an anteriorly and inferiorly positioned maxillary complex due to the anterior inclination of the middle cranial fossa; (c) a downward and backward alignment of the ramus; (d) a posterior and inferior positioning of B point due to a backward rotation of the ramus; (e) a long nasomaxillary complex; (f) an increased span of the middle cranial fossa (MCF) due to an anterior inclination of the MCF. A closing of the gonial angle at c would add to the mandibular retrusive effect. (From Bhat, M., and D. Enlow. Facial variations related to headform type. Angle Orthod., 55:269, 1985, with permission.)

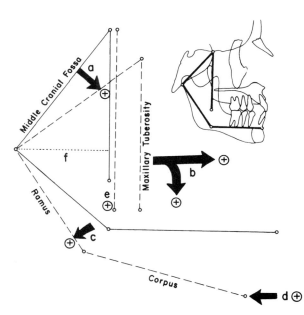

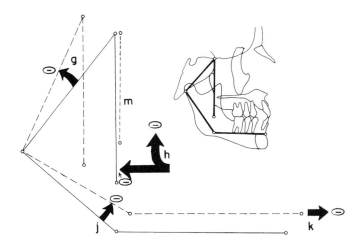

FIGURE 8–5. Mandibular protrusive/maxillary retrusive effects (−) are seen when there is (g) a posteriorly inclined middle cranial fossa; (h) a posteriorly and superiorly positioned nasomaxillary complex due to a posterior inclination of the middle cranial fossa; (j) a forward and upward alignment of the ramus; (k) an anteriorly and superiorly positioned B point due to the forward alignment of the ramus; (m) a short nasomaxillary complex. Opening of the gonial angle at j increases the mandibular protrusive effect. (From Bhat, M., and D. Enlow. Facial variations related to headform type. Angle Orthod. 55:269, 1985, with permission.)

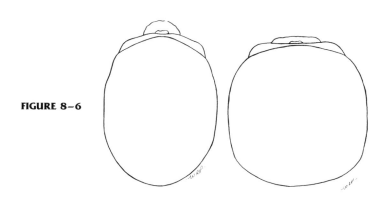

FIGURE 8–6

Iraq, and Arabia), the dolichocephalic headform tends to predominate. In central Europe (the Alpine headform) and the Far East (Oriental), brachycephaly is predominant. In many worldwide areas, however, massive population migrations, wars, and the ease of travel interchanges have led to a much muddled distribution of the historical map of headform types just outlined. In each headform category, a **range** typically exists, from less to more, for the expression of features. See Chapter 10 for a morphologic evaluation of the overlaps and mixes of features.

The Dinaric Headform

Interestingly, at certain geographic interfaces between the dolicho- and brachycephalic regions of the world, a "third" and quite distinctive type of headform commonly occurs, the **dinaric** (after the Dinaric Alps, in former Yugoslavia). The resultant admixture has, according to one theory, resulted in a "brachycephalized dolichocephalic" having a long face and large nose but with a brachycephalic cranial index. Such interface areas include regions located between middle and northern Europe, between central and southern Europe, and between Europe and the Near East. Thus, several geographically separate evolutionary lines of this headform have independently appeared and have become fairly common, although separate lines all share a number of similar craniofacial features. Admixtures of different headform types do not, thus, necessarily produce a consistent "mesocephalic" result, although this as well as pure "dolicho/brachy" offspring (mendelian-type) ratios can occur in an individual family. Rather, quite a different anatomic "blend" occurs in the dinaric. Although technically brachycephalic because it is anteroposteriorly short, it is primarily the **posterior** part of the dinaric head that has been brachycephalized (Fig. 8–3). Two basic variations exist, both of which involve **bossing** of the skull roof. First, the occipital or lambdoidal regions become widened and markedly **flattened**, with bilateral peaking (bossing) of the parietal region. The skull often has a distinctively triangular configuration when viewed from the top. Second, another common variation occurs in which the bossing is directed more upward than bilaterally, thereby forming an elevated hump or peak in the posterosuperior part of the skull dome. Cranial configuration is less triangular when viewed from the top. Whatever the manner of bossing, it accommodates the volumetric mass of a brain that has undergone alteration in overall shape. The cranial index is often hyperbrachycephalic (i.e., 90 or greater).

The old practice of "cradling"† causes or at least intensifies occipital flattening by the external force acting on the skull. Indeed, the sleeping posture of an infant, whether or not cradled as such, is likely a factor in "dinarizing" a growing head to some greater or lesser extent. It has been argued that such mechanical influences during early infancy represent the dominant reason for causing the dinaric form if the sleeping position is predominately on the back and sustained through childhood. Interestingly, it has been shown that American descendants of Old World dinaric grandparents can lose the dinaric features because cradling is not practiced. It is also argued, however, that a "genetic" dinaric form also exists because dinaric individuals certainly exist who have not been cradled as infants and who have mixed sleeping positions. Observations suggest that the "biparietal bossing" type is a product of cradling or, at least, early back-position sleeping habits. The "peaked dome" type, in contrast, may be a more "genetic" type, although formal studies are now needed to test these

---

†Immobilizing an infant on its back with a wrap of swaddling clothes on a hard palate.

hypotheses. The matter is significant because the dinaric headform, with its variations and degrees of magnitude (see below) shows different malocclusion tendencies and responses to different treatment procedures.

The ears of the dinaric characteristically appear much closer to the back of the head because of the occipital flattening, as noted in Figure 8–3. Of course, it is not the ears themselves that are back, but rather the posterior flattening making them appear so. The anterior part of the skull retains the relative narrowness that characterizes the dolichocephalic pattern. The narrow face from the dolichocephalic side of the ancestral heritage has perhaps "constrained" the anterior cranial fossa, or perhaps the converse, thereby sustaining a narrow dimension in this part of the basicranium. Even though the headform is technically brachycephalic, the form of the face itself is distinctively leptoprosopic, quite unlike the typical eurosopic brachycephalic pattern. The posterior facial parts (such as the mandibular ramus and temporomandibular joint [TMJ] region) tend to flare laterally in the "biparietal" (triangular) headform type of dinaric because they grade farther back on the widening cranial triangle. The forehead is often quite sloping in many individuals of all dinaric types, the supraorbital ridges are prominent, and the face is long and topographically protrusive. The nose tends to be very large and often aquiline (this occurs in many females as well as males), and the nasal bridge is high. The mandible tends to be less retrusive, the face less retrognathic, and the profile tending more toward orthognathic. This is because the basicranial flexure is compressed and more closed (see page 127). The midface, however, tends to be vertically long in proportion, even more so than among dolichocephalic leptoprosopics. These various leptoprosopic features often appear exaggerated in character in the dinaric headform, almost as though the brachycephalized, flattened posterior part of the cranium "pushed" the face even more protrusively than in a routine dolichocephalic headform. Any malocclusion in a dinaric will have a combination of structural features different from that in a dolichocephalic. Both, in turn, are different in malocclusion anatomy from a brachycephalic, and treatment responses and rebound tendencies will also be different. (See Bhat and Enlow, 1985; Martone et al., 1992.)

While the dinaric headform has been historically perceived as a "brachycephalized dolichocephalic," it is probable that **any** headform type, including the brachycephalic and mesocephalic, is susceptible to this modification, whether by sleeping habits or through hereditary mix. Intermediate variations, further, certainly exist, but have yet to be studied and catalogued. "Partial dinarization" is commonly observed in individuals having, for example, a mesocephalic index. This general area is a particularly inviting research opportunity. Another needed study is the possible lasting effects of various sleeping positions by an infant and young child on facial form and malocclusion tendencies.

Extraoral and functional appliances have divergent responses in the different headform groups and subgroups (Enlow et al., 1988; DiPalma, 1983; Martone et al., 1992). Because clinical procedures harness "growth" by activating regional modifications in the directions and amounts of histogenesis that lead to the different headform types, awareness of headform variations and facial differences is a fundamentally important consideration for orthodontic treatment planning.

Male Versus Female Facial Features

A talented artist can effectively render male versus female faces, and the viewer has no problem recognizing either gender from sketches or portraits of adults. (Children are another matter, as will be seen.) However, many artists, as well as the average citizen, are not really conscious of the actual, specific anatomic differences involved. They just "know." In our mind's eye, we have all subconsciously associated, over the years, the topographic characteristics that relate to facial dimorphism.

The overall body size of the male tends to be larger than that of the female, and the male lungs are correspondingly more sizable to provide for the relatively more massive muscles and body organs. This calls for a larger airway, beginning with the nose and nasopharynx. A principal sexual dimorphic difference, therefore, is the size and configuration of the nose, and this, in turn, leads to collateral differences in other topographic structures of the face, since the airway is a developmental keystone (see Chapter 1).

The male nose is proportionately larger than the female nose (Fig. 8–7). This is a "population" feature based on general comparisons among large numbers of people; any given individual female or male, of course, can display a smaller or larger nose. The male nose, in general, tends to be more protrusive, longer, wider, more fleshy, and tends to have larger and more flaring nostrils. The interorbital part of the nasal bridge in the male tends to be much higher. All of this is in contrast to a relatively thin and less protrusive female nose. The male nose usually ranges from a straight to a convex (aquiline) profile, whereas the female nose tends to range from a straight to a somewhat concave profile. The tip of the male nose is often more pointed and has a greater tendency to turn downward, and the somewhat more rounded female nose often tips upward. The external nares in the female are more often visible in a face-on view for this reason. A variation of the aquiline (Roman) type of nose, which is also much more prevalent among males than females, is the classic "Greek" nose, in which the nasal profile drops almost straight downward from a protruding forehead (Fig. 8–8). The reason for the multiple male variations in nasal configu-

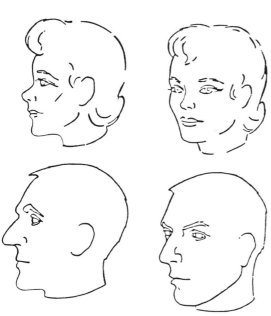

FIGURE 8–7

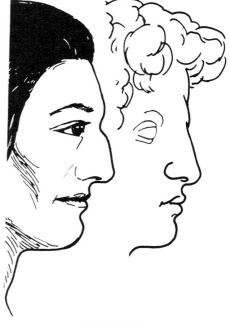

FIGURE 8–8

ration lies in the more protuberant nature of the whole nasal region. Both the upper and lower parts of the whole external nose are protrusive, but the lower part can be constrained to a degree by the septopremaxillary ligament, palate, and maxillary arch. The contour of the nose thus "rotates"; it either "bends" to give an aquiline configuration or rotates into a straight, but more vertical, alignment.

Because of the larger, more protuberant character of the male nose, the part of the forehead contiguous with it also necessarily remodels into a more protrusive position. Therefore, the male forehead tends to be more sloping, in contrast to a more bulbous, upright female forehead. The supraorbital and glabellar parts of the male forehead tend to be **quite** protrusive, as compared with the much **less** Neanderthal-like character of the female forehead. This, together with the differences in the relative size and vertical alignment of the nose, provide the features most readily recognizable in our subconscious perceptions of male and female faces.

In Figure 8–9, note the dashed line passing vertically along the surface of the upper lip perpendicular to the neutral orbital axis. In the female, this line usually crosses about midway along the upper nasal slope, and the forehead generally lies behind but seldom at the line. Conversely, in the male, the nose and forehead are often so protrusive that the forehead bulges out as far as this line or sometimes even beyond it, and the greater part of the nose often lies ahead of it.

Because of the greater extent of protrusiveness of the male forehead and nose, the eyes appear more deep-set. In the female the eyes appear more proptotic and "closer to the front" of the face. Female cheekbones also "look" much more prominent for the same reason; that is, the malar protuberances seem more apparent because the nose and forehead are less prominent. Indeed, "high cheekbones" are a classic feature of femininity, much emphasized by beauty analysts. Of course, the malar protuberances are not actually "higher;" they are just more conspicuous. This topographic feature of the female face is better seen in a 45-degree view of the face (see Fig. 8–7). In addition, the temporal region along the side of the forehead tends to be more sloping and less bulgy in the female.

The composite of all these regional, topographic distinctions render the female face flatter, proportionately (not actually) wider in appearance, and more delicate in general character. The male face, in contrast, appears

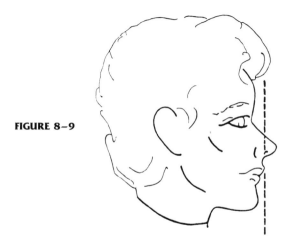

FIGURE 8–9

deeper, more irregular and knobby, and more coarse. The astute clinician will keep these general tendencies in mind when planning treatment to achieve aesthetic goals. For example, the male patient with a prominent chin may be more likely to accept an orthodontic compromise of his prognathism than a female with the same degree of mandibular prognathia.

The protuberant supraorbital part of the more sloping male forehead (because of the larger nose) is produced by a greater extent of remodeling separation of the outer table of the frontal bone beyond the earlier-stabilized inner table. In both sexes, the growth of the inner table stops when the enlargement of the frontal lobes of the cerebrum ceases around 5 to 6 years of age. The outer table, however, continues to remodel forward until contiguous nasal growth ceases, which is some years later. The inner and outer tables thereby diverge, and the cancellous bone between them is hollowed into the frontal sinus. Because the nasal part of the male face continues to grow for several years beyond that of the female, the frontal sinus is, therefore, much larger in the male face than in the more juvenile-like female face. Also, because of the smaller frontal sinuses in a female, the temporal regions of the lateral forehead often appear less full and thus more sloping. Because the forehead and nose are less protrusive in the female face, the upper jaw tends to "look" more prominent and muzzle-like. For this reason, the female patient may be more likely to accept an orthodontic compromise for a prognathic maxilla than would a male patient with the same degree of maxillary prognathia.

Now relate these male and female features to the facial features previously described that distinguish the dolichocephalic from the brachycephalic headform. This includes the degree of supraorbital protrusion, forehead slope, cheekbone prominence, nasal configuration, orbital depth, and depth or flatness of the whole face. These headform characteristics are **the same** as those that distinguish the male from the female face. The long, narrow **dolichocephalic** basicranium and facial airway lead to facial features that essentially parallel those of the **male** face. The short, wide **brachycephalic** basicranium and facial airway set up facial features that parallel those of the **female** face. The nasal part of the face underlies much of the overall character of a person's facial form. In the "brachy/dolicho" situation, it is the width and length of the basicranium that (1) establish the basis for nasal form and size and (2) the positions of all the various facial parts and their relative vertical, sagittal, and bilateral proportions. In the male/female comparison, it is **relative whole body and lung size** that leads to corresponding nasal characteristics, which, in turn, establish the other facial features that are analogous to those also associated with headform type. Please do not misunderstand this "headform and male/female" convergence. It is not being stated that males are dolichos, and that females are brachys. These are independent variables, and all possible combinations are possible.

Then what about a female dolichocephalic? Or a male brachycephalic? Or a female dinaric? Most people naturally feel a comforting confidence that they can usually distinguish gender by a person's face. However, recognition tests have shown that it is actually not all that easy. If ancillary clues (e.g., hairstyle, cosmetics) are removed by masking from facial photographs and other kinds of clues are not available (e.g., voice, clothing, gait, presence or absence of a protruding larynx, neck circumference, breadth of shoulders), recognition tests in which facial photographs are presented can lead to dismay and despair. The chances of a correct identification for many individual faces or parts of faces are often not much better than a toss-up.

In a female **brachycephalic**, the headform characteristics of a wider and flatter face, smaller nose, squared cheekbones, and an upright forehead tend to augment and emphasize the **same** dimorphic features that also relate to gender. Conversely, in the female **dolichocephalic**, the larger-nosed, more angular face, and generally more protrusive facial characteristics associated with this headform type tend to give a more "male-like" cast to the face. Of course, these features are **not** really masculine at all, but, rather, headform-linked. Thus, a leptoprosopic female is characterized by a more sloping forehead, greater supraorbital protrusion, a higher nasal bridge, a longer nose, an aquiline or more vertically aligned nasal contour, a downturned and more pointed nasal tip, and, often, a more retrognathic mandible. The average citizen has subconsciously learned the difference between brachycephalic and dolichocephalic females, even though few have any idea what a brachycephalic or a dolichocephalic is. In a male brachycephalic, the reverse situation exists. The "female-like" characteristics of the brachycephalic headform present a flatter, wider face with more prominent cheekbones; a more bulbous forehead; a smaller, less protrusive nose with a lower nasal bridge, less deep-set eyes, and a tendency for a straight-to-concave nasal profile with a more rounded and upturned tip. One frequently sees female impersonators on TV (e.g., a detective disguised as a lady of the street); the realism of the disguise is favored if the male is a wide-faced, small-nosed brachycephalic. A male dolichocephalic, as in a female long-head, has the headform features augmenting the gender characteristics, including the nasal, forehead, cheekbone, deeper set eyeball, retrusive mandibular tendency, and so on. Female "impersonation" would be more difficult and less believable. These characteristic features do not compromise the masculine character of the face; they simply represent another facial variation that we all have learned to recognize.

Finally, a common misconception is pointed out. It is frequently heard that the female mandible, more often than in the male, has a typically retrusive set (e.g., a more "submissive" position). The extent of retrognathia is a headform feature, not a sexual dimorphic one.

Child Versus Adult Facial Features

The faces of prepubertal boys and girls are essentially comparable. How many times have you been embarrassed by calling a little boy a girl? In the female, facial development begins to slow markedly after about 13 or so years of age. At about the time of puberty for the male, however, the sex-related dimorphic facial features just described begin to be fully manifested, and this maturation process of the facial superstructures continues actively throughout the adolescent period and into early adulthood. This is a factor to be taken into account by the orthodontist and orthognathic surgeon in treatment planning for girls and boys because it often has a greater aesthetic impact on the post-treatment facial profile than the sometimes controversial decision to extract permanent teeth.

Whether a young child's headform is dolichocephalic or brachycephalic, the youthful face itself appears more brachycephalic-like because it is still relatively wide and vertically short. It is wide because the brain, and therefore the basicranium, is precocious relative to facial development. The neurocranium grows earlier, faster, and to a much greater extent that the contiguous facial complex. The wider basicranium, because it establishes TMJ positions for the mandible and the facial-to-cranial sutures for the nasomaxillary complex, is thereby a template that also paces the early **width** of the growing face. The face is **vertically** short because (1) the nasal part of the face is still diminutive (overall body and lung size still correspondingly small); (2) the primary and secondary dentition has not

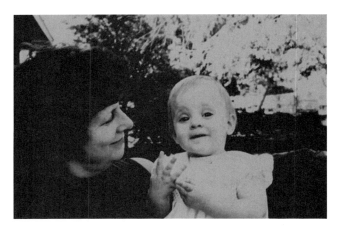

FIGURE 8–10

FIGURE 8–11

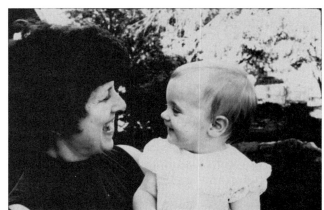

yet become fully established; and (3) the jaw bones have not yet grown to the vertical extent that will later support the full dentition, the enlarging masticatory muscles, and the airway.

Note (Figs. 8–10 and 8–11) the features of the child's face compared to the adult, regardless of sex or headform type: the nose is short, rounded, and pug-like; the nasal bridge is low; the nasal profile is concave; the nares can be seen in a face-on view; the forehead is bulbous and upright; the cheekbones are prominent; the face is flat; and the eyes seem wide-set and bulging.

The same situation, noted twice before, thus exists with regard to facial pattern: most of the **same** facial features that characterize **both** headform and sexual dimorphism **also** relate to the differences between the facial features of the child and the adult. In all three categories, the character of the nasal part of the face is a key factor that relates directly to the other facial features (forehead slope, nasal configuration, height of nasal bridge, cheekbone prominence, flatness of the face, and the general extent of facial protrusiveness). Because the facial and pharyngeal airway is yet small because of diminutive body and lung size, it thus sets up the early developmental conditions paralleling a topographic similarity with the brachycephalic headform (i.e., the basicranial template) **and** the male/female difference (i.e., the airway). The childhood situation, however, is developmentally independent of both the headform and sex dimorphic factors.

How does one recognize advancing age in an **older adult** by external facial appearance? There was a time when edentulism caused major changes in facial structure and topography. In many parts of the world, modern dentistry has effectively precluded much of this. Other facial changes, however, still occur. The velvety, soft, pink, tightly bound, resilient, and firm skin of the child becomes replaced over the years by the more leathery, crinkled, open-pored, limp, blemished skin that progressively characterizes more aged persons. As one advances through middle age, the integument begins to droop and sag noticeably. Several physical and biochemical changes are occurring in the connective tissue of the dermis and hypodermis that cause the skin to become less firmly anchored to underlying bone or facial muscles. First, if general loss of body weight occurs for whatever reason as one ages, resorption of subcutaneous adipose results in a "surplus" of skin which, with gravity, leads to sagging, wrinkling, and creasing. Loss of adipose thus exaggerates age appearance. After dieting, for example, a face often looks older. The effect can occur in children as well; the sight of a severely malnourished child with a wrinkled, lined, hollow face is not easily forgotten. Second, the distribution and character of the collagenous matrix change with advancing age. Fibers increase in massiveness, and the whole skin decreases in resilience. Third, fibroblasts decline in number as well as cellular activities. The latter includes a marked decrease in the secretion and overall amount of hydrophilic (water-bound) protein mucopolysaccharides (proteoglycans). Because of this, a widespread subcutaneous dehydration occurs that contributes significantly to shrunken facial volume and skin surplus, with consequent skin wrinkling. In advanced old age, a person's face can become an expansive carpet of noble ripples and lines. Resorption of adipose in the orbit leads to a sunken appearance of the eyes, and the more visible venous plexus in the thinned suborbital hypodermis produces a darkening of the skin below the eyes. The suborbital integument can also begin to sag perceptibly to form "bags." Something also happens to the youthful "sparkle" in many persons' eyes as they age. By waxing artificial wrinkles onto the face and blue-tinting the suborbital region, a good Hollywood make-up technician can "age" a face in minutes. Observe closely, however, and you will note that, unlike real skin, the artificial furrows are not as motile during attempts at expressive facial movements.

Facial lines and wrinkles develop in specific and characteristic locations, particularly during the middle-age period. One of the initial lines to appear is the prominent **nasolabial furrow**. This "smile line" is seen at any age when one grins, but it becomes a fixed feature of the face sometime during the late 30s or 40s in many people and continues to deepen and become more marked. It extends from the lateral side of each nasal ala down to the corners of the mouth. This is a particular facial feature that we have subconsciously learned to associate with the onset of middle age. Stopping smiling does not seem to help.

Other wrinkles and creases begin to develop as crow's feet at the lateral corners of the eyes, horizontal lines on the forehead, vertical corrugations overlying the glabella, vertical furrows along the upper lip, lines extending down from the corners of the mouth lateral to the chin, a horizontal crease just above the chin, suborbital lines, drooping jowls over the sides of the mandible, and a "turkey gobbler" bag of skin sagging down over the neck below the chin. The placement, alignment, prominence, and number of such lines and creases, as well as many other topographic facial features, are utilized as presumptive clues by the physiognomist (a practitioner of the ancient Chinese art of face reading) to judge a person's character, temperament, and ultimate fate. However, no real functional, preprogrammed, cause-and-effect relationships are likely to exist in most such correlations; there are just too many physiologic, anatomic, environmental, social, developmental, and ethnic variables involved in the biology of the human face.

How about the person who "looks younger than his or her years"? Or older? For reasons only partially understood, the onset of the smile line and some other facial wrinkles is delayed, or at least such lines look less marked, in youthful-appearing individuals. Conversely, in others, lines can appear more harsh and begin to develop at an earlier age. Intrinsic physiologic as well as environmental factors can contribute to this. For example, sun and UV damage to the facial integument, particularly in lighter-complexioned individuals, is known to accelerate the aging process of skin. Furthermore, chronic alcoholism causes the muscles of facial expression within the skin to sag because of the long-term anesthetized-like and limp state of their tone. Alcohol, further, is a dehydrator. Smoking tends to intensify wrinkling because tobacco is a peripheral vasoconstrictor. Major loss of adipose can also accelerate the onset of facial wrinkles, as previously explained. In addition, a euryprosopic (brachycephalic) type of face appears more juvenile-like because it resembles the more wide and short configuration characterizing the face of a child. A dolichocephalic adult face "looks" more mature because the nasal region is vertically longer and the face less wide in proportion. A fat face looks younger (1) because the subcutaneous adipose tends to smooth out wrinkles and (2) because it resembles the labial and buccal fat-padded face of a child. Thus, a wide-faced, more chunky, sober, nonsmoking, darker-skinned individual, particularly one protected from undue sun exposure, tends to retain a more youthful appearance somewhat longer.

The Changing Features of the Growing Face

The "baby face" has large-appearing eyes, dainty jaws, a tiny pug nose, puffy cheeks with buccal and labial fat pads, a high intellectual-like forehead without coarse eyebrow ridges, a low nasal bridge, a small mouth, velvety skin, and overall wide and short proportions. It is a cute face. It warms the cockles of parental hearts. A parent can worry, though, because the otherwise great little face "has no chin," or "the jaw is much too small," or "the eyes are too far apart." However, these and many of the other features of the baby's face gradually undergo marked changes as the face grows and develops through the years. The chin develops, jaw size catches up, and the eyes appear less wide-set. From the many possible variations that can exist among different individuals, a person's own facial characteristics take on, month by month, definitive adult form. The general features of any fully grown face can be quite different from those of the same individual as an infant and young child. Trying to decide which parent the infant "looks like" or which uncle it "takes after" is a fun game, but usually more or less futile. There is little in the general shape and proportions of the infantile face, at least topographically, to give a hint as to what form it will take in later years. Unless, of course, the adult happens to have a euryprosopic face with pudgy cheeks, wide-set eyes, pug nose, etc., all childlike features.

In general, the baby's face grows out from under the brain. Structures must grow proportionally more and for a longer period of time the further they are from the neurocranium. Therefore, growth of the mandible begins later and continues longer than midfacial or orbital development.

Growth is not merely a process of size increases. Rather, progressive facial enlargement is a "differential" developmental process in which each of the many component parts matures earlier or later than the others, to different extents in different facial regions, in a multitude of different directions, and at different rates. It is a gradual maturational process involving a complex of different but functionally interrelated organs, parts, and tissues. The growth process also involves a bewildering succession of regional changes in proportions and requires countless localized, ongoing "adjustments" to achieve proper fitting and function among all of the parts.

The child's face is not merely a miniature of the adult, as dramatically illustrated in Figure 8–12 which shows a neonatal skull enlarged to the same size as a fully grown one.

The baby's face appears diminutive relative to the larger, more precocious cranium above and behind it (Fig. 8–13). The respective proportions change significantly, however. The growth of the brain slows considerably after about the third or fourth year of childhood, but the facial bones continue to enlarge markedly for many more years to accommodate airway and masticatory growth and functions.

The eyes, which are precocious along with the brain, thus can appear large in the young child. As facial growth continues, however, the nasal and jaw regions later develop disproportionately to the earlier-maturing orbit and its soft tissues. As a result, the eyes of the adult appear smaller in proportion.

The ears of the infant and child appear to be low; in the adult they are much higher with respect to the face. Do the ears actually rise? No; they in fact move downward during continued development. However, the face enlarges inferiorly even farther, so that the **relative** position of the ears seems to rise. In an infant, note that the body of the mandible is in near alignment with the auditory meatus, thus reflecting their commonality of embryonic origin. Later, the corpus descends as the midface and ramus lengthen vertically, and this relationship becomes more obscure.

The young child's precocious forehead is upright and bulbous. The forehead of the adult, however, becomes much more sloping (the amount of slope is related to sex and headform, as already explained). The forehead region of the child seems very large and high because the face beneath it is still relatively small. The child's forehead continues to enlarge during

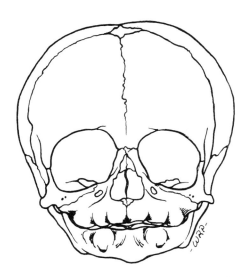
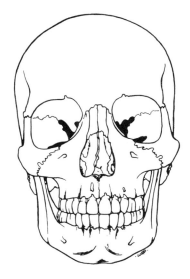

FIGURE 8–12

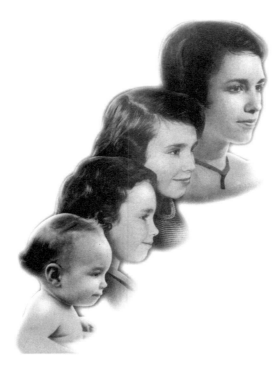

FIGURE 8–13. (Courtesy of William L. Brudon. From Enlow, D. H.: *The Human Face.* New York, Harper & Row, 1968, with permission.)

the early years, but the face enlarges much more, so that the proportionate size of the forehead becomes reduced.

The child's face appears broad because the brain and basicranium develop earlier and faster than the facial composite, as already explained. As development continues, **vertical** facial growth (enlarging airway, dentition) then comes to bypass expansion in width to a marked extent, so that a much more narrow facial proportion characterizes the adult, especially in dolichocephalics and dinarics.

The nasal bridge is quite low in the child. It rises (to a greater or lesser extent in different facial types) to become much more prominent in adults.

The eyes of the infant can seem quite wide-set, with a broad-appearing nasal bridge between them. This is because the nasal bridge is so low, and

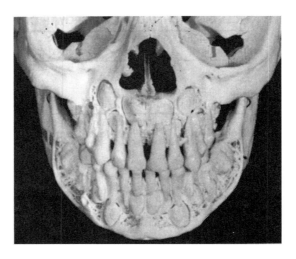

FIGURE 8–14

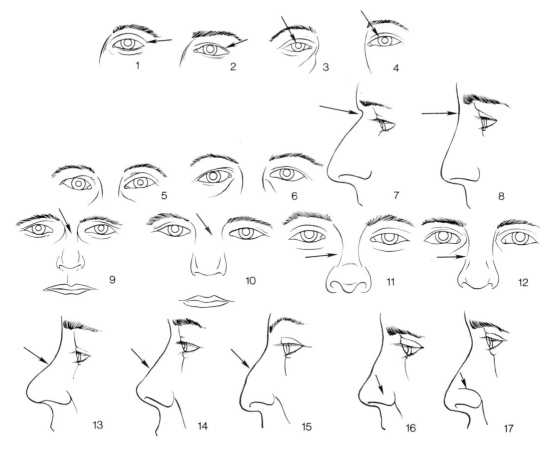

FIGURE 8–15. (Modified from Hulanicka, B.: Nadbitka Z Nru 86, Materialow 1 Prac antropologicznych Wroclaw, 115, 1973, with permission.)

also because much of the width of the bridge has already been attained in the infant. With continued growth, the eyes spread farther laterally, but only to a relatively small extent. Actually, the eyes of the adult face are not much farther apart than those in the child. Because of the larger nose, higher nasal bridge, increase in the vertical facial dimension, and the widening of the cheekbones, the eyes of the adult thus **appear** much closer together.

The infant and young child have much more of a pug nose than the adult. It protrudes very little and is vertically quite short. The shape and size of the infantile nose, however, give little indication of what will happen to it during subsequent growth. The extent of proboscis enlargement can be considerable. The lower part of the nose in the adult is proportionately much wider and a great deal more prominent.

The whole nasal region of the infant is vertically shallow. The level of the nasal floor lies close to the inferior orbital rim. In the adult, the midface becomes greatly expanded, and the nasal floor has descended well below the orbital floor. This change is quite marked because of the enormous enlargement of the nasal chambers. Note the close proximity of the young child's maxillary arch to the orbit, in contrast to their positions in the adult.

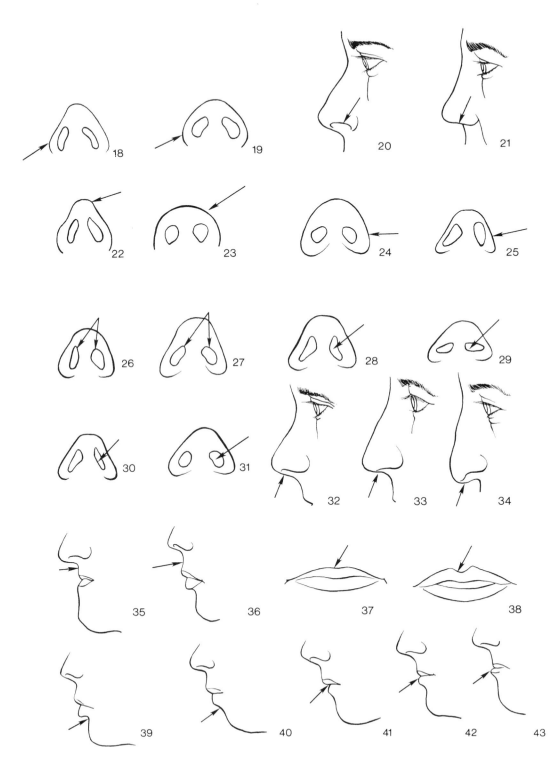

FIGURE 8–16. (Modified from Hulanicka, B.: Nadbitka Z Nru 86, Materialow 1 Prac antropologicznych Wroclaw, 115, 1973, with permission.)

The superior and inferior orbital rims of the young child are in an approximately vertical line or inclined behind (see Figs. 5–17 and 2–12). Because of frontal sinus development and supraorbital protrusion in the adult, however, the upper orbital rim noticeably overhangs the lower. The orbital opening and lateral orbital rim become inclined obliquely forward. Supraorbital and glabellar protrusion is particularly marked in the adult male because of the larger nose needed to accommodate larger lungs.

Below the orbit, the nasal chambers in the adult face expand laterally nearly halfway across the orbital floor. In the infant, the breadth of the nasal cavity inferiorly scarcely exceeds the width of the nasal bridge and interorbital space (Fig. 2–25). During subsequent growth, the inferior portion of the nose expands laterally much more than the superior part.

The tip of the infant's nasal bone protrudes very little beyond the inferior orbital rim. The area **between** the nasal tip and the inferior rim of the orbit (i.e., the lateral bony wall of the nose) is characteristically narrow and shallow. In the adult, this area becomes markedly expanded. The divergent directions of orbital, nasal, cheekbone, and maxillary arch growth "draw out" the contours among them. The facial parts become spread apart and much deeper.

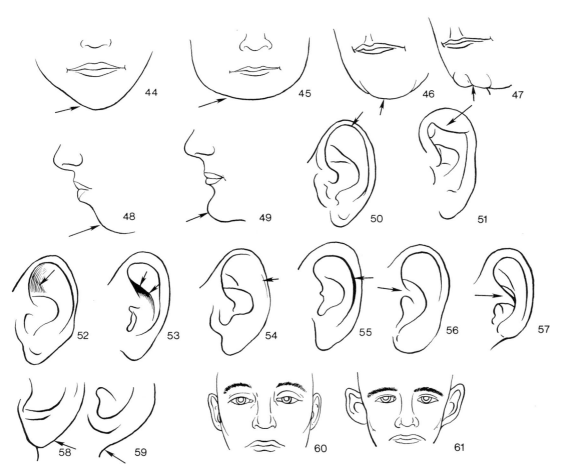

FIGURE 8–17. (Modified from Hulanicka, B.: Nadbitka Z Nru 86, Materialow 1 Prac antropologicznych Wroclaw, 115, 1973, with permission.)

The nasal region of a growing child's midface is, almost literally, a keystone of facial architecture, that is, a key part upon which other surrounding parts, and the multiple anatomic arches formed by them, are dependent for placement and stability. If this keystone is malformed for any reason, other facial parts are affected during growth, and facial dysplasia or malocclusion can occur. The facial airway, therefore, is an exceedingly significant component involved in normal versus abnormal facial morphogenesis.

The orbits and the cheekbones in the child are more forward appearing because the whole face is still relatively flat and wide. In the infant, the protrusive appearance of the cheekbones is augmented by the characteristic infantile buccal fat pad in the overlying hypodermis. Adults tending to have a relatively wide and short (thus more childlike) type of face typ-

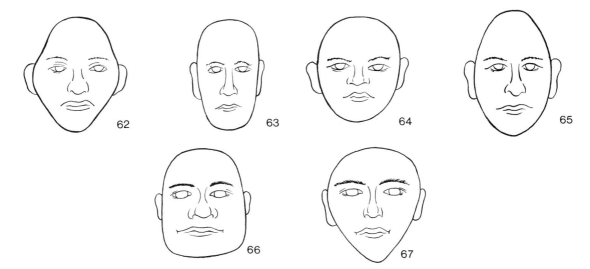

FIGURE 8–18. In Figures 8–15 to 8–18, note the following topographic facial variations: *1*, the tarsal part of the upper eyelid exposed; *2*, the eye laterally covered by an eyelid fold; *3*, the iris covered by the upper eyelid; *4*, most of the iris exposed; *5*, the lateral corner of eye higher than the medial corner; *6*, the lateral eye corner lower than the medial corner; *7*, the top of the nasal bridge (root) markedly indented; *8*, a high nasal root (so-called "Greek nose"); *9*, a narrow nasal root; *10*, a broad nasal root; *11*, a narrow nasal slope; *12*, a broad nasal slope; *13*, a concave nasal profile; *14*, a straight nasal profile; *15*, a convex nasal profile; *16*, inconspicuous nasal wings; *17*, prominent nasal wings; *18*, V-shaped nasal wings; *19*, rounded nasal wings; *20*, arched nasal wings; *21*, straight nasal wings; *22*, a narrow nasal tip; *23*, a broad, flattened nasal tip; *24*, a thick, fleshy nasal wing; *25*, a thin nasal wing; *26*, asymmetric nasal openings; *27*, symmetric openings; *28*, posterolaterally directed openings; *29*, laterally directed openings; *30*, narrow, elongate openings; *31*, rounded nasal openings; *32*, an upward nasal inclination; *33*, a straight lower nasal border; *34*, a downward inclined nasal border; *35*, a vertically short upper lip; *36*, a long upper lip (check also to see whether the upper lip profile is straight or concave); *37*, the upper lip without a midline "Cupid's bow"; *38*, a deep midline notch in the upper lip (look also for a more conspicuous philtrum above the upper lip, and check for thinness or thickness of the red part of both the upper and lower lips); *39*, an acutely curved lower border (concavity) below the lower lip; *40*, lesser concavity between lower lip and chin and a greater distance between the lip and mentolabial sulcus; *41*, the lower lip retrusive; *42*, the lips equally protruding; *43*, the lower lip protrusive; *44*, a pointed mandible; *45*, a squared mandible; *46*, no chin cleft; *47*, a bifid chin; *48*, a retrusive mandible (and chin); *49*, a prominent chin; *50*, slight rolling of the upper border of ear helix; *51*, pronounced helix rolling; *52*, a flat, shallow ear scapha; *53*, a pronounced, deep groove below the scapha; *54*, slight rolling of the middle part of the helix; *55*, pronounced middle helix rolling; *56*, a short, low crus; *57*, a prominent, long crus; *58*, a dangling ear lobe; *59*, an ear lobe fused with facial skin; *60*, slight ear protrusion; *61*, marked ear protrusion; *62*, a diamond-shaped face; *63*, a long, narrow face; *64*, a round, short face; *65*, an oval face; *66*, a square face; *67*, an egg-shaped face.

ically show an even greater "cherubic" appearance if they are overweight; the buccal region contains adipose tissue resembling the buccal fat pad of infancy.

Although the cheekbone is prominent in early childhood, it is nonetheless quite diminutive and fragile, compared with that of the adult. The malar process and the inferior part of the zygoma enlarge considerably during childhood growth, even though they actually remodel in a **backward** direction until definitive arch length is achieved. Because of the differential extents and directions of growth in other parts of the face, these growth increases by the zygoma are often masked. The **protrusive** modes of supraorbital and nasal remodeling and displacement cause the adult forehead and nose to appear progressively more prominent relative to the **retrusively** remodeling cheekbones and lateral orbital rims, thus drawing out the depth of the face due to regional developmental divergence in these contiguous facial regions. This feature is more noticeable in the male.

The entire face of the adult is thus much deeper anteroposteriorly, and the whole face is **drawn out** in many directions. The adult face has much bolder topographic features, and it is much less "flat."

As the whole face expands, the frontal, maxillary, and ethmoidal *sinuses* enlarge to occupy spaces not otherwise functionally utilized. Architecturally, the sinuses are leftover "dead" (unused) spaces (see page 154). They were not created especially to provide "resonance to the voice," nasal drip, air warming, or other special functions, although they have become secondarily involved in such roles.

The mandible of the young child appears quite small and "underdeveloped" relative to the upper jaw and the face in general. It is small not only in actual size but also proportionately, and it is retrusively placed as well. The child's anterior cranial fossae directly overlie the nasomaxillary complex suspended from them. **Because the anterior cranial fossae are developmentally precocious, the nasomaxillary complex is thereby carried to a more protrusive position than the mandible**, which articulates on the ectocranial side of the middle endocranial fossae located more posteriorly. Much of the basicranial expansion affecting forward nasomaxillary displacement thus does not affect the mandible early on. Only later does the mandible "catch up" as its ramus (together with the attached, growing muscles of mastication) matches or exceeds the development of the overlying, later-growing middle cranial fossae. Because of this, it is sometimes difficult to predict during early childhood possible skeletal malocclusions that might or might not become fully expressed during later development.

The chin is incompletely formed in the infant; indeed, it hardly exists at all. Because of remodeling changes that gradually take place, however, the chin becomes more prominent year by year. A "cleft" is sometimes formed in the **fleshy** part of the chin (not usually in the bone itself) when the two sides of the lower jaw fuse during early postnatal development. The cleft deepens when the soft tissues of the two sides then continue to expand. For some reason, this facial feature has become adopted in our society as a symbol of masculinity when it is present in the male. Its presence in the female has no social significance one way or the other.

The young child's mandible appears to be pointed. This is because it is wide, short, and more V-shaped. In the adult, the entire lower jaw becomes "squared." With the development of the chin, together with massive growth in the lateral areas of the trihedral eminence, eruption of the permanent dentition, enlargement of each ramus, expansion of the masticatory musculature, and flaring of the gonial regions, the whole lower face takes on a more U-shaped configuration, resulting in a **considerably** more full facial appearance (Fig. 2–25).

In the infant and young child, the gonial region lies well inside (medial to) the cheekbone. In the adult, the posteroinferior corner of the mandible extends laterally out to the cheekbone, or nearly so. This gives the posterior part of the jaw a square appearance.

The ramus of the adult mandible is much longer vertically (Fig. 2–12). It is also more upright (this refers to the ramus as a whole and not to the misleading "gonial angle"). The **sizeable** elongation of the ramus accommodates the massive vertical expansion of the nasal region and the eruption of the deciduous and then the permanent teeth along with masticatory muscle development.

The premaxillary region normally protrudes beyond the mandible in the infant and young child, and it lies in line with or forward of the bony tip of the nose (Fig. 2–12). This gives a prominent appearance to the upper jaw and lip. In subsequent facial development, however, the nose becomes much more protrusive, and the tip of the nasal bone comes to lie well ahead of the basal bone of the premaxilla.

The forward surface of the bony maxillary arch in the infant, with its yet unerupted dentition, has a vertically convex topography. This is in contrast to the characteristically later concave contour of this region in the adult. The alveolar bone in this area of the adult face is noticeably more protrusive and proportionately much more massive (in conjunction with the permanent dentition) (Fig. 2–12).

The whole face, vertically, is a great deal longer and more obliquely sloping as a result of the many changes outlined above (Fig. 5–17).

The quite small mastoid process of the infant later develops into the sizable protuberance of the adult. A bony styloid process is also lacking in the newborn. The ring-shaped bone around the external acoustic meatus faces downward in the infant, but is later rotated during growth into a more vertical position.

At birth, the overall length of the basicranium is approximately 60 to 65 per cent complete, and it increases rapidly. By 5 to 7 years, it reaches about 90 per cent of its full size. Also, about 85 per cent of the adult width of the cranium is attained by the second to third year.

In the newborn, six fontanelles ("soft spots") are present among the bones of the skull roof. They cover over at different times, but all have been reduced to sutures by the eighteenth month. The sutures of the cranial vault are relatively nonjagged in the baby, and the outer surface of the bone is smooth. A much rougher bone texture characterizes the surface of the adult calvaria, and the suture lines become noticeably much more dentate and interlocking (Fig. 2–12). The metopic suture (separating the right and left halves of the frontal bone) usually fuses by the second year and the premaxillary-maxillary suture is mostly fused by the first to second year, with only a trace sometimes remaining. By the third year, the principal cranial and facial suture systems still intact are the coronal, lambdoidal, and circummaxillary. Subsequent closure then begins around the twenty-fifth to thirtieth year, usually in the sequence of sagittal, coronal, and lambdoidal, with those bounding the temporal bone following. The latter can remain partially open even in the aged skull. Traces of the facial sutures can often remain through advanced old age.

In the child, the slender neck below a relatively large cranium gives a characteristic "boyish" appearance to the whole head. This gradually disappears until about puberty, when the expansion of the neck muscles and other soft tissues causes a proportionate decrease in the prominence of the head relative to enlarging neck circumference. This is less noticeable in the female.

The external appearance of the baby's face does not reveal the truly striking enormity of the dental battery developing within it (Fig. 8–14). The teeth are a dominant part of the infant's face as a whole, yet they are not even seen. The parent does not usually realize they are already even there at all, much less suspect the massiveness of their extent. In this illustration, one is almost overwhelmed by the remarkable extent of **teeth** all over the midfacial region. The average person does not appreciate that the mouth of the little child is bounded by a virtual palisade of multitiered primary and permanent teeth in many stages of development. When a crown tip first protrudes through the gingiva as it erupts, the parent naturally believes that the process is just beginning, and that the welcome new tooth is only a tiny but newsworthy addition to the pink mouth. It is not realized that the whole midface is occupied by a vast magazine of unerupted teeth hidden to the eyes. The thin covering and supporting **bone** of the jaws is a much less commanding feature of the young face.

Facial Variations

The spectrum of topographic facial variations is virtually a whole field unto itself and most interesting indeed. As pointed out earlier, relatively small features can have demanding impact on the character of a person's face. A catalog of some of these features commonly encountered is pictured in Figures 8–15 to 8–18. The spread of combinations is endless.

9

The Plan of the
Human Face

The human face is certainly different from that of other mammals. The long, narrow, functional muzzle that slopes gracefully onto the streamlined cranium of a typical mammal is in marked contrast to the muzzleless, broad, vertical, flattened human face, enveloped by an enormous balloon-shaped cranium with a bulbous forehead overhanging tiny, retrusive jaws, a small mouth, a chin, and the curious vestige of a narrow fleshy snout with an owl-eyed and wide face showing changing expressions. Although somehow beautiful to our eyes, this has to be, in the extreme, an "odd" design by ordinary mammalian standards.

Our upright posture involves a great many anatomic and functional adaptations throughout every part of the body, and no one of these would work without all the others. We have "feet," and the human foot stands by itself, as it were, as a unique human anatomic feature. The designs of the toes, foot bones, arch of the foot, ankle, leg bones, pelvis, and vertebral column all interrelate in the anatomic composite that provides upright body stance. The head is in a balanced position on an upright spine. The arms and hands have become freed. The manipulation of food and other objects, defense, offense, and so forth, utilize primarily the hands, rather than the jaws.

The enormous enlargement and the resultant configuration of the brain have caused a "flexure" (bending) of the human basicranium (Fig. 9–1). This relates to two key features. First, the spinal cord is now aligned vertically, a change that permits upright, bipedal body stance allowing free arms and hands. Second, the orbits have undergone a rotation in conjunction with frontal cerebral lobe expansion. This aligns them so that they point in the forward direction of upright (bipedal) body movement. The body has become vertical, but the neutral visual axis is thereby still horizontal, as in other mammals, which is the functional position. (Note: The muzzle of a typical animal points obliquely downward in its "neutral" position, not straight forward. This aligns the orbital axis approximately parallel with the ground and toward the direction of body movement. The cranial base of the typical mammal is flat, in contrast to the flexed human cranium, and the spinal cord passes into a horizontally directed vertebral column.)

Which particular anatomic or functional change "came first" in this evolutionary chain has long been argued. Upright stance? Brachiation? En-

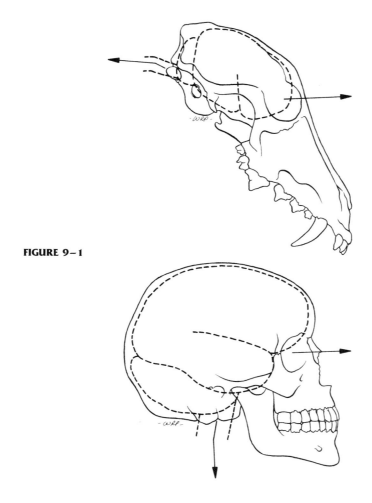

FIGURE 9–1

larged brain? Downward-rotated and decreasingly prognathic dental arches and jaws? Basicranial flexure? Development of hands and binocular vision? An important concept, however, is that the multitude of these changes are all functionally interrelated. They have developed and evolved as a phylogenetic "package," regardless of which one (or combination) actually led off as a primary step in evolution.

Although the human face is topographically "different" from the faces of other mammals, no special violations of the general mammalian plan for facial construction seem to have occurred. The face of man conforms to the same basic morphologic and morphogenetic rules complied with by most mammals in general. Differences have to do mostly with proportionate sizes of component parts and their rotational placements as related to body stance, head posture, and brain size and configuration, but not with any basic departures from the standard morphologic guidelines.

BRAIN ENLARGEMENT, BASICRANIAL FLEXURE, AND FACIAL ROTATIONS

If a short piece of adhesive tape is affixed to a rubber balloon and the balloon then inflated, it will expand in a curved manner (Fig. 9–2). The

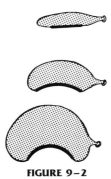

FIGURE 9-2

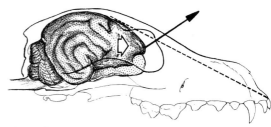

FIGURE 9-3. (From Enlow, D. H., and J. McNamara: The neurocranial basis for facial form and pattern. Angle Orthod., 43:256, 1973, with permission.)

balloon bends because it enlarges around the nonexpanding basal segment. The enormous human cerebrum similarly expands around a much smaller and lesser-enlarging midventral segment (the medulla, pons, hypothalamus, diencephalon, optic chiasma). This causes a bending of the whole underside of the brain. The **flexure** of the basicranium results. The foramen magnum in the typical mammalian skull is located at the posterior aspect of the cranium (Fig. 9-3). In man, it is in the midventral part of the expanded cranial floor at an approximate mechanical balance point for upright head support on a vertical spine (Fig. 9-4).

The expansion of the frontal cerebral lobes displaces the frontal bone upward and outward (Figs. 9-3 and 9-4). This results in the distinctive, bulbous, upright "forehead" of the human face, although it is really part of the neurocranium and not the face (viscero—or sphlanchno—cranium) proper. The frontal lobes also relate to a developmental rotation of the human orbits into new positions. As the forehead becomes developmentally rotated into a vertical plane by the enlarging brain behind it, the superior orbital rims are carried with it. The eyes now point at a right angle to the spinal cord. The spine is vertical, but the human orbital axis is still thus horizontal. Vision is directed toward forward body movement.*

The expansion of the frontal and, particularly, the temporal lobes of the cerebrum also, importantly, underlies a rotation of the orbits toward the midline (Figs. 9-5, 9-6, and 9-7). The eyes are moved closer together. **Two** separate axes of orbital rotation are thus associated with the massive expansion of the cerebrum. One displaces the orbits vertically, and the other carries them horizontally in medial directions into a full binocular position. Different extents of these two separate rotational movements are seen among different primate species. In the monkey, for example, the extent of upright orbital alignment and frontal bossing is much less than in man, as determined by the relative sizes of their frontal lobes. The simian orbits are quite close-set, however, and this relates to the proportionate sizes of the temporal lobes.

The binocular arrangement of the orbits is a feature complementing finger-controlled manipulation of food, tools, weapons, and so forth. The absence of a long, protrusive muzzle does not block the close-up vision of hand-held objects. The human **mind** directs the **free hands** that can work with **three-dimensional** perspective in an **upright** stance on feet. The enormous size of the human brain and the human basicranial flexure are key factors, but **all** these changes are required for full human expression,

---

*In some anthropoids, such as the gorilla, the massive supraorbital ridges may also rotate vertically independent of the frontal lobe. In the human face, however, the orbits **must** rotate into a vertical alignment because of the expanded size of the frontal lobes.

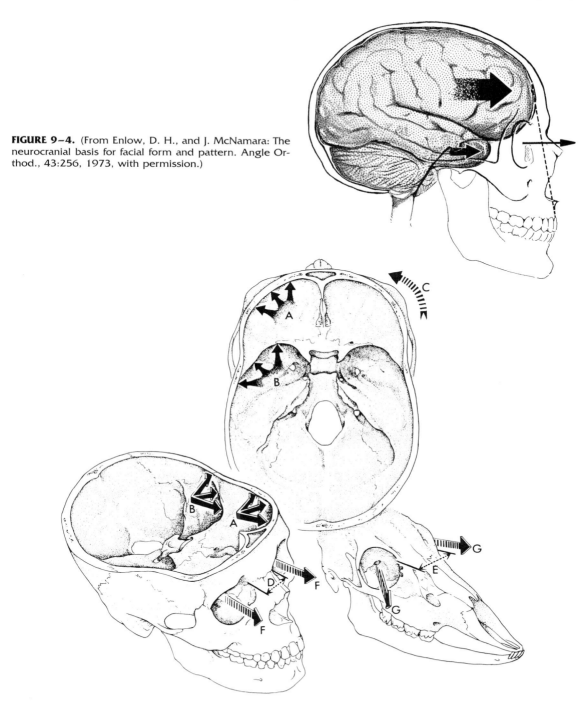

FIGURE 9–4. (From Enlow, D. H., and J. McNamara: The neurocranial basis for facial form and pattern. Angle Orthod., 43:256, 1973, with permission.)

FIGURE 9–5. Facial features related to enlarged human brain and bipedal posture compared to a smaller-brained mammal. The enlarged frontal lobes and anterior endocranial fossae (*A*), together with the large temporal lobes and middle cranial fossae (*B*), produce a wide, flat face with squared cheekbones (*C*), orbital rotation toward the midline, a reduced proportionate transverse size of the airway and nasal base (*D*), forward-pointing orbits (*F*), and a rotational placement of the facial composite beneath the cranial floor. In a typical mammal (deer), note the divergent orbital axes (*G*), the proportionately larger interorbital and nasal space (*E*), the more narrow and angular face, and the more protrusive snout and muzzle projecting forward rather than beneath the anterior cranial floor. (From Enlow, D. H.: *The Human Face*. New York, Harper & Row, 1968, p. 190, with permission.)

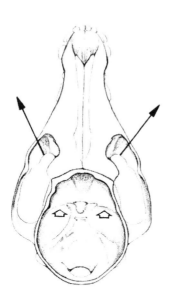

FIGURE 9–6. (From Enlow, D. H., and J. McNamara: The neurocranial basis for facial form and pattern. Angle Orthod., 43:256, 1973, with permission.)

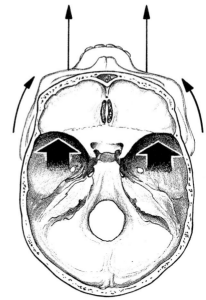

FIGURE 9–7. (From Enlow, D. H., and J. McNamara: The neurocranial basis for facial form and pattern. Angle Orthod., 43:256, 1973, with permission.)

and they are all mutually interdependent developmentally as well as functionally.

Orbital rotation toward the midline, importantly, significantly reduces the dimension of the interorbital space (Figs. 9–7 and 9–8). This is one of two basic factors that underlie reduction in the extent of snout protrusion in man and some other (but not all) primates. Because the interorbital segment is the root of the nasal region, a decrease in this dimension reduces the structural (and also the physiologic) base of the bony nose. A

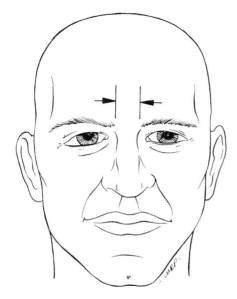

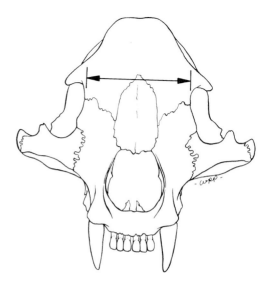

FIGURE 9–8

wide nasal base can support a proportionately longer snout. A narrow nasal base, however, reduces the architectural limit to which the bony part of the nose can protrude, and the snout is thereby shorter. The second basic factor involved in the extent of reduction of nasal protrusion deals with the rotation of the olfactory bulbs (see below).

The olfactory sense in *Homo* has become a much less dominant factor in environmental awareness and is far exceeded by many other mammalian groups. In addition to proportionate downsizing of the human nasal and olfactory mucosae, olfactory receptors in the frontal sinuses are also lacking, which is in contrast to other forms more dependent on aromatic sensations for food-getting or protection.

The nasal region above and the oral region below are two sides of the same coin, that is, the palate (Fig. 9–9). Reduction in nasal protrusion is accompanied by a more or less equivalent reduction of the upper jaw. The whole face in any mammal necessarily becomes reduced in length as a result. However, the human face has also been **rotated** into a nearly **vertical** alignment related to the massive enlargement of the brain and flexure of the basicranium. The downward rotation of the **olfactory bulbs** and the whole **anterior cranial floor** by the enlarged frontal lobes of the cerebrum has caused a corresponding downward rotation of the nasomaxillary complex (Fig. 9–10).

The nasal mucosa is ordinarily an active tissue involved in temperature regulation in most mammals. Vasoconstriction and vasodilation of the vessels in the massive mucosal spread covering the turbinates control the

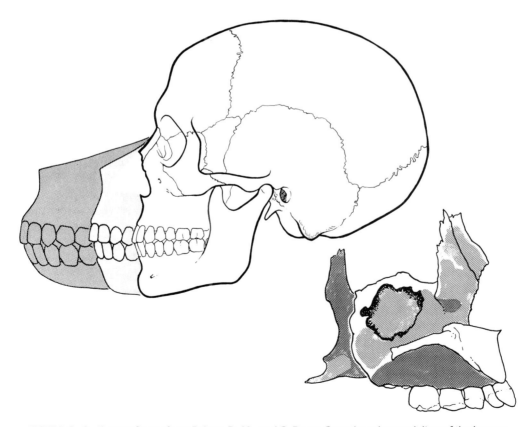

FIGURE 9–9. (Lower figure from Enlow, D. H., and S. Bang: Growth and remodeling of the human maxilla. Am. J. Orthod. 51:446, 1965, with permission.)

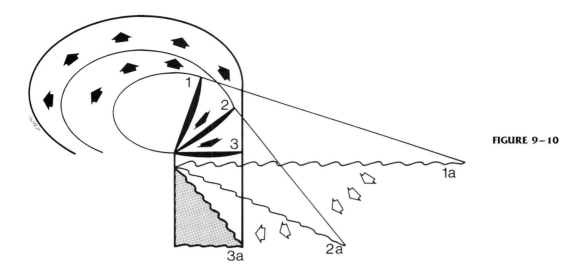

FIGURE 9-10

amount of heat retention or loss. Because of marked nasal reduction in man, however, this important function has been largely taken over by the relatively hairless and sweat gland-loaded human integument. Control of blood flow in the dermis, combined with sweat gland activity, provides the equivalent for nasal thermoregulation. This is possible in man (and in a very few other species, such as the pig) because of a near-naked skin. In thick-furred animals, thermoregulation is carried out by regulating heat transfers in the nasal mucosa, panting control to release or conserve body heat, limited perspiration in hairless areas (such as pads of the paws), and a fluffing of the fur to increase dead air insulation. The latter also makes the animal look menacingly larger to prospective enemies, and it increases the nonvital part of his anatomy for them to bite. We have only the atavistic holdover: goose bumps.

All mammalian forms have bony reinforcement "pillars" built into the architectonic design of the craniofacial complex. These pillars are parts of bones that provide a buttress for structural support and biomechanical stress resistance that balances the physical properties of the skull against the composite of forces acting within it. This includes the forces of growth itself. Although customarily described with reference to tooth positions, the nature of support goes well beyond just accommodation to masticatory forces. In the human face, one of these pillars is the "key ridge," which is a vertical column of thickened maxillary bone approximately centered above the functionally important area around the upper first molar. The mechanical support column then continues upward from this ridge into and through the lateral orbital rim and on to the supraorbital-reinforced frontal bone. The second maxillary molar is reinforced by a vertical sheet of bone, the posterolateral orbital wall, which extends directly above this tooth. Except for the very thin bone enclosing the posterior part of the large maxillary sinus, the third molar is situated behind the orbit, and it has no further bony support above this. It has thus become effectively disfranchised mechanically and phylogenetically. The incisors are supported by an arch, the bony rim of the overlying nasal opening, with which it shares a common embryonic development, and also by the vertical nasal septum. Each canine tooth is reinforced by a marked thickening of the lateral nasal wall, toward which the cuspid root points, and thence on to and through the thickened frontal process of the maxilla into the glabellar thickening of the forehead.

The human face is exceptionally wide because the brain and cranial floor are wide. However, the face has been almost engulfed by the massive brain behind and above it (Fig. 9–11). Note the wondrously, incredibly colossal size of the human cranium, in comparison with that of the typical mammal. The expanded frontal lobes of the human brain have come to lie **above** the eyes and almost the whole remainder of the face, rather than behind, and a big forehead has thus been added. This also underlies rotation of the orbits into vertical, forward-facing positions as well as to the rotation of the face as a whole into a unique downward-backward position.

Herbivores have orbits widely set to each facial side, thus providing a much greater peripheral range of vision to detect some approaching carnivore. The carnivore, on the other hand, can rotate its eyeballs into more forward-looking positions, even though the orbits are aligned obliquely laterally, thus favoring a stereoscopic chase. Carnivores generally tend to have a much shorter muzzle and snout because of the greater degree of medial rotation of the orbits, producing a more narrow interorbital nasal base. Herbivores generally tend to have greater snout and muzzle protrusion, because their orbits are much more wide-set, with a broader interorbital nasal root.

Note that the enlarged human cerebrum has caused a downward rotational displacement of the olfactory bulbs (Fig. 9–12). In all other mammals, the bulbs and cribriform plates are nearly upright or obliquely aligned, depending on the size and configuration of the frontal lobes. In man, the bulbs have been rotated into **horizontal** positions by the cerebrum. This is a significant factor in the basic design of the human face.

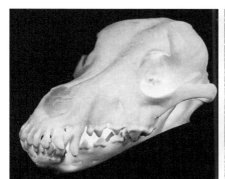 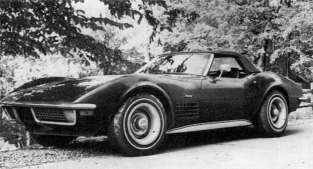

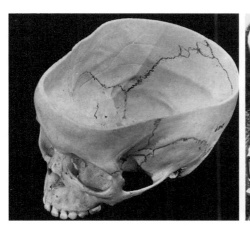 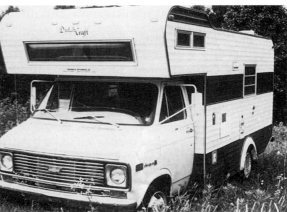

FIGURE 9–11

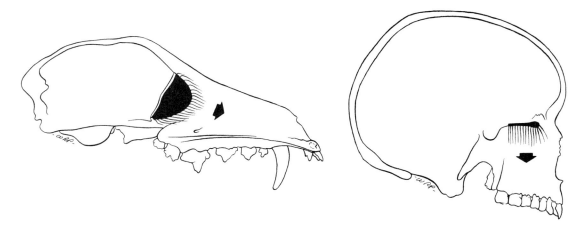

FIGURE 9-12

The olfactory bulbs relate directly to the alignment and the direction of growth of the adjacent nasal region (Fig. 9–12). The long axis of the snout in most mammals is constructed so that it necessarily points in the general direction of the sensory olfactory nerves within it. The plane of the nasomaxillary region is thereby approximately **perpendicular to the plane of the olfactory bulbs.** This is a major anatomic and functional relationship that underlies the direction of nasomaxillary development in the face of virtually any mammal. As the bulbs in the human brain became rotated progressively from a vertical position to horizontal because of increases in brain size or because of its shape (*1, 2,* and *3* in Fig. 9–10), the whole face has been similarly rotated from a horizontal to a vertically downward plane (*1a, 2a,* and *3a*). Or, stated another way, the face has become rotated down by the expanded anterior cranial floor as the floor rotates downward as a result of the enlargement of the frontal lobes.

Nasomaxillary Configuration

The maxilla of most mammals has a triangular configuration. In man, it is uniquely rectangular (Fig. 9–10). This was caused by a rotation of the occlusion into a horizontal plane adapting to the vertical rotation of the whole midface. The occlusal plane in most mammals, including man, is approximately parallel to the Frankfort plane (a plane from the top of the auditory meatus to the inferior rim of the orbit). This aligns the jaws in a functional position relative to the visual, olfactory, and hearing senses. In the human maxilla, the design change that allowed for this resulted in the creation of a new arch-positioning facial region, the unique **suborbital** compartment. Most of this phylogenetically expanded area is occupied by the otherwise nonfunctional maxillary sinus (uses such as air warming, nasal drip, and voice resonance are secondary). No prior genetic or epigenetic program for this unprecedented new area existed, no new real function caused a new tissue or organ invention, and the result, therefore, is nothing—a space. An **orbital floor** developed in conjunction with this added facial region to provide for orbital soft tissue support. This is a special feature relating to the new maxillary configuration. The middle and lower parts of the face now lie **beneath the eyes** rather than in front of them. Compare also with Figure 9–5.

The nasal region is thus **vertically** disposed in the human face (Fig. 9–12). The neutral axis of the spread of the sensory olfactory nerves is vertical, and the resultant vertical vector of nasomaxillary growth has become a major feature of human facial development. The characteristic vertical human facial profile is a composite result of (1) a bulbous forehead, (2) rotation of the whole nasal region into essentially a vertical plane, (3) reduction of snout protrusion in conjunction with medial orbital convergence, (4) rotation of the orbits into upright positions, (5) rotation of the maxillary arch downward and backward, and squaring of the nasomaxillary complex, (7) leveling of the horizontal palate and maxillary arch, (8) creation of the maxillary sinuses, (9) addition of an orbital floor and lateral orbital wall, and (10) bimaxillary reduction in the extent of prognathism matching nasal reduction. The face also became markedly widened because of the increased breadth of the brain and cranial floor and because the orbits and cheekbones are rotated into forward-facing positions. The face of man now lies **beneath** the frontal lobes of the brain; in other mammals the face is largely in front of the cerebrum. The nasal chambers are housed largely **within** the face, between and below the orbits, rather than projecting forward within a protrusive muzzle. The projecting human snout itself houses very little of the mucosal part of the nasal chambers back within the face. The whole face has been "reduced" to a quite flat topographic configuration as a combined result of these multiple alterations.

Reduction of the nasal region associated with orbital convergence and olfactory and anterior cranial fossa rotation must necessarily also be accompanied by a more or less equal reduction in maxillary arch length, as pointed out above. Only a relatively slight degree of horizontal divergence between the two can exist. If either one becomes reduced in length, so must the other. This refers only to the bony part of the nasal region; some species have a fleshy proboscis protruding beyond the jaws and palate (such as man and the elephant).

Why does the human face have an overhanging, fleshy "nose"? The protrusion of the cartilaginous and soft tissue portion of the nasal complex has a design alignment that provides for **downward**-directed external nares (Fig. 9–13). It serves to aim the inflow of air obliquely upward toward sensory nerve endings into the olfactory bulbs located in the **ceiling** of the nasal chambers. This is in contrast to the external nasal apertures of other mammals taking air into more horizontal nasal chambers having the cribriform plates and nerve endings located within the posterior wall.

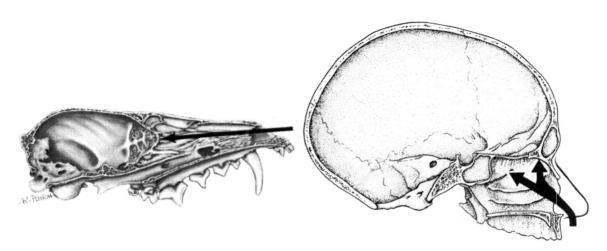

FIGURE 9–13. (Figure at right from Enlow, D. H.: *The Human Face.* New York, Harper & Row, 1968, p. 188, with permission.)

Thus, the human face has a fleshy, protuberant "nose" as a functional adaptation to the unique vertical disposition of its nasomaxillary complex.

The rotation of the whole face downward and **backward** has resulted in a facial placement within the recess (the "facial pocket") created by the basicranial flexure. What will happen if the brain **continues** to enlarge phylogenetically and thereby produce an even further extent of backward rotation? There is virtually no more room remaining to "rotate into," at least given the present design and arrangement of all the various soft tissue and skeletal parts involved. Already the face has almost reached the airway because of rotation. The posterior cranial floor, the vertebral column, and the face, as in a closing vise, are all coming together; there are important parts in between. What phylogenetic facial adjustments have occurred? See page 76 for an evaluation. (The porpoise skull shows how evolutionary craniofacial adaptations also involving an enlarged brain have taken place in yet another way that is unconventional among mammals.)

Growth Field Boundaries

The development of each part of the face involves two basic considerations. The first is the **amount** of growth, and the second is the **direction** of growth. These two factors constitute the growth "vector."

Growth proceeds according to a mosaic of regional developmental "fields." Each field as well as groups of fields have prescribed boundaries. These boundaries establish regional growth perimeters, and there is a maximum and minimum growth capacity within each. Growth does not ordinarily exceed each perimeter if a developmental equilibrium is to be sustained. However, clinical manipulation of the growing face can result in violation of these maximum and minimum boundaries. The consequences of such violations are either physiologic rebound or pathologic degeneration. Physiologic rebound occurs when the natural forces of the boundary reclaim their territory. An example of this type of rebound is the lingual collapse of lower incisors that have been pushed labially, past the equilibrium boundary of the orbicularis oris musculature. An example of pathologic degeneration is encountered when a fixed retainer is used to hold lower incisors outside the physiologic boundary. Instead of lingual collapse, fenestration of the root surface and breakdown of periodontal supporting structures occur. Since neither physiologic rebound nor pathologic degeneration is a desirable outcome, the goal of dentofacial therapeutic procedures must be to improve esthetics and function of the face in harmony with the growth boundaries of the region. Significantly, there are forward, downward, backward, and lateral growth boundaries that exist for the major parts of the face, and they are **shared** by the brain and basicranium. The regional perimeters for the fields of the brain growth and the perimeters for the major facial fields have become established in common.

The reason for this basicranial and facial relationship is that the brain has evolved in conjunction with the cranial floor. The form, size, endocranial topographic features, and angular characteristics of one conform to the other. The floor of the cranium, in turn, is the **template** upon which the face is built. The junctional part of the face cannot be significantly **wider**, for example, than the maximal width of the cranium. There would be nothing to which it could be attached.[†] Similarly, the **length** and

---

[†]Hence, there is a physiologic limit to midfacial expansion. The theoretic lateral maximum lies within the width of the basicranium, or between pace-setting cranial nerves placed by it, from which the midfacial complex is suspended. Clinically, it should be expanded past the boundary and then allowed to rebound ("develop") to the practical if not theoretical limit for jaw width.

height of specific parts of the cranial floor are projected as equivalent dimensions for the face, as described later.

The face is **not** independent of the basicranium structurally or developmentally. The whole face has often been described, in years past, as a genetically and developmentally separate region, the only tie between them being that they happen to be placed in juxtaposition, as a picture hangs on a wall. No cause-and-effect relationships were believed by some earlier workers to exist between the neurocranium and the size or shape of the face. This is certainly not the case. **Many** structural features and dimensions of the face are based on brain-cranial base-facial relationships, as will be seen. This is an important concept, because a number of normal and abnormal variations in facial form relate, at least in part, to underlying circumstances present in the cranial floor (see Chapter 10).

The floor of the cranium has developed in **phylogenetic** association with the brain. Whatever "independent" genetic control actually exists in the basicranium itself (this is historically controversial), the shape and size of the floor of the cranium have become established because its genes were especially adopted by the natural selection process to accommodate an **interdependent** association with the developing brain. Thus established, the basicranium presumably has a measure of genetic independence, since it can continue to partially develop even though the overlying brain atrophies or is removed. The face similarly develops **in conjunction with** the cranial floor (and the brain), and the control of facial development has become established in a way that accommodates its functional association with the neurocranium. In all areas, however, a developmental **latitude** exists that provides potential for **adjustments** during growth to accommodate developmental variations in one part or another. This is involved in the operation of the "functional matrix," and it is the factor that allows for a unified coexistence of the many separate, developing parts all growing and functioning in relation to one another. There are regional differences, however, in the **capacity** for such developmental adjustment. Some areas, such as the bony alveolar sockets, are extremely labile and responsive to variable and changing circumstances. Other areas, such as the basicranium, are much less sensitive and adaptable. The "intrinsic programming" for the latter is presumed to be greater than for the former because of their different levels of developmental independence and whatever the different factors are that determine and control them. The basicranium is, nonetheless, developmentally responsive and adjustive to extrinsic factors. Head position related to sleeping habits, for example, can have a marked effect on basicranial configuration which, in turn, impacts directly on facial form and pattern. (See Chapter 8.)

While the endocranial side of the cranial floor is adapted to the configuration and topographic contours of the ventral surface of the brain, the topography of the ectocranial side of the basicranium is structurally adapted to the composite of the facial, pharyngeal, and cervical components. A measure of morphogenic divergence thus occurs between these contralateral sides of the cranial floor.

The forward **boundary** of the brain is shared by the forward border of the nasomaxillary complex. The **course** of growth by the nasal part of the face relates, appropriately, to the olfactory bulbs and the sensory olfactory nerves. These two factors underlie the "vector" of midfacial growth, that is, the amount and the direction. To show this, a line is drawn from the forward edge of the brain down to the anterior-most, inferior-most point of the nasomaxillary complex (superior prosthion; Figs. 9–14 and 9–15).

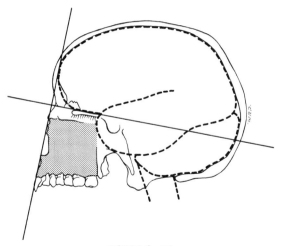

FIGURE 9–14

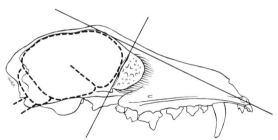

FIGURE 9–15. (From Enlow, D. H., and M. Azuma: Functional growth boundaries in the human and mammalian face. In: *Morphogenesis and Malformations of the Face and Brain.* Ed. by D. Bergsma. Birth Defects Orig. Art. Ser., Vol. XI; No. 7. New York, Alan R. Liss, Inc. for The National Foundation—March of Dimes, White Plains, New York, with permission.)

This represents the **midfacial** plane.[‡] Note that the midfacial plane is perpendicular to the **olfactory bulb** (or the cribriform plate, as seen in lateral headfilms). In the human face, this plane also frequently touches the anterior nasal spine. The development of the long axis of the nasal region thus proceeds in the same general direction as the neutral axis of its sensory nerve spread. The amount of growth is established by the prescribed perimeter of its growth field. **The nasomaxillary complex develops within a growth field out to the edge of the brain and its basicranium in a direction perpendicular to the olfactory bulbs.**

The olfactory bulb and nasomaxillary alignment relationship exists among mammals in general. In species or groups having a smaller brain and, as a result, a more upright olfactory bulb, the snout and muzzle tend to be correspondingly more horizontal and much more protrusive (Fig. 9–15). As the olfactory bulbs become rotated downward in different mammalian groups because of increasing brain size (or shape, as in more round-headed species such as the bulldog), the muzzle correspondingly rotates down with them and becomes less protrusive. In the human situation, the olfactory bulbs have become virtually horizontal because of the massive growth of the frontal lobes. The nasal part of the human face thus becomes **vertically** aligned during development in conjunction with the neutral vertical axis of olfactory nerve distribution. (Figs. 9–12 and 9–14). This is a distinctive developmental and anatomic feature. In other mammals, development of the facial airway and olfactory nerve alignment is much more horizontally or obliquely disposed.

The nasomaxillary complex, as mentioned earlier, is specifically associated with the anterior cranial fossae. The posterior boundary of these paired fossae establishes the corresponding posterior boundary for the

---

[‡]"Nasion" is often used in cephalometric studies as a point for drawing the facial plane, but this can give misleading results because nasion is so variable in relation to distinct male/female and headform differences, which are seldom taken into account. Moreover, the purpose of the **midfacial** plane described above is to show the relationship between the **brain** and the **nasomaxillary complex**. Thus, the edge of the brain is used, rather than nasion. Also, the above descriptions presume that the alignment of the nerves is the lead factor that determines the direction of midfacial growth. Of course, it may be the converse. Whichever, the important point is that they are established **together** in a constant relationship to the olfactory bulbs, which, in turn, are placed according to the size and shape of the brain.

midface. This is essentially a nonvariable anatomic relationship. The **direction** of growth in this region is established by the particular special sense located in this part of the face, which is the visual sense. The posterior maxillary tuberosity is located just beneath the floor of the orbit, and the orbital floor is the roof of the maxillary tuberosity and the sinus within it. The tuberosity is aligned approximately perpendicular to the neutral geometric axis of the orbit (Fig. 9–16). **The posterior plane of the midface extends from the junction between the anterior and middle cranial fossae (e.g., the inferior junction between the frontal and temporal lobes and the anterior-most edge of the great wings of the sphenoid), downward in a direction perpendicular to the neutral axis of the orbit.** This verticle plane passes along the posterior surface of the maxillary tuberosity.

The boundary just described represents one of the key anatomic planes in the face. This is the posterior maxillary (PM) plane (Fig. 9–17). There are many "cephalometric planes" in the face and cranium. Most of these, however, do not represent (and are not so intended) (1) key sites of growth and remodeling or (2) functional relationships among the various parts of the skull, including soft tissue associations. Most conventional cephalometric planes, such as sella-nasion, unfortunately, bypass the really important key sites of development without recognizing them. Sella itself, for example, is a "landmark of convenience" because it can be readily and reliably located. But trying to use it to determine real morphogenetic relationships would be like looking for lost keys under a lamp post because that's where the light is. The vertical PM boundary, in contrast, is a **natural anatomic and morphogenic** plane that relates directly to the factors that establish the basic design of the face. It is one of the most important developmental and structural planes in the face and cranium.

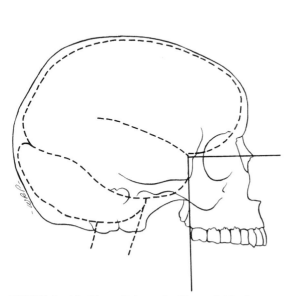

FIGURE 9–16. (From Enlow, D. H., and M. Azuma: Functional growth boundaries in the human and mammalian face. In: *Morphogenesis and Malformations of the Face and Brain.* Ed. by D. Bergsma. Birth Defects Orig. Art. Ser., Vol. XI, No. 7. New York, Alan R. Liss, Inc. for the National Foundation—March of Dimes, White Plains, New York, with permission.)

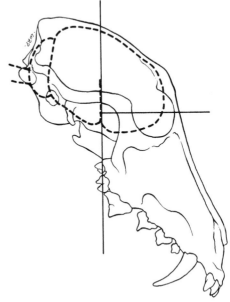

FIGURE 9–17. (From Enlow, D. H., and M. Azuma: Functional growth boundaries in the human and mammalian face. In: *Morphogenesis and Malformations of the Face and Brain.* Ed. by D. Bergsma. Birth Defects Orig. Art. Ser., Vol. XI, No. 7. New York, Alan R. Liss, Inc., for The National Foundation—March of Dimes, White Plains, New York, with permission.)

The **PM** plane delineates naturally the various anatomic **counterparts** of the craniofacial complex. The frontal lobe, the anterior cranial fossa, the upper part of the ethmomaxillary complex, the palate, and the maxillary arch are all mutual counterparts lying anterior to the PM line (Fig. 9–18, *a*, *b*, and *c*). All these parts have posterior boundaries that are placed along this vertical plane. Similarly, the temporal lobe, the middle cranial fossa, and the posterior oropharyngeal space with the bridging ramus are mutual counterparts located behind the PM plane (*d*, *e*, and *f*). The anterior boundaries of these parts are precisely positioned along this vertical line. The PM plane is a **developmental interface** between the vertical series of counterparts in front of and behind it. This key plane retains these basic relationships throughout the growth process.

The positional relationships between the frontal lobes of the cerebrum (anterior cranial fossae) and facial components, and also between part of the middle cranial fossae and the pharynx, are established early in embryonic development. In Figure 13–3, note that the cephalic flexure places the maxillary and mandibular arches in direct juxtaposition with what will become the frontal lobes and the anterior cranial fossae.

The **corpus** of the mandible is a counterpart to those parts lying in front of the PM plane. The **ramus** is a counterpart of the parts behind the PM plane. The placement of the mandible and the size of its parts, however, are more independently variable than those of the ethmomaxillary complex. The posterior boundary of the corpus **should** lie on the PM line. This is the "lingual tuberosity," which is the direct mandibular equivalent of the maxillary tuberosity. The forward boundary of the ramus, where it joins the lingual tuberosity, should also lie on the PM line. (Note: The anterior edge of the obliquely aligned ramus overlaps the lingual tuberosity, but this edge does not represent the actual forward point of the **effective** ramus dimension; the lingual tuberosity itself is the functional junction between the corpus and the ramus.) Because the mandible is a

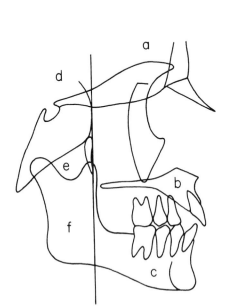

FIGURE 9–18. (From Enlow, D. H.: Postnatal growth and development of the face and cranium. In: *Scientific Foundations of Dentistry*. Ed. by B. Cohen and I. R. H. Kramer. London, Heinemann, 1975, with permission.)

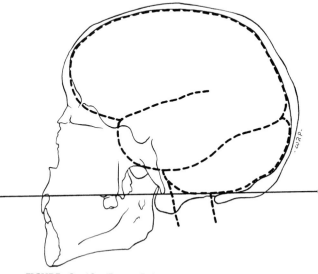

FIGURE 9–19. (From Enlow, D.H., and M. Azuma: Functional growth boundaries in the human and mammalian face. In: *Morphogenesis and Malformations of the Face and Brain*. Ed. by D. Bergsma. Birth Defects Orig. Art. Ser., Vol. XI, No. 7. New York, Alan R. Liss, Inc., for The National Foundation—March of Dimes, White Plains, New York, with permission.)

FIGURE 9–20. (From Enlow, D. H., and M. Azuma: Functional growth boundaries in the human and mammalian face. In: *Morphogenesis and Malformations of the Face and Brain.* Ed. by D. Bergsma. Birth Defects Orig. Art. Ser., Vol. XI, No. 7. New York, Alan R. Liss, Inc., for The National Foundation—March of Dimes, White Plains, New York, with permission.)

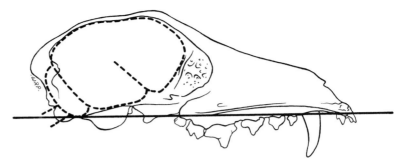

separate bone not attached directly to the cranium by sutures, its latitude for structural variation is not subject to the same degree of developmental and structural communality that occurs between the growth fields shared by the cranial floor and the maxilla. Also, ramus development relates directly to the muscles of mastication, and this requires interplay adjustments. Independent variations can thus exist in the dimensions and the placement of both the ramus and the corpus. The ramus, for example, may fall short of the PM plane, or it may protrude well forward of it. This variability in features is often **compensatory,** as described in Chapter 10. Furthermore, whole-mandible rotations are common, and these developmental "displacement" movements shift the mandible into many variable positions.

Passing from the basicranium, the maxillary nerve crosses the pterygopalatine fossa and then into the inferior orbital fissure. This segment of the nerve, prior to its downward turn through the infraorbital canal and out through the suborbital foramen, closely parallels the plane of the palate. An embryonic relationship exists, and the alignment of the nerve is usually accompanied by a corresponding upward or downward rotational alignment of the palate.

Just as other facial boundaries coincide with basicranial boundaries, the inferior nasomaxillary boundary is established, when growth is complete, by the inferior surface of the brain and basicranium (Figs. 9–19 and 9–20).[§]

If Class II and Class III headfilm tracings are superimposed on the cribriform plates (representing the olfactory bulbs), it is apparent that the anterior plane of the nasomaxillary region in both malocclusion categories conforms closely to the normal, perpendicular olfactory relationship. Note the similarity of the midfacial plane alignments (Fig. 9–21). In this particular Class II individual (and most others as well), it is not the basal bone of the maxilla itself that "protrudes" (relative to the basicranium); rather, it is the **mandible** that is actually **retrusive.** In the Class III individual, it is not always the maxilla that is retrusive; the **mandible** is **protrusive.** In both individuals, the nasomaxillary complex is located

---

[§]Some simians and anthropoids have an **established vertical hypoplasia** in the anterior part of the maxillary arch. In the rhesus monkey, for example, the premaxillary region is "high," or, at least, the posterior part of the nasomaxillary complex is vertically "long." A differentially greater extent of downward displacement takes place in the posterior part of the arch as compared with the anterior part. This in effect causes an "upward" rotation of the anterior region, and direct downward bone growth by this area does not move it fully to the inferior level attained by the posterior part of the arch. Resultant anterior open bites are quite frequent, much more so than in the human face. A similar arch rotation can, in fact, occur in the human maxilla, but the anterior part of the arch develops inferiorly to an extent that fully offsets it. (See also Chapter 10.)

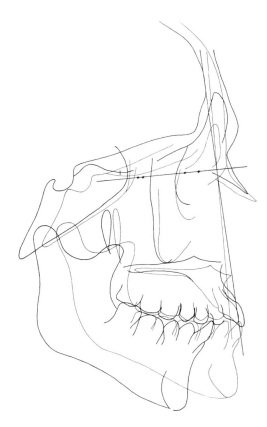

FIGURE 9-21. (From Enlow, D. H., and J. McNamara: The neurocranial basis for facial form and pattern. Angle Orthod., 43: 256, 1973, with permission.)

FIGURE 9-22. (From Enlow, D. H., and M. Azuma: Functional growth boundaries in the human and mammalian face. In: *Morphogenesis and Malformations of the Face and Brain.* Ed. by D. Bergsma. Birth Defects Orig. Art. Ser., Vol. XI, No. 7. New York, Alan R. Liss, Inc., for The National Foundation—March of Dimes, White Plains, New York, with permission.)

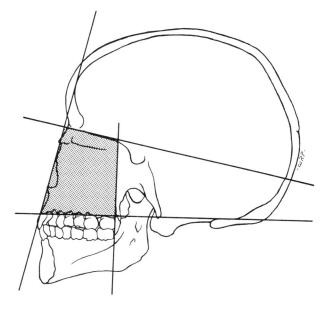

where it is supposed to be, and its horizontal dimensions are not out of line as they relate to the brain and anterior cranial fossae.

In summary, development in each region of the face involves two basic factors: (1) the amount of growth by any given part and (2) the direction of growth by that part. The brain establishes (or at least shares) the various **boundaries** that determine the **amount of facial growth**. This is because the floor of the cranium is the template upon which the face is constructed. The **directions** of regional remodeling among the different parts of the face are inseparably associated with the special sense organs housed within the face. These two factors establish a prescribed growth perimeter that defines the borders of the growth compartment occupied by the nasomaxillary complex (Figs. 9–22 and 9–23). All the many components that constitute the midface, including the bones, muscles, mucosae, connective tissues, cartilage, nerves, vessels, tongue, teeth, and so on, participate and actively interrelate in the composite expression of growth, the sum of which can produce enlargement up to a given individual's maximum, as determined by the midfacial growth boundaries. The growth of the **midface** is not limitless, and it is not independently and randomly determined entirely within itself.

Superior prosthion thus comes to lie in a predetermined position that has been programmed by the brain-cranial base-sense organ-soft tissue composite of developmental factors. Superior prosthion is composed of alveolar bone, which is a highly labile and responsive type of bone tissue. Traditionally, this area of bone is regarded as quite unstable and subject to a wide range of variations according to the many forces that act on it. This is quite true, as will be seen below. However, prosthion has a specific target location that it will occupy if the growth process is not disturbed by intrinsic or extrinsic imbalances (e.g., thumb sucking). The target point is not programmed within prosthion itself, or even just within the maxilla. It is determined, rather, by the composite of all the growth-establishing factors mentioned above. In most cases, prosthion has settled in, when growth is complete, right on or very close to its target point.

In the headfilm tracing shown in Figure 9–24, it is seen that prosthion falls short of the predetermined midfacial plane; growth is incomplete, however. In the same individual, when facial development has become largely completed, prosthion will have arrived at its place on the perpendicular adult (dashed) midfacial line. In Figure 9–25, the two headfilms are superimposed on the cribriform plane to show the "before" and "after" growth stages.

Can the brain-sense organ relationship within the face be violated? Of course; it frequently happens. For example, thumb sucking (mentioned

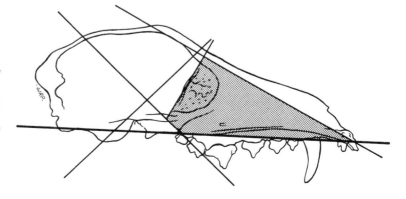

FIGURE 9–23. (From Enlow, D. H., and M. Azuma: Functional growth boundaries in the human and mammalian face. In: *Morphogenesis and Malformations of the Face and Brain.* Ed. by D. Bergsma. Birth Defects Orig. Art. Ser., Vol. XI, No. 7. New York, Alan R. Liss, Inc., for The National Foundation—March of Dimes, White Plains, New York, with permission.)

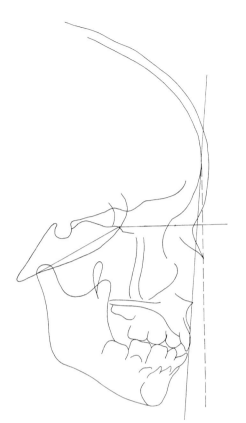

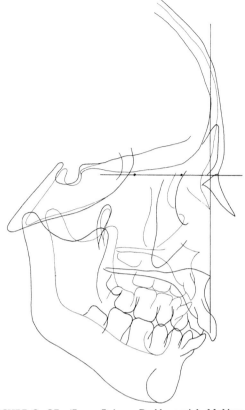

FIGURE 9–24. (From Enlow, D. H., and J. McNamara: The neurocranial basis for facial form and pattern. Angle Orthod., 43:256, 1973, with permission.)

FIGURE 9–25. (From Enlow, D. H., and J. McNamara: The neurocranial basis for facial form and pattern. Angle Orthod., 43:256, 1973, with permission.)

above), tongue thrust, and various developmental defects can move the teeth and alveolar bone to places that are out of bounds with respect to the normal growth process (Fig. 9–26). The forces and factors of ordinary growth become overridden by extrinsic forces, and the prescribed boundary and the usual limit of growth are thereby overrun. However, this produces a structural and functional imbalance. If the overriding ectopic factors are removed, the normal balance of functional intrinsic relationships work toward a greater or lesser return to the normal position, conforming with the natural anatomic boundary of the growth field. This is the reason most children who suck their thumb during early childhood, but later stop the habit, do not have the typical "thumb sucker's" malocclusion. Once the abnormal force has been removed, physiologic rebound seeks equilibrium (Chapter 1), and subsequent development returns the component parts to a balanced relationship.

Because many anatomic boundaries, large and small, exist throughout the face and cranium, the factor of boundary "security" is a major and important consideration to the clinician. If one given facial growth field is made to overrun the boundary of another field, either by clinical intervention or because of a developmental abnormality, one or the other will necessarily become compromised. A competition for the same space by the two overlapping growth fields occurs, and one field will necessarily become subordinate. This has great meaning with regard to the **stability** of a region and the functional "equilibrium" among different structural parts.

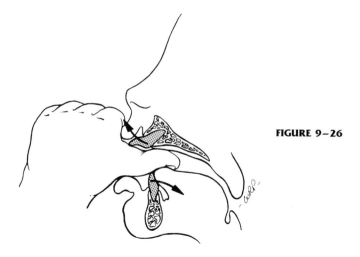

FIGURE 9–26

If, for example, a given treatment procedure causes a violation of some growth boundary, will hard-earned treatment results subsequently be lost because functional stability and balance have been disturbed? Or, perhaps, will results be lost because the activity of a growth field that has been imposed upon subsequently causes a return ("rebound") toward the original structural pattern when treatment is stopped? Another similar question is whether a treatment procedure can actually **change** the long-term growth program. If it does not, subsequent growth, after treatment is ceased, can erase the treatment results, because growth then proceeds along its original unaffected course. This may be one of the reasons for "relapse" of early treatment of malocclusion during periods of rapid growth. Periods of rapid change are more easily harnessed by the clinician "working with growth." However, physiologic factors involved in rebound must also be biologically active at this time. Therefore, the clinician contemplating early treatment must be aware that interventions that address "cause" will be more effective during periods of rapid growth, and interventions that address "effect" will be more successful during periods of slower growth and adaptation. This factor is often overlooked when comparing the stability of surgical manipulations of facial bones in the adult with orthopedic modification of facial bones in the young child. These are fundamental clinical questions, and they have to do with priorities of growth control among the many fields of growth and the natural integrity of their regional boundaries.

There are many theoretically possible alternatives with regard to stability versus rebound/relapse as summarized in Figure 1–1. Some alternatives seem more feasible than others, and still more possibilities probably exist that are not included. Some may hold true for one given clinical or growth circumstance, and others for different circumstances. All, however, must be included as considerations in the "big picture".

10

Normal Variations in Facial Form and the Anatomic Basis for Malocclusions

Variation is a basic law of biology. The pool of structural, functional, and genetic-based variations always present within a population of any species provides the capacity for adaptation to a changing environment. This increases the probability of survival for those individuals having features most suitable for the needs of the time. The human face certainly has its share of variations. Indeed, there are probably more basic, divergent kinds of facial patterns among humans than among the faces of most other species. This is because unusual facial and cranial adaptations have occurred in relation to human brain expansion. A great range of facial differences exists because the brain, proportionately, is so large and so variable in configuration. There is also a much greater likelihood for different kinds of malocclusions in the human face than in the faces of most other species for the same reasons. In fact, actual tendencies toward malocclusions are **built into** the basic design of our faces because of the unusual relationships inherent in their design.

A comprehensive taxonomic system for cataloging and naming facial types based on developmental variations does not presently exist. However, three general classification categories are in common use. One relates to headform type (see Chapter 8), another deals with malocclusions (see below), and the third is based on topographic profile (Fig. 10–7). All three systems are directly interrelated with regard to underlying and predisposing morphogenic and morphologic characteristics.

Headform and Malocclusion Tendencies

In individuals (or whole populations) having a **dolichocephalic** headform, the brain is horizontally long and relatively narrow (see Fig. 10–1). This sets up a basicranium that is somewhat more flat; that is, the flexure between the middle and the anterior parts of the cranial floor is more open (Figs. 10–1, 10–2 and 10–18). It is also horizontally longer. These factors have several basic consequences for the pattern of the face. First, the whole nasomaxillary complex is placed in a more **protrusive** position relative to the mandible because of the forward basicranial rotation and, also,

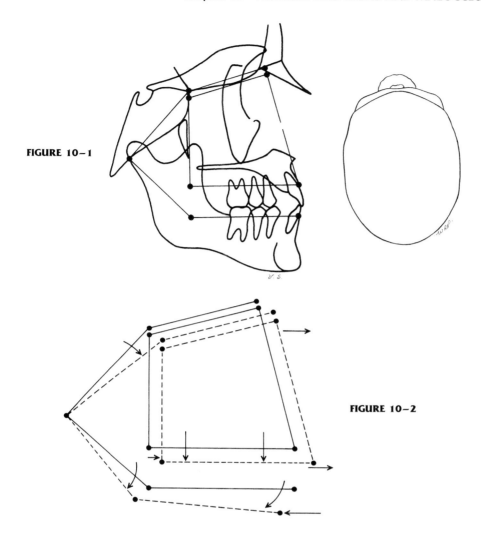

FIGURE 10-1

FIGURE 10-2

the horizontally longer anterior and middle segments of the cranial floor. Second, the whole nasomaxillary complex is lowered relative to the mandibular condyle. This causes a downward and **backward** rotation of the entire mandible. The vertically long face of the dolichocephalic adds to this, as described later. Third, the occlusal plane becomes rotated into a downward-inclined alignment. The **two-way** forward placement of the maxilla and backward placement of the mandibular corpus results in a tendency toward mandibular retrusion, and the placement of the molars results in a Class II position. The resultant profile is retrognathic (Figs. 10–3 and 10–7). However, compensatory changes are usually operative, as explained later. Because of the more open cranial base angle and the more oblique trajectory of the spinal cord into the cervical region, this type of face is associated with individuals having a greater tendency toward a somewhat stooped posture and anterior inclination of the head and neck.

Individuals or ethnic groups with a **brachycephalic** headform have a rounder, wider brain. This sets up a basicranial floor that is more upright and has a more closed flexure, which decreases the effective anteroposterior dimension of the middle cranial fossa (Figs. 10–4 and 10–5). The facial result is a more posterior placement of the maxilla. Furthermore, the hor-

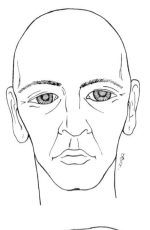

FIGURE 10–3

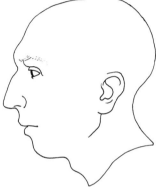

izontal length of the nasomaxillary complex is also relatively short. Because the brachycephalized basicranium is wider but less elongate in the anteroposterior dimension, the middle and anterior cranial fossae are correspondingly foreshortened (not shown in the schematic diagram). The anterior cranial fossa sets up the template for the horizontal length and bilateral width of the nasomaxillary complex, which is thereby also

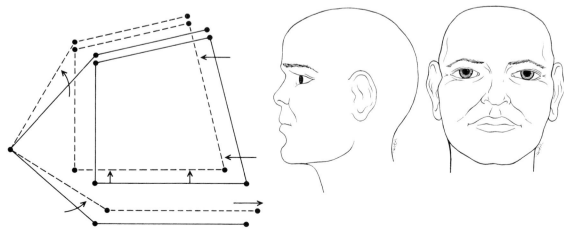

FIGURE 10–4

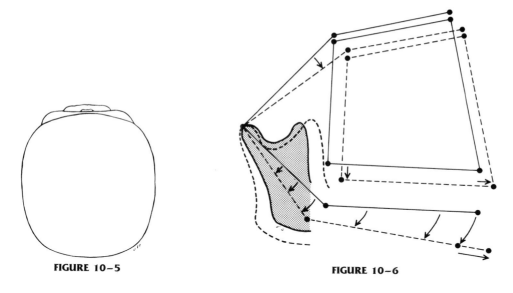

FIGURE 10–5   **FIGURE 10–6**

shorter, but wider. The composite result is a relative retrusion of the nasomaxillary complex and a more forward relative placement of the entire
mandible. This causes a greater tendency toward a prognathic profile and
a Class III molar relationship. The occlusal plane may be aligned upward,
but various compensatory processes usually result in either a perpendicular or a downward-inclined occlusal plane. Other compensatory changes
are also operative, as explained next, and these tend to counteract the
built-in Class III tendencies. Because of the more upright middle cranial
fossa and the more vertical trajectory of the spinal cord, individuals with
all these various facial features also have a tendency for a more erect
posture with the head in a more "military" (at braced attention) position.
    The basic nature of interrelationships among (1) brain form, (2) facial
profile, and (3) occlusal type predisposes characteristic facial types and
malocclusions among different types of populations. Some Caucasian
groups with a tendency for a dolichocephalic headform have a corresponding **tendency** toward Class II malocclusions and a retrognathic profile.
Far-Eastern populations, having mostly a brachycephalic headform, have
a correspondingly greater tendency toward Class III malocclusions or bimaxillary protrusion and a prognathic profile. These respective tendencies
are built into the basic plan of facial construction. However, most of us
also have intrinsic structural features that have compensated for these
tendencies (the growth process itself working toward balance, Chapter 1).
If we have such compensatory features, the built-in tendencies are offset,
to a greater or lesser extent, and we thereby have a Class I occlusion, even
though the reasons for the underlying tendencies are still present. **If** these
compensatory features are less than complete, however, the built-in tendencies then become more fully expressed, and we have a malocclusion
but less severe than the tendencies otherwise could produce.
    How does a face undergo intrinsic compensations during its develop-
ment? One example that is very common is shown here. In the situation
described above, the mandible was placed in a retrusive (retrognathic)
position owning to its downward and backward rotation resulting from the
more open type of cranial base flexure (and/or a vertically long nasomaxillary complex). The mandibular **ramus**, however, can compensate by an
increase in its horizontal dimension (Fig. 10–6). This places the whole

mandibular arch more anteriorly beneath the maxilla, and it positions the teeth in a "normal" or a Class I type of molar relationship. The extent of mandibular retrusion that would otherwise be present thus becomes partially or completely eliminated, and a profile in which the chin lies on or close to the orthognathic profile line results. The downward placement of the dental arch, caused by the downward-backward mandibular rotation described above is offset by an upward drift of the anterior mandibular teeth and a downward drift of the anterior maxillary teeth. This causes a curved occlusal plane, the curve of Spee (see following pages).

The face on each of us, virtually without exception, is the composite of a great many regional "imbalances." Some of these offset and partially or completely counteract the effects of the others. The wide ramus cited above, for example, is actually an imbalance, but it serves to reduce, as a normal adjustment process, the effects of some other angular or dimensional imbalances caused by the built-in tendencies toward malocclusions. The particular feature of a wide ramus is very common among the dolichocephalic Caucasians. When this and other compensatory factors are present, the underlying stacked deck toward retrognathia and a Class II malocclusion is removed or made less severe. Thus, many of us have a slightly retrognathic profile and a little anterior tooth crowding.

Three general types of facial profile exist: **orthognathic, retrognathic,** and **prognathic** (Fig. 10–7). The orthognathic ("straight-jawed") form is the everyday standard for a good profile, and it is the type common to most Hollywood and television big names. It is easy to "eyeball" a person's face, without actual need for headfilms or precision anthropometric instruments, to see what his or her profile type is. Simply visualize a line extending from the center of the orbit looking straight forward (*a*). Now visualize a **vertical** line **perpendicular** to the orbital line extending down along the surface of the upper lip. This line will just touch the lower lip and the tip of the chin in a person with an orthognathic profile. Time otherwise thrown away waiting around air terminals, sitting out classes, or standing in lines can be put to interesting use quietly studying people's profiles and the facial patterns described herein.

The retrognathic face has a characteristic convex-appearing profile. The tip of the chin lies somewhere behind the vertical line, and the lower lip is retrusive. The chin may be 2 or 3 cm behind the line in a severely retrognathic face (*b*). Among many Caucasians, however, it is common to have about a half centimeter or so of chin retrusion (*c*). The profile is retrognathic, but the extent is reduced because the growth process itself has provided a number of adaptive adjustments that partially offset "built-in" tendencies that can exist toward mandibular retrusion. "Facial development" is one's own personal orthodontist.

The "Effective Dimension"

In this section, specific cause-and-effect relationships underlying differences in facial pattern are explained. Each regional area throughout the face and cranium is considered separately. To evaluate the structural and developmental situation for each given region, a simple test is used: that region is compared with other regions with which it must "fit." If they have a variance of respective fit, the result is appraised by noting whether it causes (1) a mandibular retrusive or (2) mandibular protrusive effect. As will be seen, imbalances in many parts of the head are passed on, region by region, and in turn affect the placement of the jaws and the resultant nature of the occlusion.

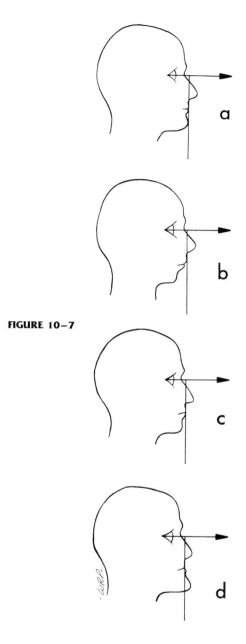

FIGURE 10–7

Two basic factors must be considered for each region. The first is the **dimension** of a particular part. Is it "long" or is it "short" with regard to its assembly with other parts?

Great care must be used to evaluate only that particular span or dimension of a bone specifically involved in actual, direct fitting. This is the **effective dimension**.

The second fundamental consideration is the **alignment** of any given part. This must also be included (although many cephalometric studies do not), because any rotational change either increases or decreases the **expression** of a dimension.

The relationship between effective mandibular length and vertical maxillary dimension is very important to the clinician because patients often present with combined anteroposterior and vertical facial disharmony. For example, individuals with mandibular prognathia can also have increased lower vertical facial height due to increased maxillary vertical dimension. This increased vertical masks the extent of the prognathism. When the vertical height is corrected surgically, the degree of prognathism is unmasked. Often patients with orthognathic profiles and long faces need both maxillary and mandibular surgery to harmonize the facial components. This is a critical factor for the clinician to consider because it dramatically affects the treatment plan.

The Dimensional Factor of Alignment

To illustrate the important effects of **alignment** as a basic factor involved in determining facial pattern, in Figure 10–18 the alignment of the middle cranial fossa in a Class I child was changed (on paper) to a less upright position. All the other facial regions, including the mandible, maxilla, and the anterior cranial fossa, were then reassembled around the realigned middle cranial fossa. **No** changes in the actual dimensions of any parts were made. The horizontal and vertical **expression** of the middle cranial fossa dimension, however, resulted in a change from the Class I pattern into a Class II pattern, even though all the individual bones were exactly the same size.

In Figures 10–8 and 10–9, if the horizontal dimension of the mandibular corpus (b) is short relative to its counterpart, the bony maxillary arch (a), the effect is, of course, mandibular retrusion (probably with anterior crowding of the teeth). Note that this does not necessarily cause a Class II molar relationship, because the **posterior** parts of the upper and lower bony arches can still be properly positioned. It is emphasized that these are **relative** comparisons between two contiguous parts within the **same** individual. The mandible is not being compared with a norm or an average value derived from a population sample. Whatever the actual value of this mandibular dimension happens to be in millimeters, or regardless of how it compares with some statistical mean, it is short when compared with

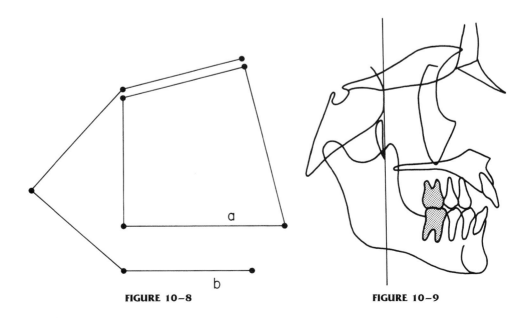

FIGURE 10–8   FIGURE 10–9

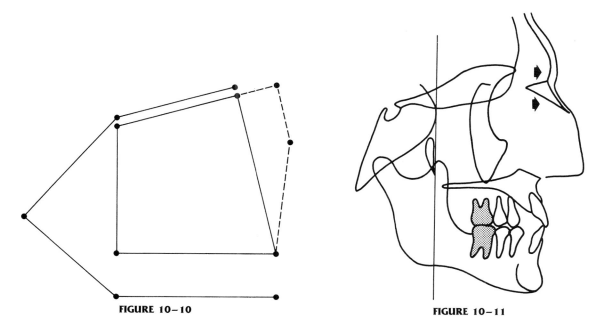

FIGURE 10–10   FIGURE 10–11

the dimensional value that really matters—its counterpart, the horizontal dimension of the maxillary body in that particular individual.*

DIMENSIONAL AND ALIGNMENT PATTERN COMBINATIONS

The remainder of this chapter describes, first, **regional** anatomic features that have a (1) mandibular retrusive or (2) mandibular protrusive effect. Throughout the face and neurocranium, each local region, one by one, is considered. The "counterpart" principle is often applied (Chapters 3 and 9). Second, regional **combinations** as they affect mandibular retrusion or protrusion are described. Third, how built-in malocclusion tendencies can be partially or almost totally compensated by the growth process itself are outlined. Fourth, the typical anatomic composite patterns underlying malocclusions are explained. Finally, the continuous spectrum of facial and malocclusion types involving all these morphologic and morphogenic features is highlighted.

If the mandibular corpus is dimensionally long, the effect, of course, is mandibular protrusion. A horizontally short maxillary arch has the same effect. (There are anatomic ways to tell which is long and which is short, as explained in Chapter 9). Whether or not a long corpus produces a Class III molar relationship depends on whether it is long mesial or distal to the first molars.

In Figure 10–10, the upper part of the nasomaxillary complex is horizontally long **relative** to its counterparts, the anterior cranial fossa, the palate, and the maxillary and mandibular arches. Note that this has no effect on the occlusion. The individual can **appear** retrognathic, but this

---

*See also Figure 9–18. Evaluation of headfilms utilizing this concept is the "counterpart analysis," a procedure that determines morphologic and developmental features **within** a given individual and which does not require tracing superimpositions or comparisons with population norms. See Martone et al., 1992 for references.

is a result of the protrusive nature of the upper part of the face and not the jaws themselves. Because the superior part of the ethmomaxillary region is protrusive, the outer table of the frontal bone remodels with it. The result is a sizeable frontal sinus, heavy eyebrow ridges and glabella, sloping forehead, high nasal bridge, and long nose. The cheekbone area appears retrusive because of the prominent nasal region and forehead, and the eyes are deep set.

If this upper part of the nasomaxillary complex is quite protrusive, as it usually is in the dolichocephalic face, the slope of the nose will often be curved or bent into a classic aquiline (eagle beak), Roman nose, or Dick Tracy configuration **if** the nose is **also** vertically long (Fig. 10–11). The longer the vertical size of the nose, the more its slope must bend. This nasal shape is quite common in leptoprosopic males, and it typically has a rather narrow and sharp configuration. The ventral edge surrounding the nares may be horizontal, but often has a tendency to tip downward. This is in contrast to the vertically and protrusively shorter type of nose in which the lower margin can angle upward. In another type of nasal bending, the **middle** part of the nasal region may be quite protrusive; this produces a characteristic and gracefully recurved (sigmoid) configuration of the nasal slope as the lower portion grades and curves back onto the less protrusive upper part. The cheekbone area in this type of face is often notably prominent because this entire level of the midface also tends to be prominent.

The above facial features, in general, characterize the long, narrow-faced, dolichocephalic headform found among many (but not all) Caucasian groups and also the dinaric type of headform. These features affect characteristics such as the extent of frontal sinus expansion and the slope of the forehead, and are thus sex and age related.

If the upper part of the nasomaxillary complex is **not** protrusive, so that its anteroposterior size more nearly matches counterpart dimensions in the anterior cranial fossa, palate, and maxillary and mandibular arches, quite a different facial pattern results. The frontal sinuses are comparatively smaller, the forehead is more upright, the eyebrow ridges and glabella are not as prominent, the nose is not nearly as protrusive, and the nasal bridge is much lower. The jaws appear more prominent because the upper nasal region is less protrusive. The cheekbones also appear more prominent for the same reason. The whole face is much flatter and wider appearing. This composite of facial features is typically found in the broad-faced, brachycephalic type of headform that characterizes many Far-Eastern individuals. Some Caucasian populations are also broad faced, with a shorter nose, more prominent mandible, lower nasal bridge, and so forth, including, for example, many individuals having a facial heritage from middle regions of Europe, parts of southern Ireland, and a scattering of geographic locations elsewhere in the world. It has become a common type of Caucasian face in North America. A shorter, but wider nose and nasal chambers provide approximately equivalent airway capacity in comparison with the narrower but longer and more protrusive nose of the dolichocephalic type of headform.

If the effective anteroposterior (not oblique) breadth of the ramus is narrow relative to its counterpart, which is the effective horizontal (not oblique) dimension of the middle cranial fossa, a mandibular retrusive effect is produced (Fig. 10–12). Note that the mandibular arch lies in a resultant **offset position** relative to its counterpart, the maxillary arch. Even though the upper and lower arches themselves are, in this example, actually matched in dimensions, the profile is retrognathic. The arches are in offset positions because the parts **behind** them are "imbalanced." Note

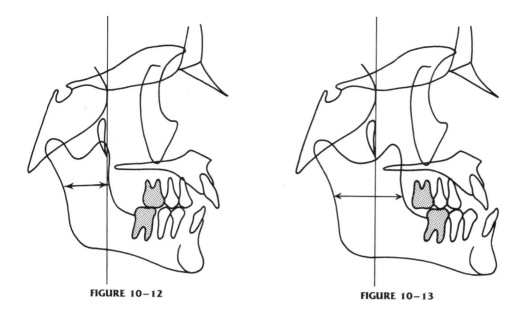

FIGURE 10-12   FIGURE 10-13

that the posterior part of the maxillary arch lies well anterior (mesial) to
the posterior part of the mandibular arch. This is one (of several) of the
basic skeletal causes that underlie a **Class II molar relationship.** Remember, the "real" anatomic junction between the ramus and corpus is
the lingual tuberosity, rather than the oblique "anterior border" where it
overlaps the corpus because of muscle attachment. Because the lingual
tuberosity cannot be directly visualized in headfilms, it is not represented
here. However, it is located distal to the vertical reference line because of
the narrow ramus in this individual.

In Figure 10–13, the effective horizontal (not oblique) dimension of the
ramus is broad relative to the middle cranial fossa. Or, the cranial fossa
is horizontally narrow relative to the ramus (either way because this is a
relative comparison). The effect is mandibular protrusion due to the resultant offset positions between the upper and lower arches, even though
the horizontal dimensions of the arches themselves can match. This is one
(of several) of the basic skeletal causes for a **Class III molar relationship**. The lingual tuberosity (not shown) is mesial to the vertical reference
line.

If the mandible as a whole has a downward-backward alignment (as a
result, for example, of a vertically long nasomaxillary region), the effect is
mandibular retrusion (Fig. 10–14). While this increases the expression of
its vertical ramus dimension, the horizontal is necessarily decreased at
the same time. The mandible is rotated downward and **backward**. As a
result, the mandibular arch becomes offset relative to the upper arch. The
profile is retrognathic, and the offset placement of the arches causes a
Class II molar relationship. Note that the mandibular corpus is rotated
downward, causing a downward-inclined mandibular occlusal plane (see
page 184 for an explanation of dental compensations).

If the mandible has a more forward and upward inclined alignment (as
a result of a vertically short midface), the effect is mandibular protrusion
(Fig. 10–15). The arches are offset, and the molars have a resultant Class
III relationship. The occlusal plane has an upward inclination relative to
the neutral orbital axis or to the vertical posterior maxillary (PM) line.
The posterior maxillary teeth can drift inferiorly and/or the gonial angle

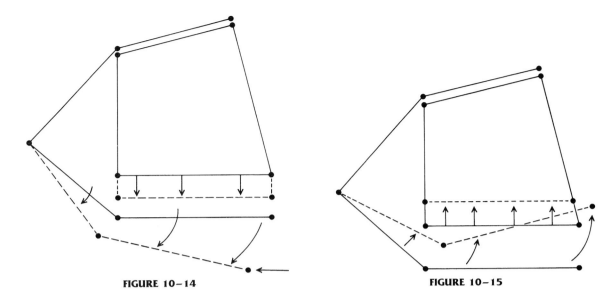

FIGURE 10-14   FIGURE 10-15

can open (compensatory adjustments) to provide proper occlusal fit. Otherwise, a posterior open bite can result.

If the ramus has a closed alignment with the corpus (i.e., a closed "gonial angle"), a mandibular **retrusive** effect is produced. A more open alignment ramus-to-corpus relationship produces a mandibular protrusive effect. These various alignment relationships can be misunderstood and the whole subject of mandibular "rotations" has been perplexing because there are two basic and separate kinds of mandibular skeletal rotations (exclusive of dental arch rotations, which will be described separately).

1.   The alignment position of the **whole mandible** can be up or down at the condylar pivot. The primary reason that this kind of developmental rotation takes place is to adjust to whatever vertical size exists for the midface **and** the alignment of the middle cranial fossa. The mandible rotates forward and upward to meet a short midface and/or a closed basicranial flexure (Fig. 10–16), and it rotates down and back (Figs. 10–14,

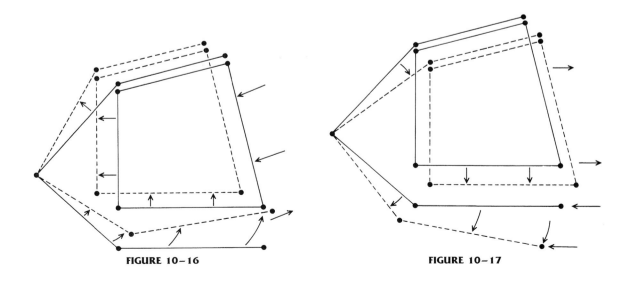

FIGURE 10-16   FIGURE 10-17

10–17 and 10–18) to accommodate a vertically long midface and/or a more open basicranial flexure. These are a **displacement** type of rotation (see page 34).

2. The angle between the ramus and the corpus also can become increased or decreased as a separate kind of rotation (Fig. 10–19). This does not refer merely to the conventional "gonial angle" but, rather, to the alignment between the whole of the ramus and the corpus. This is a **remodeling** type of rotation, in contrast to the displacement type (page 35). The oblique axis of the ramus can thus be **more upright,** with the ramus-corpus angular relationship thereby "closed." (See also Fig. 10–20.) Or the converse can occur by an opening of the ramus-corpus angle. In either case, the corpus thereby becomes positioned up or down **relative** to the ramus. While the corpus and its dental arch can participate to a limited extent in the opening and closing of its angle with the ramus, it is necessarily the **ramus** that carries out most of developmental remodeling involved. It would not be possible, for example, for the entire corpus (not merely the dentoalveolar portion) to rotate upward by its own remodeling to close the gonial angle.

There are two basic reasons ramus-corpus remodeling rotations occur. The **first** was described on page 74 and deals with the need for a progressively more upright ramus to accommodate a vertically lengthening midface. The remodeling changes that carry this out were also outlined.

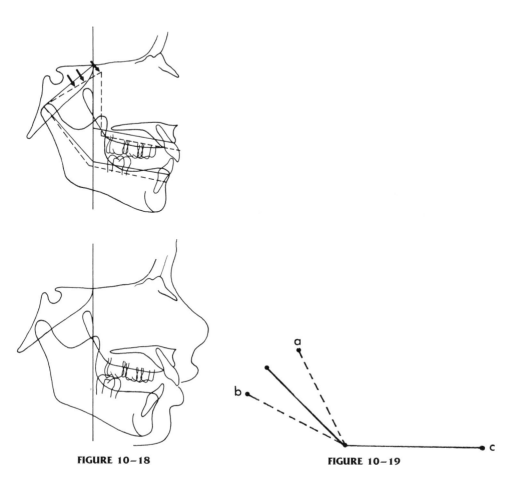

FIGURE 10–18   **FIGURE 10–19**

The result is a ramus-corpus alignment that naturally and normally becomes more closed as the midface grows. The **second** reason is to accommodate the results of whole-mandible (displacement) rotation. When the
entire mandible rotates forward and upward, the mandibular corpus is
normally rotated downward by ramus remodeling to some extent in order
to compensate. This helps to keep the mandibular dental arch in a constant functional relationship. In addition, the posterior maxillary teeth
may drift inferiorly. The occlusal plane can be brought to a perpendicular
position relative to the PM plane, or it may still have slight upward inclination. When the ramus (and whole mandible) is rotated backward and
downward by displacement, the ramus-to-corpus angle can be closed by
ramus remodeling, thereby compensating. The respective amounts of these
counteracting rotations are not always equal, however. If they are equal,
or if no rotations at all occur, the occlusal plane will be almost exactly
perpendicular to the vertical **PM** plane. Often, however, the occlusal plane
has a noticeable downward angulation because the amount of ramus remodeling realignment falls short of the downward displacement rotation
of the whole mandible. One can "eyeball" how much downward occlusal
plane rotation exists by visualizing it relative to the neutral horizontal
axis of the orbit. If the two are parallel, the occlusal plane is perpendicular

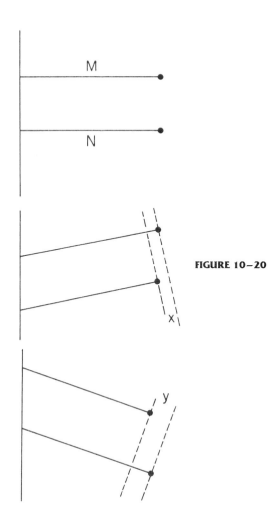

FIGURE 10–20

to the **PM** plane. In many individuals the occlusal plane angles downward, to a greater or lesser extent, and in a few it will angle upward. Persons with a vertically shorter nasal region tend to have a perpendicular or an upward occlusal plane alignment, or at least a much lesser amount of downward rotation. The occlusal plane in long-faced and long-nosed individuals tends to be downward-rotated to a greater extent.

A closed alignment between the ramus and the corpus **shortens** overall mandibular length and thereby has a mandibular retrusive effect (Fig. 10–19*a*). An open alignment increases it and has a protrusive effect (Fig. 10–19*b*). There are two ways to illustrate why this occurs. First, the straight-line dimension (overall mandibular length) from *a* to *c* is decreased; the dimension from *b* to *c* is increased. Second, if the upper and lower arches *M* and *N* in Figure 10–20 are aligned upward, *M* protrudes beyond *N* by the distance *x* relative to the **occlusal plane** (not the vertical facial profile). When aligned downward, *N* protrudes by the distance *y* relative to the downward-inclined occlusal plane.

If the ramus-corpus angle is opened, the prominence of the antegonial notch is increased. This is caused by the downward angulation of the mandibular body at its junction with the ramus. If the ramus-corpus angle is **closed**, the size of the antegonial notch can be reduced or obliterated entirely because of the upward alignment of the corpus relative to the ramus. (See Fig. 4–20.)

Note especially that the effects of whole-mandible rotations and ramus-to-corpus rotations are **opposite**. This is why the subject of mandibular "rotations" can be confusing. When the entire mandible is aligned downward, a mandibular retrusive effect is produced; but when just the corpus is aligned downward relative to the ramus, a mandibular protrusive effect results (Fig. 10–21). An upward whole-mandible alignment is mandibular protrusive, and an upward alignment of the corpus only is mandibular retrusive.

An individual can have a retrognathic profile and **not** have a Class II malocclusion, even though many of the underlying skeletal factors are the same for both. This is because different planes of reference relate separately to the profile and to malocclusions.

A forward-inclined middle cranial fossa has a two-way maxillary protrusive and a mandibular retrusive effect (Figs. 10–17 and 10–18). Because the expression of the effective horizontal (not oblique) dimension of the middle fossa is increased, the maxilla becomes offset anteriorly with

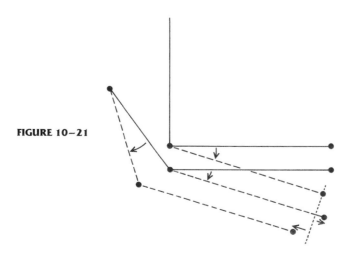

FIGURE 10–21

respect to the mandibular corpus. The midface is also lowered, and this causes the whole mandible to rock down and back. The maxilla thus is carried forward, and the mandible is rotated backward in this composite, two-way movement. Mandibular retrusion results, even though the arch lengths of the upper and lower jaws can have equivalent dimensions, as shown here. These changes in skeletal pattern cause a Class II molar relationship because the lower bony arch is posteriorly offset.

A backward-inclined middle cranial fossa[†] has a mandibular protrusive effect. This contributes to a Class III type of molar relationship. The maxilla is placed backward, and the mandible rotates forward into a protrusive position. Note that the mandibular occlusal plane is rotated into an upward-inclined position. To compensate, as mentioned above, the posterior maxillary teeth can descend (drift inferiorly) or the ramus-corpus angle is opened, or both.

It was pointed out above that if the nasomaxillary region is vertically long relative to the ramus and middle cranial fossa, the result is a downward and backward placement of the whole mandible to varying degrees in different faces (Figs. 10–14 and 10–22). Note the resultant mandibular retrusive effect, the retrognathic profile, and the skeletal basis for a Class II molar relationship. A forward alignment of the middle cranial fossa also causes a similar kind of mandibular rotation. If **both** occur in the same individual, the total extent of mandibular rotation is the sum of the two. (Dental changes can preclude an anterior open bite; see discussion of curve of Spee on page 186.)

If the nasomaxillary region is vertically short, as noted earlier, a mandibular protrusive effect is produced (Figs. 10–15 and 10–23). The mandible rotates forward and upward, and the resultant offset positions between the maxillary and mandibular arches can contribute to a Class III type of molar relationship. Note that a **vertical** imbalance has resulted in a **horizontal** structural effect.[‡] It is, of course, incorrect to assume that malocclusions are based, essentially, only on horizontal dysplasias. A closed basicranial relationship is also mandibular protrusive and adds to the extent if involved together with a short midface.

All the above relationships illustrate the various effects of changes in the dimensions or the alignment of any **one** given region, as for the ramus, middle cranial fossa, maxillary arch, and so on. The skull of any given individual, however, is a composite of many combinations of such relationships among **all** the regional parts. Outlined below are examples of several different combinations of various regional dimensional and alignment imbalances and balances.

[†]Note this important point. The conventional way to represent the "cranial base angle" is by a line from basion to sella to nasion. Although useful in conventional cephalometrics, this is not the anatomically meaningful way to do it. The **real** relationship (so far as the face is concerned) involves the contact between the condyle and the cranial floor (thus not basion), and the junction corner between the cranial floor and the nasomaxillary complex (thus not sella). **This** is the relationship that **directly** determines the anatomic effects of the three-point contact among the cranial floor, the mandible, and the maxillary tuberosity. Basion-sella-nasion only indirectly reflects this and these three traditional landmarks have nothing to do with the actual anatomic fitting of the key junctions involved. They are removed **midline** structures that do not relate directly to the **lateral** positions of the upper and lower arches, the lateral contacts between the mandibular condyles and the cranial floor, and the lateral effects of the angle between the lateral parts of the floor of the middle and anterior cranial fossae relative to the maxillary tuberosities. Sella, basion, and nasion themselves can be almost **anywhere** among the midline axis, within normal variation limits, and not affect the "angle" that really counts: the angle from the temporomandible joint (TMJ) articulation to the point of junction between the middle and anterior cranial fossae, that is, the point where the nasomaxillary complex joins the cranial floor.

[‡]This is important clinically because ideally the vertical **imbalance** must be addressed, not the horizontal **effect**. (See Fig. 10–23.)

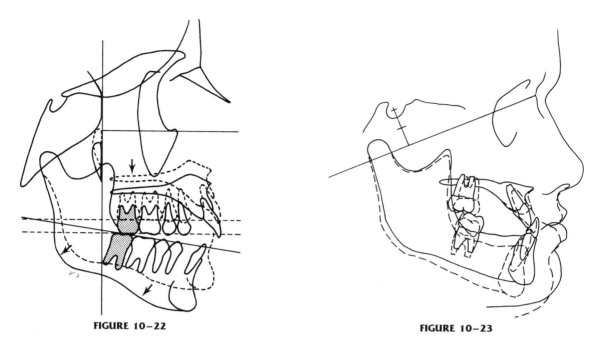

FIGURE 10–22

FIGURE 10–23

In the combination shown in Figure 10–24, the horizontal dimension of the maxillary arch exceeds that of the mandibular arch (*a*). The middle cranial fossa has a forward-inclined alignment (*b*), and the midface (*c*) is also vertically long. The mandible is rotated downward and backward (*d*). **All** of these features have mandibular retrusive effects, and their combined sum (*e*) results in a severe Class II malocclusion and severe retrognathia. Idealized treatment for this individual would require a treatment plan that addressed each imbalance. The development of a problem list (imbalance list) and intervention to address each problem is the essence of orthodontic diagnosis and treatment planning. For example, in the case shown in Figure 10–25, in a young child, the protrusion and vertical ex-

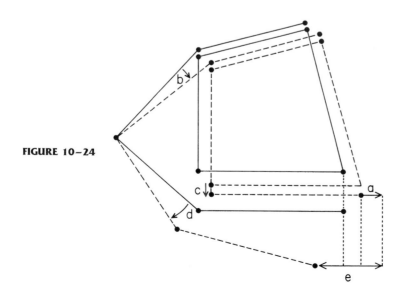

FIGURE 10–24

cess of the maxilla might be addressed using a high pull headgear and lower bite block (*b*). The headgear would be designed to redirect maxillary forward development and the bite block used to modify vertical facial relationships. As the vertical imbalance improves, treatment may then address the mandibular shape using a vertical chin cup or Frankel FR IV appliance (*c*). In the adult, a treatment plan might include extraction of upper first bicuspids (to address the maxillary protrusion) followed by maxillary LeForte I surgery (to address the vertical) with autorotation of the mandible (to address displacement rotation of the mandible). A vertical reduction and advancement genioplasty (to address the remodeling rotation of the mandible) may also improve the final aesthetic result.

The combination schematized in Figure 10−26 illustrates a horizontally short mandibular corpus (relative to the individual's maxillary arch) in combination with a backward-rotated middle cranial fossa, a forward-rotated mandible, and an opened ramus-corpus angle. The composite result is an individual with a Class II type of lower arch, a Class III molar re-

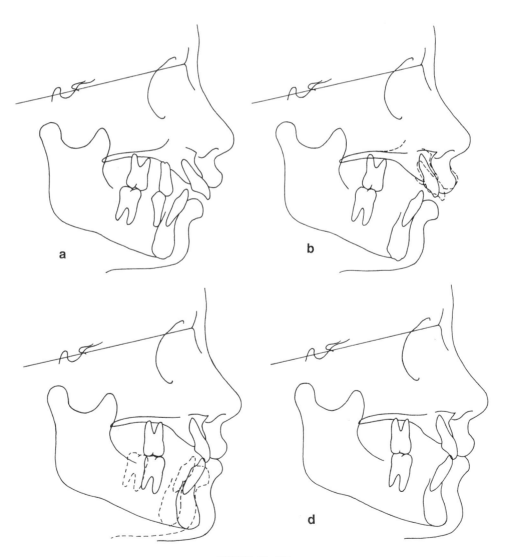

FIGURE 10−25

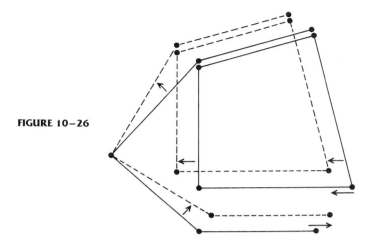

FIGURE 10-26

lationship, a Class III type of basicranial alignment, and a Class I (or-thognathic) type of profile because of the contrasting retrusive/protrusive combination.

Growth "Compensations"

A more biologic heading for this intrinsic growth process is "developmental adjustments working toward balance," as outlined in Chapter 1. The factor of morphologic adjustment during facial development is a basic and important biologic concept. The compensatory process involves latitudes of morphogenetic give and take among the various regional parts as all grow in close interrelationship. The composite result is a state of functional and structural equilibrium. Indeed, growth is a constant, ongoing, compensatory process striving toward ultimate homeostasis as a bone grows in relation to its developing muscles, as connective tissue grows in relation to both bone and muscle, and as blood vessels, nerves, epithelia, and so forth all develop in relation to everything. When the growth process is "complete," a state of compromise equilibrium has been achieved, even though a malocclusion or some other dysplasia may exist. There nearly always exist a number of regional morphologic imbalances to greater or lesser degrees of severity, but the aggregate construction of the craniofacial composite as a whole is functional, albeit with multiple regional variations, some of which likely depart from a population mean.

A frequently encountered compensatory combination involves the ramus of the mandible. When the nasomaxillary complex is vertically "long" and/or the middle cranial fossa has a forward-downward rotational alignment, the whole mandible consequently becomes rotated into a downward-backward placement. As described previously, these are significant factors that underlie the skeletal basis for a retrusion of the mandible and a Class II molar relationship. However, developmental processes can respond by a widening of the horizontal breadth of the ramus. This compensatory adjustment places the mandibular arch more protrusively, thereby partially or totally counteracting the extent of its backward rotation. What would have been a Class II malocclusion and a retrognathic profile have been converted into a Class I occlusion, and the severity of the potential malocclusion has been reduced. Should compensation fail entirely, the malocclusion becomes fully expressed.

Understand that, in carrying out this compensatory role, the ramus does not itself respond as though it has a brain of its own and somehow elects to do something good. As pointed out earlier, growth is a prolonged process striving toward functional and structural equilibrium. The skeletal response by the ramus is a result of continuous remodeling actions by its "genic" tissues receiving instruction signals paced by the growth and function of the masticatory muscles; the airway; the pharyngeal muscles, and mucosa, tonsils, tongue, lips, cheeks, connective tissue, and so on, all of which develop in a composite, interrelated manner that has a latitude for adjustment to the growth and morphology of other, contiguous regions (e.g., the basicranium, nasal region, and oral complex). If such latitude is not exceeded, at least a partial compensatory relationship can be achieved during the growth period. When growth has become completed, the capacity for compensation by parts remodeling to adjust to other parts, as a component of growth, becomes diminished. The potential in the adult, thus, is less (Fig. 1–1).

Other examples of compensatory developmental adjustments, including palatal rotations, anterior crowding, gonial angle remodeling, and occlusal plane rotations, are described elsewhere in this and other chapters. It is apparent that a Class II malocclusion is **not** merely caused by a "long maxillary arch" or a short mandible. Malocclusions are quite multifactorial because of the complex architectonics involved.

Dentoalveolar Compensations

During the development and establishment of the occlusion, ongoing and intensive adjustments occur involving dentoalveolar remodeling as well. The functional placement of the teeth is very much a part of growth. The mobility of the teeth allows responses to the many skeletal and soft tissue growth processes taking place throughout the face and cranium. A basic point to keep in mind is that, unlike bone, a tooth is not self-mobile by its own remodeling process. It must be moved by forces extrinsic to it. Figures 10–27 to 10–31 explain some common changes involved.

In the first diagram (Fig. 10–27), the vertical and horizontal dimensions among the various skeletal parts and counterparts are in balance. The alignments of all the parts also are in "neutral" positions. That is, the nature of the alignments is such that neither protrusion nor retrusion of the upper or lower jaws is produced; the angular relationships are balanced so as not to increase or decrease the "expression" of any of the various key dimensions. Note that the occlusal plane is perpendicular to the vertical reference line (the PM plane) and parallel to the neutral orbital axis (shown here below the orbit, rather than within its geometric center).

The nasomaxillary complex in the next stage (Fig. 10–28) has become lengthened vertically to a greater extent. This is common, as described earlier. The amount of midfacial growth has **exceeded** the vertical growth of the ramus-middle cranial fossa composite. The result is downward-backward alignment of the whole mandible to accommodate the longer nasomaxillary complex. A vertical "imbalance" has thus been introduced, and the expression of the vertical ramus height has been increased to match it by a downward mandibular rotation. (This same effect on the mandible can also be caused or augmented by a proclination of the middle cranial fossa, as previously described.) Note especially that the mandibular corpus, and with it the lower teeth, now has a consequent downward inclination relative to the vertical **PM** line. This "opens" the anterior bite; only

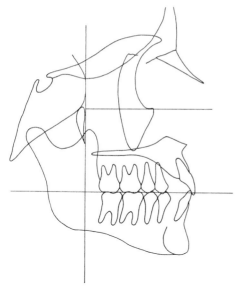

FIGURE 10–27 (From Enlow, D. H., T. Kuroda, and A. B. Lewis: The morphological and morphogenetic basis for craniofacial form and pattern. Angle Orthod. 41:161, 1971, with permission.)

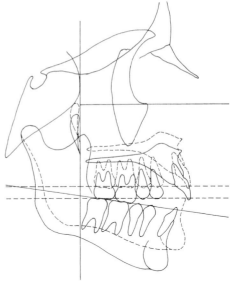

FIGURE 10–28 (From Enlow, D. H., T. Kuroda, and A. B. Lewis: The morphological and morphogenetic basis to craniofacial form and pattern. Angle Orthod., 41:161, 1971, with permission.)

the second molars are in occlusal contact. The amount of occlusal separation increases toward the incisors.

Note also the retrusion of the mandible, overjet, and the Class II molar relationship caused by the mandible's rotation. The upper teeth "drift" (**not** simply erupt) inferiorly until each comes into contact with its antagonist (Fig. 10–29). The last molars were already in contact; the second

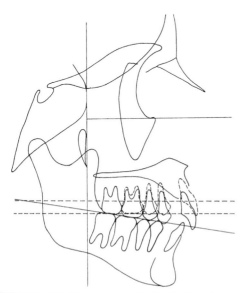

FIGURE 10–29 (From Enlow, D. H., T. Kuroda, and A. B. Lewis. The morphological and morphogenetic basis for craniofacial form and pattern. Angle Orthod., 41: 161, 1971, with permission.)

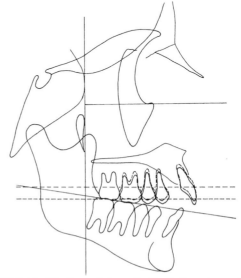

FIGURE 10–30 (From Enlow, D. H., T. Kuroda, and A. B. Lewis. The morphological and morphogenetic basis for craniofacial form and pattern. Angle Orthod., 41: 161, 1971, with permission.)

premolar must drift downward only a short distance. The first premolar drifts inferiorly even more because of the greater gap involved. The central incisors move down the greatest distance. As a final result, full arch-length occlusal contact is attained. The occlusal plane is **straight** (not curved, as in other variations described below). The occlusal plane bisects the upper and lower incisor overlap, just as it did in the first, "balanced" stage. The occlusal plane, however, is now inclined obliquely downward.

Another common adjustive combination may occur. The upper teeth drift inferiorly, but the canines and incisors do not move down to the full extent needed to completely close the occlusion, only to about the same extent that the premolars drift inferiorly (Fig. 10–30).

The anterior **mandibular** teeth, however, drift superiorly until full arch occlusal contact is reached (Fig. 10–31). The lower incisors must move upward much more, however, than the cuspids and premolars. Note that the roots of the anterior teeth have become realigned as all of the teeth are repackaged, and that the cusps of the lower incisors and canines are **noticeably much higher** than the premolars and molars.

Dentoalveolar Curve (of Spee)

There are two ways to represent the **occlusal plane.** The traditional method is to draw a line along the contact points of all the teeth to the midpoint of the overlap between the upper and lower incisors. In the first two examples cited above, this line is straight. In the last, however, note how the line is curved as it exactly bisects the overlap of the upper and lower incisors. This is called the **curve of Spee** or the dentoalveolar curve, and the reason for its development was just outlined above. A second way to represent the occlusal plane is to run a line from the posterior-most molar contact point straight to the anterior-most premolar contact point. The incisors are not considered. This is termed the "functional occlusal plane," and it is always a straight line whether or not a curve of Spee exists.

In the first and second examples of occlusal development (Figs. 10–28 and 10–29), a curve of Spee did not develop, and the two methods for

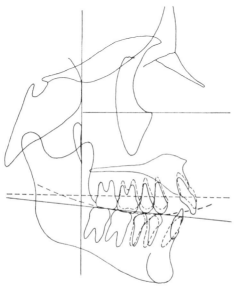

FIGURE 10–31 (From Enlow, D. H., T. Kuroda, and A. B. Lewis: The morphological and morphogenetiuc basis for craniofacial form and pattern. Angle Orthod., 41:161, 1971, with permission.)

representing the occlusal plane result in the same line. In the last example, however, the curved occlusal plane bisecting the incisor overlap and the straight functional occlusal plane are divergent. Note how the mandibular incisors rise considerably above the level of the functional occlusal plane. The maxillary incisors, however, fall well short and do not even touch this straight-line functional occlusal plane. In individuals having a marked curve of Spee, the alveolar region of the mandible just above the chin is characteristically more elongate because the incisors have drifted superiorly for several millimeters or more.

The dentoalveolar curve (of Spee) is a common developmental adjustment that provides intrinsic compensation for an **anterior open bite**. A combination of several factors underlies the skeletal tendency for this type of malocclusion. If (1) normal long-faced development or, also, if airway (or other) problems lead to an opening of the ramus-corpus (gonial) angle; (2) if the whole mandible is displacement-rotated down and back as explained previously; and/or (3) if a counterclockwise rotational alignment of the palate and maxillary arch occurs because of displacement by the anterior cranial fossa, the conditions predisposing an anterior open bite can converge to cause this developmental variation. The vertical drifting (not simply eruption) of the anterior mandibular teeth can then close what would otherwise be a skeletal (not merely dental) gap. Should this intrinsic process fail, the open bite thereby expresses itself fully. Relapse is a frequent problem because these predisposing conditions are not fully eliminated by treatment, and the resultant imbalance activates the growth process to return to a state of balance. Conversely, if a **deep overbite** occurs, it is often in patients who have a horizontally short mandible in conjunction with a closed ramus-corpus angle, a clockwise rotational alignment of the palate and maxillary arch, and a deep curve of Spee.

Another kind of dental compensation also commonly occurs. It was underscored earlier that the teeth have only a very limited capacity for remodeling (particularly after they have become fully formed). That is, a tooth cannot become markedly reshaped by selective remodeling resorption and deposition of dentin and enamel throughout its various areas to accommodate spatial and functional relationships; only a relatively limited extent of root resorption, deposition of cementum, trajectory of root growth, and crown wear is possible in this regard. This means that most adaptive adjustments for a tooth must be carried out by the "displacement" process. While extensive resorptive and depository remodeling is a basic growth function for the housing alveolar bone, it is not a factor for the tooth itself. If, however, the capacity for this bone remodeling is exceeded, as for example, by an alveolar arch that is too small for the teeth it must support, the developmental and functional recourse then is displacement of some of the teeth. Thus, **anterior crowding** is, in effect, a compensatory means by which the teeth are housed beyond the limit (growth field) provided by the available bone and its growth and remodeling potential. The treatment options for alignment of crowded lower teeth are (1) to increase the available alveolar bone for tooth alignment or (2) to reduce the number of teeth to compensate for the lack of alveolar bone. Importantly, since the anterior mandibular alveolar surface is resorptive and its growth field boundary constrained, option 2 is often the biologically sound treatment decision.

SUMMARY OF CLASS II AND CLASS III SKELETAL FEATURES

In the Class II individual (Fig. 10–32), note that the mandibular arch is short relative to the maxillary arch. The mandibular arch in the Class

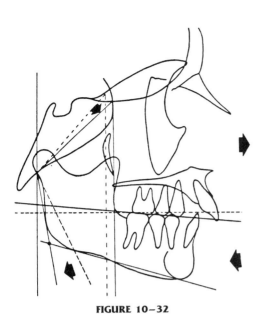

FIGURE 10–32

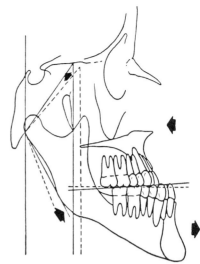

FIGURE 10–33 (From Enlow, D. H., T. Kuroda, and A. B. Lewis: The morphological and morphogenetiuc basis for craniofacial form and pattern. Angle Orthod., 41: 161, 1971, with permission.)

III individual (Fig. 10–33), conversely, is horizontally long relative to the maxillary arch, its counterpart.

The middle cranial fossa in the Class II individual has a forward and downward-inclined alignment. In the Class III individual the middle cranial fossa is aligned backward and upward. The nasomaxillary complex is thereby placed more retrusively in the Class III individual and more protrusively in the Class II individual. Rotations of the mandible are also involved (see below).

The nasomaxillary complex in the Class II individual is vertically long relative to the vertical dimension of the ramus (or the ramus is short relative to the maxilla). This long midface, together with the downward-forward alignment of the middle cranial fossa, causes a downward-backward rotational alignment of the whole mandible in the Class II individual.[§] The Class III mandible is rotated forward in conjunction with an upward-backward middle cranial fossa rotation and a vertically short nasal region. The midface is short relative to the vertical dimension of the ramus (or the ramus is long relative to the maxilla; either way, since it is a relative comparison). Although the face of the Class III individual "looks" quite long (Fig. 10–33), it is the lower face (mandible), not the nasal region, that causes this (see below).

In Class II individuals, the headform type is often dolichocephalic or mesocephalic. The anterior cranial fossa is thereby relatively long and narrow; and because it is the template for the nasomaxillary complex, the palate and maxillary arch are correspondingly elongate and narrow. In Class III individuals, conversely, both the anterior and middle cranial fossae tend to be wider and shorter (brachycephalic), and this thereby establishes a foreshortened, but wider palate, maxillary arch, and pharynx.

The ramus-corpus (gonial) angle is more closed in the Class II, but open in the Class III face, thereby shortening and lengthening, respectively,

---

[§]The dashed lines in the figures represent "neutral" alignment positions. See Enlow et al., 1971a, for the biologic rationale involved.

overall mandibular length. In the Class III face this produces the characteristic steeply angled alignment of the mandibular corpus.[∥] Note that the anterior mandibular teeth in the Class III individual have drifted upward to a considerable extent (a compensatory adjustment to close the open ramus-corpus angle), so that the occlusal plane itself is not angled as sharply downward. This causes the characteristically elongate, high alveolar region above a prominent-appearing chin observed in many Class III faces.[¶] It is interesting to note that, although the anterior mandibular teeth drift markedly superiorly in the Class III, they do not rise above the functional occlusal plane to form a dentoalveolar curve. A marked extent of compensatory downward drifting of the maxillary dentition may also occur in many cases (as seen in Figure 10–33) to compensate for the vertically short nasal region. In the Class II face, conversely, it is the **nasal region** that appears relatively elongate vertically, with a much shorter appearing vertical depth in the region of the chin. Note that the Class II maxillary apical base is **much closer** to the palate compared to the **more downward-drifted** maxillary teeth in the Class III. However, some Class II individuals may show a steeply inclined mandibular plane causing a lengthened, but still retrusive, appearance of the lower face. This results when the downward-backward alignment of the whole mandible (a displacement rotation produced by the Class II long face/short ramus/open middle cranial fossa relationships described earlier) is not accompanied by closure of the gonial angle. A deeper compensatory curve of Spee often develops.

To date, the combination of these multiple features contributes to the composite skeletal basis for mandibular retrusion in the Class II individual and mandibular protrusion in the Class III individual. However, note that the Class II ramus is horizontally broad and that the Class III ramus is narrow. These are, as explained earlier, compensatory features that partially counteract the other characteristics that combine to cause Class II mandibular retrusion and Class III protrusion, respectively. The resultant malocclusions are thereby less severe than they would have been had the ramus in each been of "normal" dimension. Had the ramus actually been narrow in the Class II individual and wide in the Class III individual, they would, of course, have added to (rather than subtracting from) the composite basis for the malocclusion.

Most Class II individuals thus have an anterioposteriorly short mandibular corpus, a vertically long nasomaxillary complex, a whole maxillary dental arch that drifts inferiorly much less than in Class III but in which the anterior teeth drift down more than the posterior teeth, a downward-and backward-aligned mandible, a forward and downward middle cranial fossa alignment, a closed ramus-corpus (gonial) angle, and (in severe malocclusions) a narrow ramus and a long fore-and-aft middle cranial fossa.

[∥]Note this significant point. The Class II face can have a steep mandibular plane angle, thereby appearing similar to the downward-inclined mandibular corpus of the Class III face, which also is a "steep plane" (Fig. 10–31). The underlying reasons, however, are different and should not be confused. In the Class II, it is a **whole-mandible displacement** rotation. In the Class III, it is a **ramus-to-corpus remodeling** rotation. The former relates to a **long** midface, whereas the latter relates to a **short** midface, a significant distinction often overlooked!

[¶]An interesting and not uncommon Class III variation occurs in the **dolichocephalic**, rather than the usual brachycephalic headform. It is related to Class I individuals having a strong Class III tendency, except that underlying mandibular protrusive features dominate over the long, narrow (leptoprosopic) maxillary protrusive features also present. The result is an elongate, narrow head with a long, pointed nose, but also with a contrasting protrusive, rather than retrusive, mandible (as in the classic "wicked witch"). See Martone et al., 1992.

The **converse** of all these regional relationships characterizes the Class III malocclusion. Each such feature occurs in about 70 per cent or more of Class II and III individuals respectively. What about the other 30 or so per cent? This is where "offsetting penalties" come into play. Instead of a forward-inclined, dolichocephalic type of middle cranial fossa and/or a long midface causing mandibular retrusion, for example, a given individual can have a **backward**-aligned, brachycephalic type of fossa and a more pug-like nasal region. These features may then combine with one or more other regional mandibular **protrusive** features, such as, perhaps, a broad ramus, a long corpus, or an open gonial angle, to partially counteract the various mandibular retrusive factors also present. In any given individual, the sum of the dimensional values for all the mandibular protrusive features weighs against the sum of the values for all the mandibular retrusive features. Either they come into a effective balance that zero's out, or one or the other wins. If the mandibular retrusive features dominate, the **severity** of the resultant Class II malocclusion and retrognathic type of face depends, first, on how much (in millimeters) the total of these retrusive features amounts to, and second, how much the counteracting features subtract from this total.

Each of us has a natural, normal predisposition toward either mandibular retrusion (Class II) or protrusion (Class III). A fundamental concept is that there is no such thing as a "separate" Class I facial category. A pervasive misconception is that the Class I craniofacial composite is essentially "all normal and balanced except for minor irregularities." All Class I individuals, however, have a predominant **tendency** one way or the other toward a composite retrusive or protrusive malocclusion. Most narrow- and long-faced Class I individuals have the **same** underlying facial and cranial features that are present in the long-faced Class II individuals. The same percentage of the various mandibular retrusive relationships described above occur in both. This is why a Class II predisposition usually exists to a greater or lesser extent. The difference between the Class I and II malocclusions, however, is the extent and magnitude of the imbalances and the number and extent of counteracting features. If the compensating characteristics are adequate, a more or less balance of imbalances in a Class I face results. If they partially or totally fail, marginal to severe malocclusion and facial disproportion results. A person having an attractive, well-proportioned face, with an orthognathic (or nearly so) profile and only relatively minor occlusal irregularities **also** has, unsuspected by him or her and deep within the face and cranium, the **same** underlying characteristics that caused a cousin to have a noticeably retrognathic profile and a Class II malocclusion. Our hero, however, has a particularly broad ramus and some other happy offsetting characteristics that are winners for him as an individual. Most of us have at least a reasonable-appearing face, although somewhat short of perfect, for the same reasons.

A fundamental principle to keep always in mind is that the growth process is continuously creating imbalances as the muscles and the airway, for example, continue to develop. At the same time, however, the growth process is **working toward** an aggregate state of composite functional and developmental equilibrium among all the separate multitudes of parts. (See Chapter 1.)

THE FACIAL SPECTRUM

The conventional perception of pattern variation is that there are essentially three principal facial types, each associated with one of the three chief malocclusion categories. These are, simply, mandibular protrusion (Class III), mandibular retrusion (Class II), and normal or nearly so (Class I). Even as a generalization, however, this perception bypasses significant morphologic and key developmental points and precludes a much more basic biologic awareness of the factors underlying facial form and pattern. It is not possible, for example, **not** to have underlying malocclusion tendencies in the Class I, whether or not fully masked by the growth process, considering our unique craniofacial character.

As already described in the other chapters and in the pages above describing facial component combinations, the multiple structural reasons for the wide variations in facial form are cataloged. How the nature of the anatomic combinations leads to a **spectrum** of facial patterns is now outlined.

The Continuous Facial Sequence and Developmental Intergrades

If **all** of the regional anatomic conditions (1) having a mandibular **protrusive** effect should exist in a given person, and (2) each regional effect is **severe** within the bounds of workable function, and (3) no significant compensatory adjustments occur, **then** the aggregate result would be a severe pattern of mandibular protrusion and an extreme Class III malocclusion. This is one end of a continuous morphologic spectrum. It extends on to the other (opposite) anatomic end representing retrognathia and severe Class II malocclusion in which all of the opposite regional features exist and without significant developmental compensatory adjustments. Between these opposite extremes lies an infinite spectrum of **mixes** that grade from each end toward the middle. Facial taxonomists have divided the whole into the three general groups, I, II, and III. An important point is that the middle span (Class I) **is not** comprised of individuals in which no retrusive or protrusive regional features exist at all—that is, everything is actually quite neutral and nearly perfectly constructed with only minor misfits among parts. Quite the contrary, as described next.

Working toward a retrusive/protrusive overlap in the middle of the spectrum, two factors are in play that create **gradations**. First, the severities at both ends decrease for some (not necessarily all) of the regional "trusive-causing" relationships. Second, a contrasting **mix** of relationships, with compensations added, occurs in a progressive direction toward the middle overlap. The result is a gradation away from "severe" until both ends meet at the transition crossover from one side to the other. This point is different in every individual person because of the infinite variability of the magnitudes and character of the mix.

In all cases, it is important to understand that the built-in, underlying protrusive/retrusive tendencies relating to headform variations (Chapters 1, 8, and 10) **are still present**, but are masked because of the offsetting combinations of contrasting local features. For example, palatal and ramus remodeling can help offset a maxillary displacement; or, upward dentoalveolar remodeling (curve of Spee) offsets a downward-backward mandibular alignment relating to an elongate nasomaxillary complex.

Just where the central crossover point exists is subject to a taxonomist's definition and a value judgment. Then, an arbitrary boundary is designated on either side of the point as definition of the Class I span. The serious misconception arises, however, that no significant malocclusion-causing factors now exist within this middle span because everything is virtually neutral or nearly so and within the bounds of our definition of normal. What, in fact, does indeed exist within this middle span is a composite of regional variations that are protrusive or retrusive-causing but, in combination, balance each other out.[#] This is a point that needs really serious consideration.

The Class I category, thus, is not in itself an anatomically discrete group. It is, rather, a blend of contrasting features that more or less nullify each other to an extent that is intermediate between the groups on either side having blends weighted either more toward retrusion versus protrusion.

An important point, as a bottom line, is that **Class I is not a homogeneous grouping**. To regard it as so is to mask significant variations within it. Most individuals are either on the Class II or the Class III **side**, depending on their personal mix of regional features. Thus, some persons are Class I with an underlying Class III tendency, others with a Class II tendency. Each will likely respond quite differently to treatment procedures (Enlow et al., 1988).

Interestingly, a Class I more on the Class II side is actually more closely related morphologically to a Class II than to a Class I on the Class III side.

To regard all Class Is, thus, simply as a single, structurally neutral and homogenous group, without taking these contrasting anatomic factors fully into account, is most regrettable. It disguises significant underlying morphology and developmental tendencies. This is a clinically **most** relevant point because divergent vectors of growth are involved. Since the clinical objective is to "work with growth" (i.e., to understand what is happening in order to manage it), the contrasting conditions involved are obviously fundamental factors.

Another and most significant point is that clinical and research studies **not** taking these anatomic and developmental distinctions into account yield nondiscriminating findings because results are mixed into a common pot and all simply cancel each other out with no decisive trends established. This is a most important consideration and merits strong emphasis. Please consider this point carefully, since it has almost never been a factor in most clinical and research studies.

A final and significant point is drawn from the spectrum of these morphogenic and facial assembly patterns. It is significant because of the great potential for clinical fine-tuning. The point is that, because of the structural spectrum involving mixes of the retrusive and protrusive original combinations, Class I, II, and III *subgroups* can be distinguished. Although not yet named or formally designated, their existence is real. That subgroupings demonstrate different developmental lines is known (Enlow et al., 1988; Martone et al., 1992, Choi, 1993). Different morphogenic responses to treatment procedures, thus, is the knowledge to be gained.

[#]This factor might help "explain" the clinical case that "appeared" to be a simple Class I and during treatment "turned into" a Class II or III. The Class II or III components were there all along, and they became more fully expressed during treatment.

11

The Structural Basis for Ethnic Variations in Facial Form

Age, sex, and population differences in the pattern of facial structure have been pointed out in the preceding chapters. The purpose of this section is to summarize this information briefly and add to it as a separate topic. Although this is an interesting subject in its own right, it is quite important for the clinician to realize that population norms derived from a given sample are not necessarily valid or accurate for other samples or groups, especially if ethnic and geographic variations are involved.

The phylogenetic basis for the unique construction of the human face was outlined in Chapter 9. It will be recalled that both the shape and size of the brain are key factors relating to the structure of the face. Because the basicranium is the bridge between them, and because the floor of the cranium is the template upon which the face is constructed, variations in the shape of the brain in **any** species are associated with corresponding variations in the form of the face. For example, the junctional part of the midface can only be as wide as the floor of the cranium. It cannot be wider because there is nothing to attach it to. Thus, narrow-brain species or subgroups are correspondingly narrow faced. Compare the face of the long, narrow-brained collie dog with that of the short, round-brained boxer or bulldog. Proportionately, man has an exceptionally wide face, in comparison with the typical mammal, because of the colossal size and the shape of the brain. The various rotations of the olfactory bulbs, orbits, and so forth (caused by the brain's characteristics) combine with the boundaries of the brain to establish, in all species, the amount and the principal directions of facial growth. Because of these factors, the shape and size of the brain are involved, also, in the variations of facial pattern **within** any given species or population group, as well as between them. There are, however, other factors that come into play, as will be seen.

Human population groups having a dolichocephalic headform naturally have a proportionately more narrow and longer face than those with a brachycephalic type of headform. The wider brain (with no special difference in overall volume) has the proportionately wider face. It has been claimed that there is an evolutionary (secular) trend toward the brachycephalic type among human groups. If this is happening, there will also be, as well, related long-term population distribution changes in facial structure, the nature of built-in tendencies toward malocclusions, and profile features.

The more open ("flat") cranial base flexure that usually characterizes the dolichocephalic headform in many Caucasian groups sets up a more protrusive upper face and a more retrusive lower face (Figs. 11–1, 11–2, and 11–3, bottom). The whole nasomaxillary complex is placed in a more forward position, and it is lowered relative to the mandibular condyle. Because the midface is relatively long, there is the tendency for a downward and backward rotation of the whole mandible. The posteroanterior dimension of the pharynx is large because of the longer and more horizontally aligned middle cranial fossae. Because the anterior cranial fossae are elongate and narrow, the palate and maxillary arch are correspondingly long and narrow. The extent of nasal protrusion is quite marked, and the outer cortical table of the forehead remodels anteriorly contiguous with a high nasal bridge. A large frontal sinus is thereby formed between the inner and outer tables. The forehead is much more sloping as a result, and the glabella becomes noticeably protrusive. The eyeballs are deep-set. The cheekbones often appear less prominent and more "hollow" because the remainder of the upper and the middle face are so protrusive. Because the mandible is rotated posteriorly, it tends to be retrusive, and the whole profile takes on a characteristic convexity for all these reasons. A Class II tendency (i.e., maxillary protrusion and/or mandibular retrusion) is **built in**. There is also a high incidence of a broad ramus to compensate, at least in part, for the tendency toward mandibular retrusion.

The more closed, upright basicranial flexure that usually characterizes the brachycephalic head sets up a correspondingly wider, flatter, more upright type of face (Figs. 11–3, top, and 11–4). The rounder, horizontally shorter brain and correspondingly foreshortened anterior cranial fossa establish a wider but anteroposteriorly shorter upper and midfacial region. The palate and dental arches are thereby also foreshortened, but relatively wide. The whole upper and midfacial region is also placed less protrusively

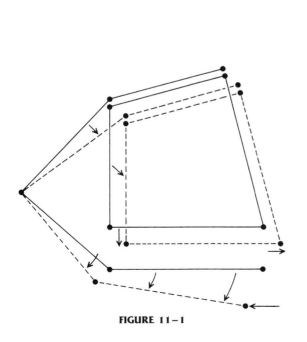

FIGURE 11–1

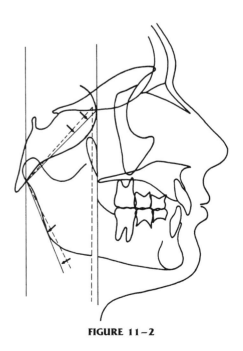

FIGURE 11–2

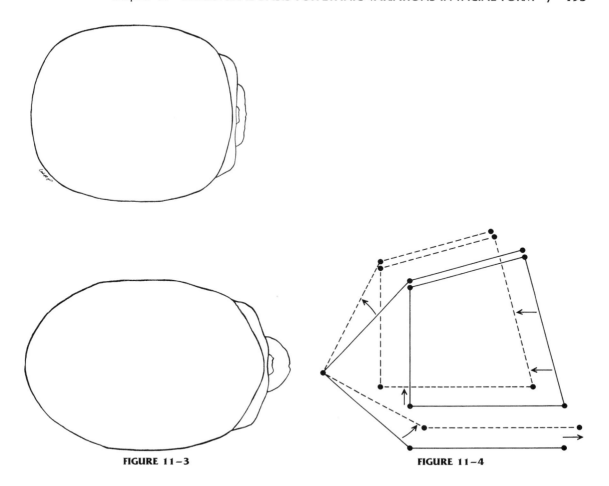

FIGURE 11–3   **FIGURE 11–4**

because of the more upright middle cranial fossa. The middle cranial fossa, and, therefore, the pharyngeal region, is anteroposteriorly shorter for the same reasons. This further decreases the relative extent of the upper and midfacial protrusion. In addition, the upper part of the ethmomaxillary complex does not expand anteriorly to nearly the same extent described for the previous facial type. The wider, shorter nasal and pharyngeal airway is approximately equivalent in capacity to those of other facial types having a much greater extent of nasal and maxillary protrusion but with a more narrow passageway. The composite result is a more upright and bulbous forehead, a lesser protrusion of the glabella and eyebrow ridges, a thinner frontal sinus, a much lower nasal bridge, a shorter pug-type nose, more shallow orbits and less deep-set eyeballs, and a tendency for a forward rotation of the entire mandible (unless offset by a vertical lengthening of the midface, and vertical drifting of the dentoalveolar arch, which is a feature in some, but not all, individuals.) The face appears flatter, broader, and squared. The cheekbones are more prominent appearing because the remainder of the upper and middle face is not as protrusive. There is a greater likelihood for an orthognathic (straight) profile, and the chin appears prominent and the mandible quite full. A greater tendency for bimaxillary protrusion or a Class III type of malocclusion and a prognathic mandible exists. In the brachycephalic (euryprosopic) face, the eyes can "look" wide-set because the nasal bridge is low. In some sub-groups, the nasomaxillary complex can be relatively long vertically, and the man-

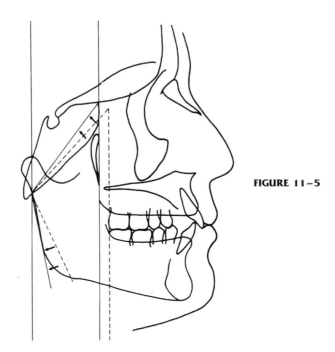

FIGURE 11–5

dible can thus rotate downward and backward (Fig. 11–5) rather than anterosuperiorly (Fig. 11–4). The mandibular corpus tends to be shorter relative to the maxillary arch in some groups, and these mandibular features contribute to a compensation for the built-in tendency toward prognathism and bimaxillary protrusion.

It is important to realize that any predominantly brachycephalic population embodies a great range of variation from the "typical," as outlined above, to a mix of underlying facial features that grade toward the dolichocephalic/leptoprosopic form. The Far-Eastern (Oriental) populations, for example, do not represent a single, homogeneous grouping, but, rather, a composite assemblage of many geographically, environmentally, and morphologically diverse subgroups that have evolved into quite distinctive and variably dissimilar craniofacial types. In contrast to the very round and flat-faced pattern, a more leptoprosopic, angular, long, and thin-nosed form also exists. The extent to which such facial variation relates to different anatomic types of malocclusions, and responses to different clinical procedures, is presently not at all well catalogued. Thorough anatomic and morphogenetic descriptions of these variations are yet very scant.

The above features characterize the Oriental face,* as well as certain Caucasian groups that also have a rounder brachycephalic ("Alpine") type of headform with many of these same facial features. (This does not include the dinaric headform, which is a fundamentally separate brachycephalic category.) The brachycephalic Caucasian type of face, like many Oriental faces, is wider, the nasal bridge lower, the nose flatter and shorter, the midface variably shorter, the forehead more upright, and the mandible more prominent. There are fewer underlying Class II tendencies in this basically different type of Caucasian face. Class I individuals having this composite facial structure tend toward a more orthognathic type

---

*The information in this section is based on investigations carried out by the author in collaboration with Dr. Takayuki Kuroda of the Tokyo Medical and Dental University.

of profile. When a Class II malocclusion does develop, however, it is a different kind (see Enlow et al., 1988). Care must be taken by the orthodontist because there are often stronger mandibular protrusive factors within this face. For example, the use of Class II elastic traction to establish a Class I molar relationship may be delayed in these individuals until mandibular growth has been more fully expressed.

Black individuals, as with some Caucasians, tend to have an elongate, dolichocephalic headform, although there also occur wider faced individuals, just as among some Caucasian individuals and subgroups. The middle cranial fossa has an anteriorly inclined (open) alignment, even more so than in Caucasians. This factor causes the whole mandible to rotate markedly down and back (Fig. 11–6). The mandibular corpus tends to be horizontally long relative to the bony (not dental) maxillary arch. Unlike the typical "long-headed" Caucasian facial type, the upper part of the face in the black expands much less and is, therefore, not nearly so protrusive. In this respect, the face of the black corresponds to that of the Oriental. The forehead is more upright and bulbous than in most Caucasians, the frontal sinus proportionately less expanded; the nasal bridge lower; the nose flatter, wider, and less protrusive; and the cheekbones more prominent. Although the upper part of the nasal region in narrow-faced black individuals tends to be correspondingly narrow, approximately equivalent airway capacity is achieved by a wider dimension in the more inferior part of the nasal passageway in conjunction with a flaring of the nasal alae.

One special feature characterizes the black face; the mandibular **ramus is quite broad** proportionate to the middle cranial fossa. In a previous chapter, it was pointed out that the horizontal dimension of the ramus is a site that commonly participates in compensations for structural imbalances in other parts of the face and cranium. The forward inclination of the middle cranial fossa that characterizes many Caucasian groups, for example, is partially or completely counteracted by the development of a wider ramus, thereby offsetting or reducing the intrinsic tendency for mandibular retrusion and a Class II malocclusion. The mandible of the black also has this feature, but the amount is characteristically **much** greater. The very broad ramus places the mandibular corpus (which can also be long relative to the bony maxillary arch) in a resultant protrusive

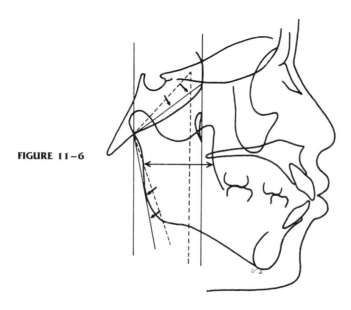

FIGURE 11–6

position. This, in turn, causes the maxillary incisors to tip labially, and a **bimaxillary** protrusion is thereby produced. This is an advanced feature that for the dolichocephalic black often precludes severe Class II malocclusions. If present at all, they are usually of the Class II "B" type. That is, mandibular B point lies well ahead of maxillary A point, in contrast to the more severe Class II "A" type, in which A point is the more protrusive relative to the occlusal plane (see Enlow et al., 1971a). Class I variations can also be problematic, especially when mandibular retrognathia is associated with a Class I molar occlusion. These "tooth/face" discrepancies require careful consideration of the treatment alternatives to achieve the optimal compromise between esthetics and function, and stability. Surgical augmentation of the bony chin is often a necessary procedure if optimum aesthetic balance of the profile is to be achieved.

The anatomic basis for the Class III type of malocclusion in blacks has a different structural pattern compared to other population groups. The basicranium of the black Class III (or the related bimaxillary protrusive tendency) does not usually have a posterosuperior alignment of the middle cranial fossa in contrast to the brachycephalic Oriental and Caucasian Class III (and bimaxillary protrusion). Rather, the black Class III malocclusion tends to have an actual forward-downward rotated middle cranial fossa, and the ramus is aligned backward, not forward. This reduces the extent of the mandibular protrusive features. The nasomaxillary complex is thereby placed more anteriorly, not posteriorly. The basicranium, thus, is not a principal factor among blacks that contributes directly to the protrusive placement of the mandible in Class III malocclusions, as it does in the other population groups. The basicranium, rather, is a counteracting feature. As pointed out above, the **wider ramus** of the black is a key anatomic compensatory feature that effectively offsets and largely precludes Class II malocclusion tendencies that otherwise relate to an anteriorly inclined middle cranial fossa. However, the same broad nature of the ramus **also** exists in most black Class III individuals as well as in the Class I. In Orientals and Caucasians, the Class III ramus is often "narrow" and reduces the extent of, and thereby partially compensates for, lower jaw protrusion. In the black Class III individual, conversely, not only is the ramus noncompensatory, its broad relative dimension adds to rather than subtracts from the extent of mandibular prognathism. Thus, the mandibular ramus of the black is an effective feature that minimizes one type of malocclusion, but that tends to aggravate another type. (See Enlow et al., 1982; Martone et al., 1992 for additional descriptive information.) Nonetheless, it is an advanced craniofacial factor that has eliminated a real threat in human evolution, which is the entrapment of the lower jaw caused by brain expansion and upright, bipedal body posture. (See Chapter 8.)

The combination of the tendency for bimaxillary protrusion and wide mandibular ramus often makes treatment planning for the black patient with anterior dental crossbite a challenge for the clinician. Two points are worthy of consideration in the treatment planning process. First, bimaxillary protrusion allows the clinician a greater range of dental compensation in treating anterior crossbite. Because the vertical facial relationships are often favorable, individuals with bimaxillary protrusion can often be dentally compensated by removal of upper second and lower first bicuspids. This often produces an aesthetically acceptable dental compromise, because the length of the mandibular corpus and position of the bony chin are acceptable. The second factor that needs to be considered concerns the individual with skeletal mandibular prognathia, secondary to an increase in ramus width.

In this group the clinician should consider surgical reduction in overall mandibular length by narrowing the ramus rather than the corpus. Procedures such as the internal vertical sliding osteotomy may be more effective in reducing mandibular prognathism in an individual with a wide ramus. However, the impact of malocclusion tendencies on treatment response is an area that desperately needs further study.

12

Control Processes in Facial Growth

There was a time, not long ago, when attempts to understand how facial growth is regulated were at a much simpler level. Most of the discussions seemed to settle on intrinsic "genetic" control versus everything else, such as biomechanical forces and hormones, and the lability of intramembranous versus the presumed preprogrammed (i.e., genetic) control of endochondral growth. A common approach was, and often still is, the naming of some special part or process that has the master power to control growth and thereby explain what can't be explained; a kind of theological disclaimer. From primitive civilization to today, if some particular phenomenon is not understood, a "deity" can be contrived to account for it, that is, a graven image, a fanciful invention of the mind. Thus, we have "condylar growth," and there has been abiding faith. Genetics itself has been such a deity, often misused to cover our insightful shortfall and to delude ourselves into believing that we understand what we fully do not. A common variation is the giving of descriptive titles, quite legitimate as far as they are intended to go, but which can be misused to try to explain the "how" when only the "what" is partially revealed (e.g., the functional matrix and Wolff's law of bone transformation). With regard to genetics, the old and compelling idea that there exist specific genes for virtually every structural detail throughout the craniofacial complex has been yielding to the newer concepts outlined herein. Furthermore, how selective gene activations are in **response** (effect, rather than cause) to extracellular signals is a direction receiving increasing understanding and emphasis.

The explanations of the growth control process that prevailed until just a few years ago were straightforward, easy to understand, and so plausible that they were adopted and used for many years as the basis for a number of clinical concepts. Most seemed to center on control of **bone** growth, probably because the bones are what are seen in headfilms and because any basic clinical change in the face requires a reshaping and resizing of the underlying bones. The entire process of growth control seemed no particular puzzle and readily explainable. First, the growth of bone tissue by cartilage growth plates was presumed to be regulated entirely and directly by the intrinsic genetic programming within the cartilage cells. Intramembranous bone growth, however, was believed to have a different source of control. This latter mode of the osteogenetic process was known to be particularly sensitive to biomechanical stress and strain and responds to tension and pressure by either bone deposition or resorption. Tension, as traditionally believed, specifically induces bone formation. Pressure, if it exceeds a relatively sensitive threshold limit, specifically triggers resorption. When tension is exerted on a bone, as at places of muscle attachment, the bone grows locally in response. Thus, sites of muscle insertion are usually marked by tuberosities, tubercles, and crests that form because of direct, localized fields of muscle traction. Because many muscles attach near the ends of a bone, rather than on its shaft, the epiphyses are much larger than the diaphysis, because this is where the muscles apply the most tension and where the bone thereby expands. As long as a muscle continues to grow, the bone is also stimulated to grow. This is because of the continuing biomechanical imbalance between them due to the expansion in muscle mass and resultant increasing force. The growing muscle would exceed the capacity of the bone to support it, and the osteoblasts are thereby triggered to form new bone in response. When muscle and overall body growth is complete, the bones attain biomechanical equilibrium with the muscles (and body weight, posture, and so forth). The forces of the muscles are then in balance with the physical properties of the bone. This turns off osteoblastic activity, and skeletal growth ceases. If any future circumstances cause departure from this sensitive state of bone–soft tissue equilibrium, such as major changes in body weight, loss of teeth, or the fracture of a bone, the process is revived until once again mechanical equilibrium subsequently becomes attained.

It is easy to understand why such up-front and reasonable explanations were attractive and almost universally adopted by earlier workers. For one thing, there is much basic truth in some of these concepts, as far as they go. They served to explain almost everything then known about bone and its growth. More recently, the realization that a number of shortcomings exist led to a reevaluation of the whole process of growth control. The subject has become a "new" frontier in facial biology. It is perhaps the most important clinical and research arena that now faces us.

First, there is no one-to-one correlation between places of muscle attachment and the pattern of distribution of resorptive and depository fields (Fig. 12–1); remodeling control is more biologically complex. Moreover, it is now known that there is no direct one-to-one correlation between tension deposition and pressure resorption (this old pressure versus tension concept is greatly oversimplified; see pages 113 and 117). This is important. About half of all craniofacial bone surfaces to which muscles attach are actually **resorptive**, not depository. Many muscles have widespread attachments, and within these surface areas, some growth fields are resorptive and others are depository. Yet these contrasting remodeling surfaces are subject to the same pull by the same muscle, supplied by the same blood vessels, and innervated by the same nerves. The temporalis muscle, for example, inserts onto the coronoid process of the mandible (Fig. 12–2). As shown in Chapter 4, parts of this mandibular region have external surfaces that are resorptive. The muscle exerts tension, but the bone to which it directly attaches undergoes resorption. Other surfaces of temporalis muscle attachment are characteristically depository.

Furthermore, some muscles pull in one direction, but the bone surfaces into which they insert grow in other directions. The pterygoid muscle, for example, attaches onto the posterior part of the ramus. The muscle pulls anteriorly, but this part of the bone remodels posteriorly.

Growth control involves a cascade of graded feedback chains from the systemic down to the local tissue, cellular, and molecular levels and back again. The problems at hand deal with the **local** control process in all the

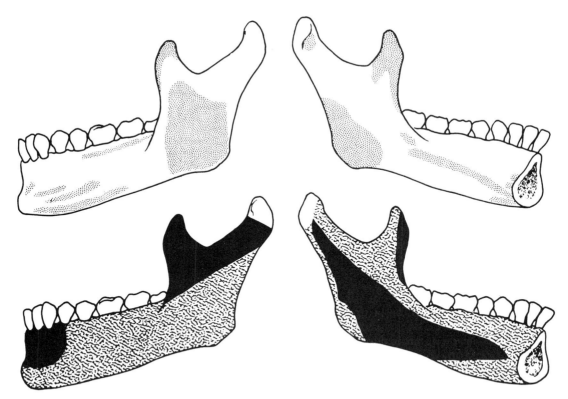

FIGURE 12–1. The top figures show the distribution of muscle attachments on the buccal and lingual sides of the mandible. The bottom figures illustrate the pattern of surface resorptive (dark) and depository (light) growth and remodeling fields. Note that there is no one-to-one correlation between these respective patterns. As described in the text, this does not mean that muscle forces are not involved in growth control; it does show, however, that the old "muscle-tension—direct bone deposition" concept is invalid. (From Enlow, D. H.: Wolff's law and the factor of architectonic circumstance. Am. J. Orthod., 54:803, 1968, with permission.)

regional parts everywhere. How each local area responds to the local activating signals involved in the local anatomy with local functions, and how each local region grows in concert with all other regions—this is the complex biologic holy grail. Learning to better control all this is the ultimate clinical objective.

SYNOPSIS OF CRANIOFACIAL GROWTH CONTROL THEORIES

Several alternative explanations attempting to address the questions on the ultimate basis of growth control, or some of its component aspects, have historically dominated the attention and thinking of leading biologic theoreticians. Although each such working theory is separate, a trend has always been to merge some of them selectively into a composite scheme in order to help account for the baffling array of poorly understood issues.

The Genetic Blueprint

Always at the forefront of any growth control discussion is the old and perplexing question of the real extent of "genetic" control. The role of ge-

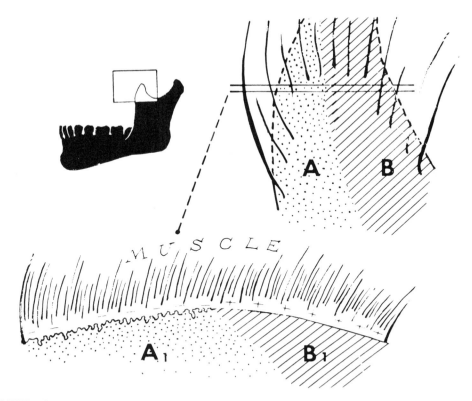

FIGURE 12–2. The temporalis muscle attaches to surface *A* and *B* on the lingual side of the coronoid process. In microscopic sections, it is seen that the attachment on A_1 involves a resorptive bone surface; the same muscle is also inserted on surface B_1, which is depository. (From Enlow, D. H.: Wolff's law and the factor of architectonic circumstance. Am. J. Orthod., 54:803, 1968, with permission.)

netic preprogramming has long been presumed by many to have a fundamental and perhaps overriding influence in establishing basic facial pattern and the features upon which internal and external "environment" then begins to play at some yet-to-be-understood levels. Contemporary researchers, however, have not been able to accept the idea that, simply stated, genes are the exclusive determinants for all growth parameters, including regional growth amounts, velocities, and minute details of regional configuration. Fully realized, of course, is the understanding that genes are indeed a basic participant in the operation of any given cell's organelles leading to the expression of that cell's particular function. For example, an osteoclast, a prechondroblast, or a contractile fibroblast each does its cellular function when activated, and it then ceases when signals deactivate it. Its own internal genes are not the actual "starter and stopper." In fact, the DNA content of all cells in the body is identical. It is the RNA being expressed by each cell type that determines the cell's intracellular and extracellular proteins and ultimately the functions of that cell line. At issue is the mechanism by which intercellular conditions **activate** an intracellular process, and just how the complex array of many different cell types and tissue combinations can manage to interact as a composite whole. **Selective** and **regulated** activation of specific genes within a cell's full genetic complement from without, however, is presumed to be one answer. A key factor is the recognition that **epigenetic** regulation can determine, to a substantial extent, the behavioral growth activities of "genic" tissue types. This means that these developmental "genic" tissues do not actually govern their own functions; rather, their role in growth is controlled by epigenetic influences from **other** tissue groups and their functional, structural, and developmental input signals.

Biomechanical Forces

A powerful line of reasoning has historically focused on the play of physical forces acting on a bone to regulate its development, morphologic configuration, histologic structure, and physical properties. Wolff's law of bone transformation, introduced in the late 1800s, quickly became a leading and most useful working concept, and is still quite valid **if** it is not overextended. Essentially, an application of the old and trusted idea that form interrelates with and is inseparable from function, this cornerstone principle states the biologic truism that a bone grows and develops in such a manner that the composite of physiologic forces exerted on it are accommodated by the bone's developmental process, thereby adapting structure to the complex of functions. This descriptive perspective, however, has often been overstated; it has been presumed that the actual biologic process of developmental control is explained, that is, **how** control of development is carried out, rather than simply a description of what is happening. One principal omission (and a major flaw) in many old attempts to apply Wolff's law has been a lack of distinction between physical forces acting on a bone (i.e., its hard part) and forces acting on the osteogenic connective tissues (periosteum, growth cartilages, sutures, etc.) that actually produce and remodel the bone.

Many experiments have been carried out in which muscles were severed, or the soft tissues otherwise altered, and in which artificial mechanical forces were experimentally exerted on a living bone. Because such procedures always produce some kind of response with resultant changes in the form of the bone, it has often been concluded that stress is, therefore, the principal factor controlling bone growth. Such experiments, however, do not "prove" such a role for the mechanical forces, since certain critical variables necessarily exist that cannot be controlled in the experimental design. These include vascular and neural interruption, temperature changes, alterations in pH and oxygen tension, and so on, all of which are known to affect bone growth. The fundamental question must then be asked: Do extrinsic or unusual factors that can affect the course of a bone's development also necessarily represent the same intrinsic factors that actually carry out the direct, primary control of the basic histogenic processes of growth and differentiation? That key question is simply not addressed. Nonetheless, there can be no doubt whatsoever that mechanical forces, indeed, represent one (of many) of the "messengers" (see below) involved in the activation of osteogenic connective tissue. What **regulates** the complex **balance** of "genic" activities among all the multitude of cell and tissue participants is the key issue.

Sutures, Condyles, and Synchondroses

In the 1920s, a then new model for growth control began to emerge that flourished through the 1940s and 1950s, with some holdover yet even today. Many of the groundbreaking ideas within these pioneering explanations have since been set aside and replaced by more biologically tuned and complete understandings. They did, nonetheless, introduce issues that led to much basic research and new, more on-target questions to be asked. History was served.

It was presumed, quite reasonably at the time, that the growth, form, and dimensions of a bone are governed by intrinsic genetic programming residing within that bone's own bone-producing cells of the periosteum, sutures, and bone-related cartilages. While influences such as hormones and muscle actions could augment these gene-dominant growth determinants, bones such as the mandible or maxilla, and all of their morphologic features, were held to be largely self-generated products. The displacements of bones as they enlarge were also attributed to the expansive forces residing within their osteogenic sutures and cartilages and a "thrust" by the new bone tissues they produce. The idea expanded to include a concept of growth "centers" that were presumed to provide inclusive growth regulation for each of the whole bones they serve. Today, most front-line researchers discount the notion of such "master growth centers," replacing it with a concept of regional "sites" of growth, each of which is a localized area having its own regional circumstances and conditions and which operates under its own regional process of growth control. A feedback system allows reciprocal growth interactions and developmental adaptations with the other sites.

The Nasal Septum

It became understood (albeit slowly, historically) that "centers," such as the facial sutures, cannot actually **drive** the nasomaxillary complex into downward and forward displacement. This is because a suture is a traction-adapted (not a "pushing" and pressure-adapted) type of tissue. To try to resolve the dilemma that then arose, James Scott, a well-known Irish anatomist, reasoned that the cartilaginous nasal septum has features and occupies a strategic position that might answer the question of what "motor" causes the midface to displace anteriorly and inferiorly as it grows in size. Because cartilage is a more pressure-tolerant tissue than the vascular-sensitive sutures, it presumably has the developmental capacity to expansively **push** the whole nasomaxillary complex downward and forward. With this thought, Scott's famous nasal septum theory was born.

The laboratory testing of this theory has been a concerted target of many researchers for many years since, but the idea has encountered formidable laboratory obstacles because of difficulties in controlling the multiple developmental variables involved. This has led to differing interpretations of the experimental results. One problem is that animal experiments of the kind here relevant almost always involve conditions in which functions normally carried out by some given anatomic structure, when that anatomic part is altered or excised, can be compensated to some extent by other structures. Or, it cannot be presumed that, if some structural part is experimentally removed, what happens as a consequence, therefore, reflects the actual function of that part in situ. Then, too, importantly, it cannot be simply assumed that any given structure's function is the same when conditions have been experimentally altered as when they existed in an undisturbed (nonexperimental) state. Moreover, the actual physical force for the maxillary displacement movement may be, at least in part, a pulling action of the septopremaxillary ligament resulting from septal enlargement, rather than a pushing action (Latham, 1970). Such an effect can be noted in a bilateral palatal cleft: the embryonic nasomedial process ("premaxilla") is displaced protrusively, but without maxillary-to-premaxillary sutural attachment, the maxillae are not drawn forward and thus left behind retrusively. Other concerns are outlined in Chapter 1.

Whether or not the nasal septum operates as the essential pacemaker for maxillary displacement, it nonetheless has membership as a component of the "functional matrix," and it thereby contributes its own share of developmental participation in combination with all the other components necessarily also involved.

An important and most fundamental conceptual advance is that the old notion in which any single, presiding agent, such as the nasal septum or condyle, has sole responsibility for pacesetting the growth process has been preempted by concepts involving **multifactorial** interrelationships. This is highlighted later as well as discussions in several previous chapters.

The Functional Matrix

Basic form/function principles proposed by van der Klaauw were greatly elaborated by Melvin Moss and evolved into a landmark concept having great impact among practicing clinicians and craniofacial theoreticians alike. Although some of the deeper issues involved were heatedly controversial for a time, one very valued outcome was a most intensive and productive debate on important questions and a great deal of new research.

Simply stated and omitting some details, the "functional matrix" concept deals primarily with the ultimate source of osteogenetic regulation. Although many aspects were clouded historically by operational uncertainties as to "**how**" it operates, the core of the idea is straightforward and not in itself controversial.

The role of genes in cellular organelle functioning (e.g., production of specific tissue protein types, enzymes) in response to extracellular messengers that activate a given cell's physiologic role in the grand scheme is not an issue. Stimuli emanating from the **growth** and the **actions** of all the multiple sources within the growing head and body (the functional matrix), directly or indirectly, function to turn on or turn off cellular organelle activity in each and all of the "genic" tissues. This yields growing, changing, custom-fitted bones having regional dimensions and changing configurations that update constantly to accommodate the changing developmental conditions and biomechanical circumstances in each localized region of each separate bone and the aggregate of all in an interrelated system. Each bone becomes **continuously** and precisely adapted to these multiple developmental conditions because it is the composite of these conditions that regulate a bone's ongoing configuration, size, fitting, and the timing involved.

The functional matrix concept is not intended to explain **how** the actual morphogenic process works, but, rather, describes **what** happens to achieve the combination of actions, reactions, and feedback interplay that occurs. This is important. The nature of the signals involved and how they operate are separate but quite significant issues dealt with later.

A basic consideration, also, is that the term "functional matrix" can be misleading, because it connotes primarily the function of a soft tissue part (e.g., muscle contraction). **Growth enlargements** are also directly involved in giving the signals that activate osteogenic connective tissues, and this is an equally significant factor (see Fig. 1–7). Also, the functional matrix concept was developed primarily for bone growth; the biologic principles involved can be extended effectively to soft tissues as well.

Composite Explanations

Many experimental studies, together with observations of certain congenital craniofacial dysplasias ("nature's experiments") and much theoretical reasoning, led to combinations of various growth control theories attempting to account for the complexities of development. Some were grouped by van Limborgh, for example, into a model that distinguishes factors influencing chondrocranial versus desmocranial (intramembranous) craniofacial development. With the chondrocranium serving as an early but ongoing pacer, intrinsic genetic cell multiplication capability, general epigenetic influence (e.g., hormones), and general environmental factors (food and oxygen supply, etc.) were all proposed as agents within an interplay scheme for the endochondral part of basicranial developmental control. Desmocranial development, separately, was described as a morphogenic response to some balance among most of these factors, but with local epigenetic and local environmental factors (mechanical forces) playing a dominant regulatory role.

The elegant studies of Petrovic and his colleagues have had great impact on the directions of thinking among contemporary craniofacial biologists. Emerging from their long-term experimental work have been elaborate cybernetic models that illustrate, in extensive detail, many of the complex developmental interrelationships among almost all of the multiple cellular and tissue elements involved in growth control. Professional students going beyond the present chapter's introduction on "control" will need to utilize their insight as a springboard.

Control Messengers

Growth control is essentially a localized developmental process working with local function as it responds to multiple developmental interplay with other growing parts. It is complemented all the while by systemic support. Growth is carried out by specific, restricted, regional **fields**, each of which has differing growth activity in amounts, directions, velocities, and timing (described in earlier chapters). The diverse cell populations within each of these fields respond to activating intracellular or extracellular signals. "First messengers" are extracellular activators for which specific cell-surface receptors are selectively sensitive. They include biomechanical, bioelectric, hormonal, enzymatic, oxygen, carbon dioxide, etc., factors. A reception signal then fires a cascade of "second messengers" within a given cell that results in the function of that cell and its organelles, such as fiber production and proteoglycan production, calcification, acid or alkaline phosphatase secretion, and rate and duration of mitotic cell divisions. Adenyl cyclase and cyclic adenosine monophosphate (cAMP) are second messengers leading to cytoplasmic and nuclear DNA-RNA transfers.

In the **immediate** environment enclosing an osteoblast or osteoclast, a first-messenger hormone or enzyme, a bioelectric potential change, or a pressure/tension factor acting on the cell's outer sensory membrane receptors can activate a second messenger (membrane-bound adenyl cyclase), which in turn accelerates the transformation of adenosine triphosphate (ATP) to cAMP within the cytoplasm, which then activates the synthesis of other specific enzymes relating specifically to bone deposition or resorption. Ionic calcium is mobilized from mitochondrion storage, and inner and outer membrane permeability is altered that selectively controls the flux of other ions in the synthesis and discharge of the products secreted by the cell.

During bone formation, the osteoblast takes in amino acids, glucose, and sulfate for the synthesis of the glycoproteins and collagen in the formative organic part of the bone matrix. The cytoplasmic organelles within the osteoblast participate in the formation, storage, and secretion of tropocollagen, the mucopolysaccharide ground substance, and also ions that form the inorganic (hydroxyapatite) phase of the bone matrix. Alkaline glycerophosphatase is related to bone formation (in contrast to acid phosphatase, which relates to resorption) and is associated with the collagen fibril as it is released from the osteoblast. High levels of alkaline phosphatase are also involved in the formation of the hydroxyapatite. The citric acid cycle and glycolytic enzymes provide generalized energy sources for all these activities.

The osteoclast contains an abundance of mitochondria in addition to lysosomes and an extensive endoplasmic smooth membrane system. The osteoclast produces, stores, and secretes enzymes (such as collagenase) and acids that relate to the breakdown of both the organic and inorganic components of bone. The lysosomes are involved in acid phosphatase storage and transport. First messengers, such as parathyroid hormone or bioelectric charges, stimulate receptor sites on the cell membrane. This activates adenyl cyclase, which in turn causes increases in cytoplasmic AMP. The latter then increases the permeability of the lysosomal membrane. By an exocytosis of the lysosomal contents, the resorption of both the organic and inorganic parts of the bone is carried out through the activity of the acid hydrolases, lactates, and citrates. The endoplasmic smooth membrane system is also involved in this process of enzyme transport and release.

Bioelectric Signals

The piezo factor has been one of the great bone growth-control hopes since the mid-1960s and has promised to clarify just how muscle and other biomechanical force actions can be translated into precisely regulated bone remodeling responses. The idea, in brief, is that distortions of the collagen crystals in bone, caused by minute (ultramicroscopic) deformations of the bone matrix due to mechanical strains, generate bioelectric charges in the immediate area of deformation (i.e, the piezo effect). These altered electrical potentials appear to relate, either directly or indirectly, to the triggering of osteoblastic and osteoclastic responses (see page 119).

To put this factor in perspective, one key point must be understood. There are two separate **target categories** for the mechanical actions of muscles, and also the effect of muscle and soft tissue growth enlargements, gravity, and all other such physical sources. One target is the cellular component of the osteogenic **connective tissues** that cover a bone. The outer surfaces of these cells are loaded with receptors that are sensitive to the **direct** effects of first messenger agents and forces. The second basic target category is the calcified part of the bone itself, the matrix, in contrast to the covering connective tissues just mentioned. Mechanical forces produced both by growth and by function acting on the calcified matrix cause minute distortions that generate positive and negative polarities. While response thresholds of regional force levels are still poorly understood, a minute **concavity** under active distortion is known to emanate a negative (−) bioelectric charge, and a **convexity** generates a positive (+) charge. (Figure 7−9 shows a schematic "bone" responding to a force, producing a convex side and a concave side, and the resulting bioelectric potentials created.) Negative charges then transmit to the osteogenic cells within the connective tissue on the concave side firing osteoblasts into depository activity. A positive charge on the convex side activates an osteoclastic response. The result is **coordinated regional** remodeling, inside and outside surfaces alike, that shapes the bone and enlarges its overall size. When mechanical equilibrium is achieved between the bone and the composite of growth and functional forces playing on it, the polarities are neutralized, and the remodeling activities are turned off.

This scheme appears to explain nicely the actual basis for remodeling **coordination** between the periosteal side and the contralateral endosteal surface in a given region of a bone; that is, one side can be convex, and the other concave, with the common forces acting within this region thus resulting in complementary deposition/resorption responses. Also, note that the pressure/tension and deposition/resorption responses characterizing the osteogenic connective tissue membrane versus the bone matrix itself are opposites. (See pages 119 to 120 for further discussion.) While the piezo electric effect has been found to be a good model for long-bone remodeling, recent studies suggest that other factors may be involved in tooth movement and alveolar bone remodeling (Tuncay et al., 1990, 1994).

There is a key question, however, that contemporary researchers appear not yet to have asked, at least to date: an explanation of the nature of the **balance and interplay** between growth-affecting mechanical forces acting directly on a bone's **osteogenic membranes** (the first category) versus forces acting on the **bone matrix itself** (second category). Since the respective force-causing responses are actually reversed, a threshold sensitivity or some synergistic means for selectivity must be operative. There is a basic need for resolving this key question, yet the question itself has yet to be asked by researchers.

Other Factors of Growth Control

The **neurotropic factor** involves the network of nerves (all kinds, motor as well as sensory) as links for feedback interrelationships among all the soft tissues and bone. Researchers are increasingly interested in the supporting cells of the nervous system (e.g., Schwann, glial); the potential role of these cells in the growth process is mostly unexplored. The nerves are believed to provide pathways for stimuli that presumably can trigger certain bone and soft tissue remodeling responses. It is not believed, however, that this process is carried out by actual nervous impulses. Rather, it appears to function by transport of neurosecretory material along nerve tracts (analogous perhaps to the neurohumoral flow from the hypothalamus to the neurohypophysis along tracts in the infundibulum) or by an exoplasmic streaming within the neuron. In this way, feedback information is passed, for example, from the connective tissue stroma of a muscle to the osteogenic periosteum of the bone associated with that muscle. The "functional matrix" thereby operates to govern the bone's development. It is an interesting but yet incomplete hypothesis in need of more study.

A great many laboratory investigations are now being conducted in attempts to clarify relationships between, for example, AMP and biomechanical forces. Other independent studies have been underway, most not even dealing with craniofacial biology per se, on the role of important substances such as the cascade of prostaglandins, somatomedins, osteonectines, leukotrienes, possible neurotropic balancing agents, and intercellular communications involving "G" proteins. Still other work is ongoing seeking out possible chalone-like agents in bone (i.e., localized tissue-level, hormone-like substances believed to affect the magnitude of cell divisions). Day by day, new information and new links are being added. A real problem is that such frontier research is proceeding quite separate from our own craniofacial mainstream, and with very little input. However, to help place all these old and new factors in some kind of working perspective, one can use the following relative simple "test" to classify their respective roles:

1.   Is a given factor held to be the sole, primary agent that is directly responsible for the master control of growth? Of course, such a single, ubiquitous agent does not exist. Historically, bone investigators have

searched for such a master control factor, perhaps a special "hormone" or special "inductor," that does it all. However, it is now realized that the control process must necessarily be multifactorial and control involves a multidirectional chain of regulatory links. Not all of the individual links participate in all types of growth changes. Rather, selected directional combinations exist for different specific control pathways that follow many objective routes and involve many different agents.

2. Does a given factor function as a "trigger" that induces or turns on other specific, selected agents that then launch the process of control response? Is it the first link in the lengthy chain? Is it the initial agent in the process of "induction"? Is it a "first messenger"? Biomechanical forces presumably represent such a trigger. It is still justifiably believed that pressures and tensions are indeed among the basic agents involved in eventual growth control (although not following the traditional but over-simplified historical explanations). Different kinds of bone, however, appear to have variable thresholds of response to physical forces (e.g., basal bone versus alveolar bone in the mandible and maxilla, which are relatively nonsensitive versus quite labile, respectively, to physical strain). It is also evident that biomechanical forces are not the sole agents participating in control. Even when involved, many other links are also required as second and third level messengers. Oxygen tension at the intercellular level may be another example, since this factor is known to be involved in "genic" cell differentiation.

3. Is a given factor, in effect, the **title** for some biologic process without accounting for the actual operational mechanism involved? This is an important category. **Such a title describes what happens, but not how it happens.** It does not explain the implementation and mechanics of the control process it is presumed to represent. It is just, in effect, a synonym for "control process" without explaining how it actually works. The reason an awareness of this category is so important is that we all often tend to use such titles as though they do indeed explain the mechanism involved. With continued use, we delude ourselves into believing that we actually understand the real basis for the control process itself. "Wolff's law," "functional matrix," "genetics," "induction," and even "development" itself are all such descriptive labels for biologic control systems. While each has a legitimate and valid place in describing the events that occur during growth, they do not, of course, explain how the system works (each was never intended for this ultimate purpose, even though all of us have often misused them as such). Be ever alert to this common and deceptive conceptual pitfall. (See also the "graven image" analogy used to explain what we do not fully understand, page 210.)

4. Does a given factor function essentially in a supportive role or as a catalyst? Many nutrients would be examples of this category.

5. Does a given factor accompany the control process, but not actually take part in a determinative way? It has been necessary for laboratory researchers studying the piezo effect, for example, to establish whether bioelectric potentials are actually first messengers or whether they simply "occur" in a by-product and non–remodeling-activating role.

6. Is a given factor an actual cause, rather than an inert effect, in the growth control process? The piezo factor also serves as an example of this category. Do bioelectric charges in bone directly trigger remodeling responses, or are the responses merely the incidental result? Is there an intermediary role for this factor? Whatever future research answers this question, the replacement ideas will be subject to the same tests.

One fundamental feature of the control process is now clear. No given tissue, such as bone, grows and differentiates in an isolated, independent manner by a wholly intrinsic regulatory process. Control is essentially a system of complex intercellular feedback pathways, informational interchanges, and reciprocal responses. Tissues, organs and parts of organs all necessarily develop as packages, all differentiating in close interplay. A given bone and all its muscles, nerves, blood vessels, connective tissues, and epithelia is an interdependent, developmental composite. Bones have specific mechanisms for increasing in length (e.g., an epiphyseal plate, synchondrosis, condyle), and they have another specific mechanism for increasing in width (subperiosteal intramembranous remodeling). Correspondingly, muscles also have a specific growth mechanism for increases in length and another, separately, for increases in width. Both of these conjoint muscle growth processes proceed in concert with respective linear and diametrical growth mechanisms for the bone. There are reciprocal feedback interrelationships between the muscle and bone, as well as the various other tissues, and they all enlarge together, not as "separate," independent, and self-contained units. For example, input to the sensory nerve endings in the periodontal membrane can trigger alveolar remodeling responses to occlusal signals from the teeth. These same signals can be passed on through an arc to motor nerves supplying the muscles of mastication. In conjunction with muscle adaptations to the individualized nature of the occlusion, then, the bones of the face undergo widespread, regional remodeling in association with the muscles and soft tissue matrix. The old concept that a "growth cartilage," simply, serves as the primary self-contained regulator for the overall development of the facial and mandibular musculoskeletal composite is now regarded as an unacceptable explanation. This is because many input factors are now known to be involved. However, we still have a long way to go in understanding the whole of the growth control system. History will probably judge this as one of the great problems of our time.

THE ARCHITECTONICS OF GROWTH CONTROL: A SUMMARY

A diverse collection of factors that need to be taken into account whenever dealing with facial "growth control" has been drawn from previous chapters. These are presented below as a series of separate points and issues with emphasis on the "architectonics" of growth control—simply, the dynamics of the developmental interrelationships among all of the growing parts, soft and hard tissues alike, and how this enters into the Big Picture.

1. Growth is a **differential** process of progressive maturation. Different parts have different schedules in which changing growth velocities occur at different times, by different regional amounts, and in different regional directions. For example, vertical facial development has a quite different morphogenic timetable than the transverse because bilateral basicranial width is precocious, compared with facial airway enlargement and tooth eruption. The airway relates to whole body and lung development, whereas the bicondylar and bizygomatic dimensions relate to the earlier transverse maturation of the cerebral temporal and frontal lobes with their basicranial fossae. This creates many developmental complexities. For example, the architectonics of mandibular growth control must thereby provide for a differential timing of whole-ramus (not just condylar) development to adapt to differences in vertical versus anteroposterior maturation of the pharyngeal compartment as well as, at the same time, dif-

ferential anteroposterior versus vertical growth enlargements, remodeling, and displacement of the nasomaxillary complex, including its airway and erupting dental components. This indeed requires fancy developmental footwork on the part of the growing ramus if precision of dimensional changes, fitting of separate parts, and proper timing are to be collectively achieved. The developmental complexities here cannot be overstated.

2. **Development is a process working toward an ongoing state of aggregate, composite structural and functional equilibrium.** Growth, of course, involves constant changes in size, shape, and relationships among all of the separate parts and the regional components of each part. Any change in any given part must be proportionately matched by appropriate growth changes and adjustments in **many** other parts, nearby as well as distant, to sustain and progressively achieve functional and structural balance of the whole. In short, growth anywhere in any region, local area, or part, is **not isolated.** This seems quite obvious; yet the complex of **interrelations** that exist is often bypassed in our thinking and in the literature. "Balance" is a developmental aggregate involving close interplay throughout. For example, the shape and size of one's external nose and facial airway are not determined solely by blueprint (or any other kind of control) just within these parts themselves, since many other parts elsewhere establish rigid developmental conditions. Interorbital width and nasomaxillary boundaries presented by the basicranium, for example, require reciprocal compliance of any genetic, epigenetic, or soft tissue growth determinants acting on the separate "genic" tissues that produce the growing nasal region.

Certain regional **imbalances** exist in everyone that are natural and architectonically inescapable (Chapters 1, 9, and 10). Individual or population differences in headform configuration, for example, establish corresponding differences in the basicranial template for many facial dimensions, growth field boundaries, and component alignments. These variations set up many different kinds of facial configurations within which some "imbalances" have necessarily been introduced because of architectural complexity. However, growth and development work toward a state of aggregate architectonic equilibrium, so that emerging from the process of development are certain other regional "imbalances" that are offsetting and compensating. Groups of localized imbalances thus can balance other groups of imbalances as a normal part of the growth control process, the composite of which is more or less in functional equilibrium. Nonetheless, virtually limitless morphologic variations have been introduced, most of which we regard as more or less normal. For some others, the latitude for developmental adjustment is exceeded, and a malocclusion or some other structural dysplasia results, even though "balanced" in itself. In a sense, the process of growth and development is nature's own clinician, and it usually works quite well, even though various malocclusion **tendencies** exist in all of us because of established, normal headform type variations.

In addition to different phylogenic lines (e.g., headform variations) leading to developmental facial variations, ontogenic factors are involved as well. Mouth breathing is an example. A broken lip seal requires different muscle actions for mandibular posturing, and an open-jaw swallow similarly requires different muscular combinations. These factors produce different signals to the osteogenic, chondrogenic, myogenic, and fibrogenic components that revise the course of development, thus leading to adjustive morphologic variations to create a developmental balance among parts that had become morphogenetically imbalanced. (See Fig. 1–7.)

3. The goodness of fit among contiguous anatomic parts and groups of parts is remarkable. Consider the extreme precision of shape and size

fitting between, for example, the temporalis muscle and its bony coronoid process; or the fit between a tooth's root and its alveolar socket; or one bone in sutural articulation with another. Developmental interplay establishes this, while all the time sustaining continuous growth and function. This requires a kind of "servo" system to create the architectonic exchange of signals that turn on or off, up or down, the cytogenic responses that drive the remodeling progression. Consider a cranial nerve and its basicranial foramen. The size and shape of the foramen must **precisely** match its nerve and perineural connective and vascular tissues. As the latter grow and develop, so must the foramen with no mismatch whatever. Then, as the nerve **moves** with the developing brain, the foramen must likewise remodel in **precise** lockstep. This is one example of the many delicate, very significant kinds of developmental relationships that all too often have gone unsung in our appreciation of the Big Picture.

4.   If we consider only bony components, we see that each bone and all of its regional parts participate directly and actively. Most of us readily acknowledge this. Why, then, do we persist in highlighting just a mandibular condyle, for example, while largely ignoring the rest of the ramus, which is just as significant and developmentally noteworthy in the Big Picture. It is the **whole** ramus that is a respondent to the massive growth-influencing muscles of mastication, and it is the development of the **whole** ramus and all of its parts, in teamwork, that places the mandibular arch, and establishes mandibular fitting with the maxilla on one side and the basicranium on the other.

It is important to understand that there is no common, overriding, **centralized** control force that regulates the developmental and anatomic details for each individual region throughout any given whole bone. Rather, the different regional areas have different **local** developmental, functional, and structural conditions and circumstances that generate appropriate regional signals activating all local osteogenic connective tissues (periosteum, endosteum, cartilages, sutures, periodontal membranes) for precision operation of their responses as a part of the overall growth control system. This provides the **regional** balances and goodness-of-fit among parts, as highlighted herein.

5.   The nature and capacity for interrelated growth adjustments among separate parts vary among different tissue types. Bone, for example, has a wide latitude for responsive remodeling adaptations through intrinsic manipulation of the osteogenic connective tissues to produce size and shape conformation in precision fitting. A tooth, in contrast, has a much lower potential for adjustive remodeling and, hence, teeth undergo posteruptive growth movements and location changes mostly by a displacement process. An **occlusal curve** is another such intrinsic developmental adjustment of the dentition and its alveolar bone to developmental conditions imposed on the dental arches from without. **Anterior crowding** is another and, while a "malocclusion," is actually an adjustive compensation to provide fitting of the dentition within a prescribed growth field as established by other, multiple architectonic and morphogenic relationships. One imbalance has balanced others to achieve a kind of aggregate structural equilibrium. This concept of dental crowding as a biologically necessary compensatory mechanism to allow adjustment to changes in regional and global growth fields has important implications for the orthodontic clinician. Currently, lifelong retention of dental alignment is advocated by many clinicians. This recommendation is often thought to have no associated risk. However, if changes in dental alignment occur to maintain a healthy occlusion in a changing environment, preventing those changes may lead to pathologic degeneration of the teeth or supporting

structures. This theoretical problem may indeed become a real concern as lifetime retention gains increasing popularity in the orthodontically treated population.

The capacity for remodeling of cartilage, either interstitially or by its chondrogenic connective tissue, is also much more constrained than for bone. **Condylar** cartilage can, however, undergo alterations in growth direction and magnitude by differential turning on and turning off of prechondroblastic proliferation around its periphery, thus producing adaptive growth vectors in response to changing architectonic conditions. This is in contrast, significantly, to the "primary" cartilages of the basicranium and long bones.

6.   The two principal categories of growth movement, **displacement** and **remodeling**, is one of the most fundamental concepts of growth. Yet to this day, this all-important facet, more often than not, is totally disregarded when trying to account for how a given appliance or other clinical procedure is presumed to work. The significance of this point cannot be overemphasized. Both types of movement are usually clumped together simply as "growth" without distinguishing between them. The reason distinction is very important is that each represents a separate and distinct target in the intrinsic control process utilized for different clinical procedures. Headgear, for example, manipulates directions and magnitudes of the displacement type of movement (whole-bone and soft tissue movements), with bony and soft tissue remodeling then providing adjustments to altered whole-part placements. Periodontal connective tissue responses to fixed appliances activate alveolar remodeling adjustments in response to tooth displacements. Functional appliances presumably activate altered combinations of displacement and remodeling up and down the line. Some orthognathic procedures involve the surgical moving of bones or their parts followed by osteogenic transplants, thus paralleling that which natural growth did not fully achieve—displacement (surgical movements) and remodeling (sizing and shaping by transplants). This also highlights the reason bony articulations, including sutures, movable joints, synchondroses, and tooth junctions, need a full share of attention in understanding the growth process and its control. They are the places from which displacement movements emanate as a given bone simultaneously undergoes its remodeling by the enclosing osteogenic and chondrogenic connective tissues. Displacement moves whole bones away from each other at their joint contacts, thus complementing their enlargements. Remodeling, at the same time, produces the enlargement, constructs the configuration and its progressive changes, provides precision fitting with contiguous soft tissues and with other bones, and creates the ongoing "compensations" or adjustments leading to a composite working equilibrium among all the separate parts.

Another example of the displacement/remodeling combination is the placement and development of the incisor part of the maxilla. By far, most of the actual downward-forward "growth" of the premaxillary region is by whole-maxilla movement caused by enlargements of all the other craniofacial parts above and behind, not just intrinsic remodeling growth within that localized premaxillary region itself. Localized remodeling produces the size and shape of that regional area, but most of its considerable extent of growth movement over the years is a product of secondary displacement.

7.   Variation in headform, as previously mentioned, is an important factor. The reason is that the dolicho, brachy, or dinaric types establish quite different basicranial templates for facial development. Whatever growth control resides within the mandibular and ethmomaxillary components themselves must necessarily yield and conform to a higher level of pre-

determination in a number of respects. For example, facial shape and proportions are projections of the anterior cranial fossa and can incorporate any basicranial asymmetries that exist. The apical base of the maxillary dentition, in turn, is established by the basicranial-determined configuration and size of the palatal perimeter. For another example, the middle cranial fossa establishes the anteroposterior placement of the maxilla relative to the mandible. Because it is known that (1) variations in headform set up corresponding variations in facial type and pattern, (2) headform variations predispose specific, corresponding malocclusion tendencies, (3) headform and resultant facial variations involving different anatomic combinations respond differently to different treatment procedures, and (4) that different rebound tendencies exist in different pattern combinations, **much** closer attention should be given to headform consideration than at present. A Class I dinaric has a different anatomic combination than a Class I brachycephalic, and both are basically different than a Class I dolichocephalic. The intrinsic control of facial growth, therefore, is strongly influenced by factors external to the face itself, and this must be taken into account in our Big Architectonic Picture. Predispositions for variations in mandibular retrusive versus protrusive tendencies are **built into** the phylogenetic heritage of different population groups.

Beginning students are inclined to perceived the Class I category as an anatomically separate and distinct type having good overall balance for each regional part with only minor departures from an ideal. Not so. In the assembly of all the multitude of craniofacial parts, **all** of us have a multitude of regional phylogenic and headform-established imbalances throughout the craniofacial complex, as briefly summarized above. Some of these are mandibular retrusive and others protrusive in their regional effects. If the aggregate is offsetting (i.e., a balancing of imbalances), a Class I results, but with a "tendency" one way or the other because the underlying features that are retrusive-causing or protrusive-causing still exist, but are partially nullified by the compensations. The Class I is in the middle span between the extremes of this spectrum involving multiple composites of different architectonic combinations but with two sides grading away in opposite directions.

8.   With regard to our phylogenic facial heritage, the factor of bipedal body posture interrelating with our enormous human brain and marked basicranial flexure have led to an inferoposterior rotational placement of the nasomaxillary complex. The midface has come to lie **below** the anterior cranial fossa, rather than protruding largely forward from it. This has caught the mandible in a closing vise between the midface above and the pharyngeal airway, gullet, and cervical column behind. Overjet, overbite, anterior crossbite, and an unprecedented developmental problem situation for the human temporomandibular joint (TMJ) are some consequences. The adaptive remodeling capacity of the ramus, with its condyle, is especially noteworthy in adjusting to these severe conditions. The wonder is not that so much TMJ distress as a common clinical result exists, but rather, that there is not much more.

Furthermore, the human basicranial suture growth system, inherited from smaller brained ancestors, cannot provide for the full range needed to accommodate our grossly enlarged brain. Thus, an unusual basicranial remodeling pattern, not found in any other known mammal including anthropoids, has been added to the human growth package. Still another evolutionary factor is that of orbital convergence toward the midline in conjunction with enlarged temporal lobe expansion. Together with facial rotation, nasal configuration and placement are affected, since the interorbital (nasal) compartment has become significantly reduced as well as moved into a vertical position. Human nasomaxillary development has adjusted, in many regional ways, to these major phylogenic and ontogenic conditions.

9.   With respect to growth rotations, this timely subject has justifiably become of great interest. The classification of rotation types is simple: some are "displacement" types, and some are "remodeling" rotations. (The literature is needlessly confusing on this subject.) Remodeling rotations represent one of the developmental adjustments ("compensations") emphasized above. For example, basicranial growth can predispose a nasomaxillary "displacement rotation" that would "unbalance" the alignment of the palate. By differential "remodeling rotation" of the anterior versus posterior parts of the palate, however, the palate as a whole can be progressively leveled into a functional position as the basicranium grows. Similar mandibular rotations exist in relation to variable basicranial proportions as well as midfacial size, configuration, rotations, and alignment variations. The architectonic factor of developmental rotations thus enters prominently into our Big Picture of selective, regional growth control factors.

10.   Considering architectonic feedback communication and give-and-take regional adaptations in the interrelationships involved in growth control, three examples stand out in which component parts each play a particularly significant role. One is the mandibular ramus; the second is the periodontal connective tissue membrane; and the third is the insignificant-appearing little lacrimal bone.

In a typical gross anatomy course for freshmen, the ramus is usually dismissed as just a handle (the word itself means "branch") for masticatory muscle attachments, which is surely important enough. But how much more dynamic for the student if its **other** very interesting and essential (developmental) functions were also dramatized. Consider first, that the ramus bridges the pharyngeal space to functionally position the lower arch in changing occlusion with the upper. The enlargement of this changing pharyngeal space is progressively established by its ceiling, which is formed by the enlarging middle cranial fossae and their growing temporal lobes, a morphogenic process continuing long into childhood. The antero-posterior breadth of the ramus must **match** this basicranial developmental progression, with multiple and diverse basicranial, maxillary, and mandibular rotations also taken into account, by equivalent growth amounts and with corresponding timing—an elaborate architectonic interrelationship of many separate parts. Otherwise, either excessive anterior crossbite or mandibular retrusion would ensue. Furthermore, the vertical height of the ramus must match the changing vertical increases of the nasal and dental parts of the ethmomaxillary complex, taking into account the vertical lengthening of the middle cranial fossae as well and, importantly, marked differences in vertical versus horizontal timing within the nasomaxillary complex and basicranium. Too much or too little and too early or too late sets up an anterior deep or open bite, and the latitude for mismatch is very slight. All of this requires a precision and coordination of signals given to the osteogenic connective tissues that enclose the ramus, which respond by enlarging, relocating, rotating, shaping, and constantly adjusting the whole ramus (and its condyle). This is a most remarkable complex and histogenically interplay among the separate parts involved.

The periodontal membrane (PDM) is a "genic" connective tissue that shapes, sizes, and constantly remodels and relocates the alveolar bone to match its moving, resident teeth and which also carries the teeth in vertical and horizontal drifting movements in addition to their initial eruption. The PDM is a dynamic, complex connective tissue membrane with many and diverse component elements (often demeaned as merely a connecting "ligament") responsive to the multiple signals that activate its multiple cell types to carry out these architectonic growth functions. In addition, the PDM contributes to tooth formation and provides vascular pathways and proprioceptive and other sensory and vasomotor innervations. Consider the high degree of precision required of the intrinsic control process in coordinating tooth movement and alveolar remodeling. The direction, amount, and timing must be absolutely precise, with virtually no divergence. It is the wondrous PDM that carries all this out. Clinically, this elaborately coordinated growth process is manipulated by substituting clinical control to override the intrinsic control. But the histogenic process itself is the same. The remarkable PDM and its symphony of movements are a workhorse for the orthodontist.

The tiny, thin flake of a lacrimal bone receives little, if any, attention in a standard gross anatomy course and given no special highlight at all. Yet phylogenetically this seemingly insignificant little bone has survived as a discrete part even as many of the other much more robust cranial bones have lost their individual identity through multiple mergers and fusions. The reason for its evolutionary retention is that it has a special and essential architectonic role in facial development. It is an island of bone surrounded by osteogenic (remodeling-capable) sutural connective tissue responsive to growth control signals emanating from all around it. It is strategically situated with the ethmoid, the nasal part of the maxilla, the frontal bone, the orbitosphenoid, the alisphenoid, and the orbital part of the maxilla, all of which are growing in different directions, at different times, by different amounts, and with different functional relationships. A "slide" of bones along their sutural interfaces is involved, and this is achieved through an elaborate process of relinkages by the sutural connective tissue fibers. It was pointed out that precision of fitting is an essential part of growth control; by virtue of the lacrimal bone's **adjustive suture system**, all of these separate parts can undergo their differential displacements and their own enlargements, directional relocations, and remodeling, yet continuously fit with one another as they all develop and function. Without this adaptive system, the face simply could not "grow" at all. With it, the human (and mammalian) face has successfully survived in the long course of evolution. (Refer to pages 86 and 94.)

There should be marble and bronze monuments glorifying the ramus, the PDM, and the lacrimal bone, all prominently displayed in the atrium of every dental school; and students should be expected to doff their caps in solemn reverence each morning when passing!

11. Clinical intervention into the growth process and its control is by either one of two approaches, both of which are analogous to the intrinsic growth process itself. The first approach is by surgical substitutions for the natural displacement and remodeling processes that were incomplete or derailed. The second approach is by overriding intrinsic control signals with clinically induced (e.g., orthodontic) signals that overwhelm the intrinsic regulation of osteogenic, chondrogenic, myogenic, neurogenic, and fibrogenic systems. Then, the same actual biologic operations of these systems proceed, but now under control-revised directions. However, in all cases, if the same conditions that created the original intrinsic signals still persist after treatment, then architectonic *rebound growth* naturally adjusts back to the former, balanced pattern. Interestingly, these two forms of clinical intervention are conceptually different. Orthodontic intervention attempts to augment natural compensatory changes to achieve an improved aesthetic and functional balance among facial components. For

example, for patients with mandibular retrognathia, an orthodontist will often accentuate the degree of mandibular dental protrusion (a natural anatomic compensation for mandibular retrognathia) by using Class II elastic traction of a bionator-type removable appliance. In contrast, surgical interventions require that dental compensations be removed (usually by presurgical orthodontic tooth movement) prior to surgical correction of the skeletal imbalance.*

Removal of compensation allows the surgical team to maximize skeletal balance and to improve postsurgical occlusal stability. Although conceptually different, these two clinical intervention strategies must necessarily "work with" the same set of biologic rules. This fact is often overlooked in debates concerning the clinical efficacy of surgery and/or orthodontic correction of malocclusion. Clearly, the degree and amount of change that occurs with facial development between 9 and 14 years of age far exceeds the limits of surgical manipulation of facial bones. However, the potential for posttreatment physiologic rebound is also far greater.

12.   There is another fundamental clinical consideration that, more often than not, is conceptually bypassed. When the muscles of facial expression contract (*function*), the mechanical effect is an **upward** and **backward** retrusive force exerted on the maxilla. Yet everyone knows that the maxilla "grows forward and downward." Does **this** not contradict the *functional matrix* principle? Similarly, when the masticatory muscles function, the net mechanical effect on the mandible is also upward and backward, not downward and forward. Does **this,** thereby, not also violate belief that "function" of the functional matrix is the basic driver for growth control? However, two basic factors are omitted in presenting these comments. First, the important distinction between the **displacement** type of growth movement versus **remodeling** growth movement was not made. Second, importantly, the **growth enlargements** of the respective muscles were not included, only their contractile functions.

With respect to displacement movements, the connective tissue stroma of each muscle is directly or indirectly continuous with fibers attaching to the bones, and **enlargements in diameter** of mandibular muscles such as the masseter and temporalis have an anteriorly displacing effect on the whole mandible. Their **enlargements in length** have an inferiorly displacing and mandibular-carrying effect. As the facial expression muscles, oropharyngeal soft tissues, and facial integument all undergo **outward** growth expansion, there is an outward and downward carrying movement of all the nasomaxillary and mandibular parts.

At the same time, **functioning** of all the muscles (contractions) and all other soft tissue components is proceeding. The "genic" connective tissues (condylar cartilages and the sutural, periosteal, endosteal, and periodontal membranes) respond to the signals produced by the functioning, growing systems everywhere around the mandible and maxilla. This activates remodeling to adapt regional sizes, progressive regional configurations, and ongoing adjustments involved throughout all regional parts of each whole bone and its contiguous soft tissues. The maxilla and mandible "separate" (displacement) at their sutures and at the TMJ, and this is simultaneously accompanied by overall enlargement of each bone into the "spaces" created. The coronoid process, the gonial region, the lingual tuberosity, and so forth, are all formed and continuously enlarged to **precisely fit** with

---

*It is interesting to note that by removing dental compensations prior to surgery, the clinician is creating a facial morphology that is capable of postsurgical compensation (sometimes referred to incorrectly as surgical relapse). Such postsurgical compensation is probably responsible for the occlusal stability seen with orthognathic procedures compared to gnathic procedures.

the muscles and other soft tissues they serve. They fit because of feedback control among them involving the turning on and off of the regional osteogenic connective tissues. Tooth roots fit their sockets for the same reason. Bony edges at the interdigitating sutures merge and mesh precisely. Nerves and vessels to and from a bone exactly fit their foramina in size, shape, and constantly changing locations. The condylar cartilage continues to fit its displacement-moving and remodeling fossa. And so on. To do this, (1) the growing configurations and size changes of the muscles and other soft tissues, (2) the displacements of the bones, (3) the functions of all the multitude of soft tissues, and (4) the complex bony remodeling processes everywhere, are all developmentally inseparable. All are required as an architectonic package. They are isolated here descriptively so that we can better perceive their respective roles. In real life they simply cannot be biologically separated. One of the reasons many animal experiments intended to "prove or disprove," for example, the "functional matrix" or the "condyle as a master growth center," have always been much less than fully successful, is that these four factors were not **each** recognized and taken into account. Indeed, such experiments play against a stacked deck because of the actual inseparability of these factors as independent and controllable experimental variables.

Finally, refer to Figure 1–7 for a generalized overview of the dynamic, exceedingly precise architectonic interplay among regional parts as they all develop and as all continue to function as they do so. A most remarkable developmental system indeed.

13

Prenatal Facial Growth and Development*

A 1-month-old embryo has no real face. But the key primordia have already begun to gather, and these slight early swellings, depressions, and thickenings are rapidly to undergo a series of mergers, rearrangements, and enlargements that will transform them, as if by sleight of hand, from a cluster of separate masses into a **face**.

The head of a 4-week-old human embryo is mostly just a brain covered by a thin sheet of ectoderm and mesoderm. Where the mouth will later be is marked by a tiny depression, the **stomodeum** (Fig. 13-1). The eyes have already begun to form by a thickening of the surface ectoderm (the future lens), which meets an outpouching from the brain (the future retina). The eyes are still located at the sides of the head, however, as in a fish. As the brain continues to grow and expand, the eyes become rotated toward each other by the rapidly enlarging brain and toward the midline of what is soon to become a face. Does this not greatly reduce the intervening span between the right and left eyes? Yes, but in a relative sense. **Everything** is increasing in size, including the interorbital dimension. The eyes are actually moving farther apart; but because other parts of the head are enlarging even more, the proportionate size of the interorbital area is becoming decreased. When illustrating the process of facial growth, it has always been traditional to show all of the stages as about equal in size. Keep in mind, however, that there is actually considerable overall enlargement as the process progresses. These changes are continuous and proceed very swiftly.

The mammalian pharynx is the homologue of the ancestral region that develops into the branchial chamber and gill system of fishes. The human pharyngeal pouches and clefts, however, did not "evolve from gills." More correctly, the embryonic primordia that developed into the fish's branchial system were phylogenetically converted to develop into **other** structures instead of gills. This is where many of the parts of the face come in.

As the whole developing head markedly expands, the membrane that covers the stomodeum does not keep pace with it. This thin sheet (the

---

*This brief chapter presents a digest of the basics of facial embryology, not an extended account for advanced-level study. The objective is an introductory overview or an outline intended for a refresher review.

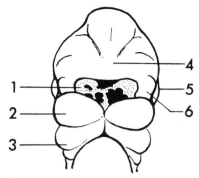

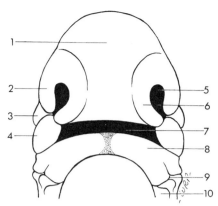

FIGURE 13–1. Human face of about 4 weeks. *1*, Stomodeal plate (buccopharyngeal membrane). *2*, Mandibular arch (swelling or process). *3*, Hyoid arch. *4*, Frontal eminence (or prominence). *5*, Optic vesicle. *6*, Region where the maxillary process (or "swelling") of the first arch is just beginning to form. (Modified from Patten, B. M.: *Human Embryology*, 3rd Ed. New York, McGraw-Hill, 1968, with permission.)

FIGURE 13–2. Face at about 5 weeks. *1*, Frontal prominence. *2*, Lateral nasal swelling. *3*, Eye. *4*, Maxilliary swelling. *5*, Nasal pit. *6*, Medial nasal swelling. *7*, Stomodeum. *8*, Mandibular swelling. *9*, Hyomandibular cleft. *10*, Hyoid arch.

buccopharyngeal or oral membrane) quickly breaks through, and the **pharynx** becomes opened to the outside (Fig. 13–2). Everything in front will become the face, and **this** is what is now about to develop. To appreciate how much facial growth is going to occur, realize that the location of the buccopharyngeal membrane in the 1-month-old embryo is at the level of the tonsils in the adult. An enormous amount of facial expansion thus will proceed in front of the stomodeum. On the internal side of this early cornerstone opening is the endodermally lined pharyngeal region. The pharynx is that part of the foregut characterized by the **pharyngeal** (visceral, branchial) **arches** (Fig. 13–3). Within the pharynx, a **pharyngeal pouch** lies between the arches, and on the outside a **pharyngeal cleft** occurs between the arches (Fig. 13–4). The ectoderm-endoderm contact between each cleft and pouch is the **branchial membrane** (Fig. 13–6).

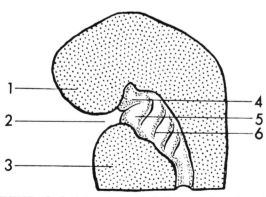

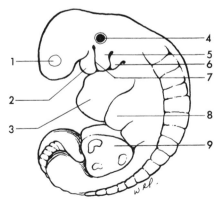

FIGURE 13–3. Internal view of pharyngeal region. *1*, Forebrain. *2*, Stomodeum. *3*, Cardiac prominence. *4*, Maxillary process. *5*, Mandibular process. *6*, Pouch between second and third arches. (Modified from Langman, J.: *Medical Embryology*. Baltimore, Williams & Wilkins, 1969, with permission.)

FIGURE 13–4. Human embryo at about 4 weeks. *1*, Optic vesicle. *2*, Mandibular arch (process or swelling). *3*, Cardiac prominence. *4*, Auditory (otic) vesicle. *5*, Hyoid arch. *6*, Third arch. *7*, Hyomandibular cleft. *8*, Hepatic prominence. *9*, Primitive umbilical cord. (Modified from Patten, B. M.: *Human Embryology*, 3rd Ed. New York, McGraw-Hill, 1968, with permission.)

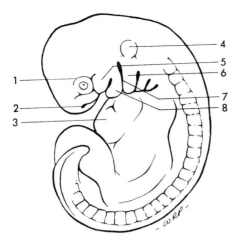

FIGURE 13-5. Human embryo at about 5 weeks. *1,* Eye. *2,* Nasal pit. *3,* Cardiac prominence. *4,* Auditory vesicle. *5,* Maxillary process. *6,* Hyoid arch. *7,* Hyomandibular cleft. *8,* Mandibular arch. (Modified from Patten, B. M.: *Human Embryology,* 3rd Ed. New York, McGraw-Hill, 1968, with permission.)

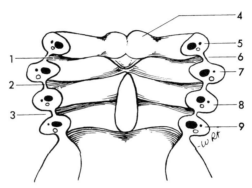

FIGURE 13-6. Internal view of pharyngeal floor and cut arches. *1,* First pharyngeal pouch between first and second arches (to become middle ear chamber). *2,* Branchial membrane. *3,* Pharyngeal cleft. *4,* Region that will develop into the anterior two thirds (body) of tongue. *5,* First (mandibular) arch containing its specific cartilage, cranial nerve, and aortic arch. The pharyngeal arch is also filled with branchiomeric mesenchyme. *6,* First pharyngeal cleft (hyomandibular) to become external ear canal. *7,* Second (hyoid) pharyngeal arch. *8,* Third pharyngeal arch with its own cartilage, aortic arch, cranial nerve, and branchiomeric mesenchyme. *9,* Fourth pharyngeal arch. (Modified from Moore, K. L.: *Before We Are Born: Basic Embryology and Birth Defects.* Philadelphia, W. B. Saunders, 1974, with permission.)

All these various pharyngeal parts are major participants in the subsequent formation of many component structures in the head and neck.[†]

Each right and left pharyngeal arch has a specific cranial nerve, a specific artery (aortic arch), and programmed mesenchyme that develops into the particular muscles and specific embryonic cartilages that identify with that pharyngeal arch (Figs. 13-5 and 13-6). Specific facial bones then develop within specific pharyngeal arches. This is a basic and important concept because, if one can understand the simple embryonic relationships involved, understanding the exceedingly complex adult anatomy is so much easier. The **muscles** that develop in relation to each arch associate directly with the **bones** forming in that arch and are innervated by the resident **cranial nerve** of the same arch as well as supplied by the corresponding artery. Embryonic pharyngeal pouches and clefts also give rise to developing parts that extend to adult derivatives. All of this has a log-

---

[†]Migrating cranial neural crest cells contribute extensively to the early primordia of many tissues developing in the face and pharyngeal region (see Johnston et al., 1973).

ical, systematic, readily recognizable developmental rationale in the embryo. Remembering these specific prenatal relationships, the far less fathomable plan for the seemingly garbled adult morphology makes sense.

In the human embryo, there are five bilateral pairs of pharyngeal arches. The first is the right and left **mandibular** arch. A bud develops from each first arch to form the paired **maxillary processes**. Both the mandibular and maxillary primordia are thus of first arch origin. The second pharyngeal arch is the **hyoid** arch (Fig. 13–5). The remaining arches are identified by respective numbers only.

The cartilage of the first pharyngeal arch is **Meckel's** cartilage, right and left (Figs. 13–1, 13–6, and 13–7). It occupies a location that becomes the core of the mandibular corpus, which forms around it. The bony mandible itself develops, independently, directly from the embryonic connective tissue that surrounds Meckel's cartilage. Most of this cartilage actually disappears, but parts of it give rise to the anlagen for two ear ossicles (the malleus and incus), and the perichondrium of Meckel's cartilage forms the beginning of the sphenomandibular ligament.

The cartilage of the hyoid (second) arch is **Reichert's** cartilage. It forms the third of the three ear ossicles on each side, the stapes. The remainder gives rise to the styloid process of the cranium, the stylohyoid ligament, the lesser horn of the hyoid bone, and a portion of the hyoid body (Fig. 13–7).

Muscles form from the mesenchyme of the arches. This mesenchyme is termed **branchiomeric** (Gr. *branchia*, gills; Gr. *meros*, segment), in contrast to mesenchyme of somite origin elsewhere in the body. From the branchiomeric mesenchyme of the first arch, the muscles of mastication, the anterior belly of the digastric, the tensor palatini, the mylohyoid, and the tensor tympani muscles all develop. From the branchiomeric mesenchyme of the second arch develop the muscles of facial expression, the stylohyoid, the stapedius, the posterior belly of the digastric, and the auricular muscles.

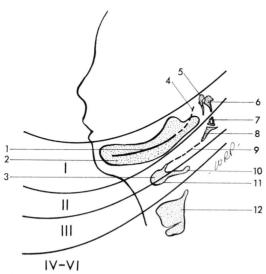

FIGURE 13–7. Pharyngeal arch derivatives (I to VI). *1,* Meckel's cartilage. *2,* Intramembranous bone developing around Meckel's cartilage. *3,* Superior part of body and lesser horn of hyoid. *4,* Sphenomandibular ligament. *5,* Malleus. *6,* Incus. *7,* Stapes. *8,* Styloid process. *9,* Stylohyoid ligament. *10,* Greater horn of hyoid bone. *11,* Inferior part of hyoid body. *12,* Laryngeal cartilages.

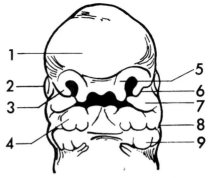

FIGURE 13–8. Facial region at about 5½ weeks. *1,* Forebrain. *2,* Optic vesicle. *3,* Lateral nasal swelling. *4,* Mandibular process. *5,* Medial nasal swelling. *6,* Nasolacrimal groove. *7,* Maxillary process. *8,* Hyomandibular cleft. *9,* Hyoid arch. (Modified from Patten, B. M.: *Human Embryology,* 3rd Ed. New York, McGraw-Hill, 1968, with permission.)

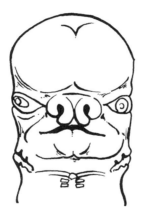

FIGURE 13-9. Face at about 7 weeks.

The specific cranial nerves that supply the first arch are the mandibular and maxillary branches of the trigeminal nerve (V). The specific cranial nerve for the second arch is the facial nerve (VII). Thus, the muscles of the first arch (muscles of mastication, and so forth) are innervated by the mandibular division of V, regardless of the anatomic position in which each muscle finally becomes located later in development. The muscles of facial expression formed by the branchiomeric mesenchyme of the second pharyngeal arch correspondingly are all innervated by the facial nerve.

Note the gathering of many structures related to the formative ear region in and around the first and second pharyngeal arches (Figs. 13-8 and 13-9). The **auditory placode** differentiates early as a surface thickening of the ectoderm just above and behind the first pharyngeal cleft. This placode rapidly invaginates to form the auditory (otic) vesicle (Figs. 13-4 and 13-5), which then differentiates into the structures of the inner ear (semicircular canals, cochlea). The first pharyngeal **cleft** (between the first and second arches) forms the external auditory meatus and outer ear canal, and the branchial membrane between the cleft and pouch undergoes remodeling to participate in the formation of the tympanic membrane (Fig. 13-10). The first pharyngeal **pouch** becomes expanded into the middle ear chamber leading into the pharynx. The ear ossicles, developing from the cartilages of the first and second arches, conveniently abut this area and soon become enveloped within the expanding first pharyngeal pouch (middle ear chamber). They function as the bridge between the tympanic membrane and the inner ear. The auricle of each external ear develops from the surface swellings around the first pharyngeal cleft, and the bumps already present on these embryonic primordia form the characteristic hillocks of the adult ear lobe (Fig. 13-9).

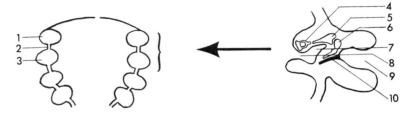

FIGURE 13-10. Developing ear region. *1,* Mandibular arch. *2,* Branchial membrane between the cleft on the outside and pouch on the inside of the pharynx. *3,* Hyoid arch. *4,* Stapes. *5,* Incus. *6,* Malleus. *7,* Middle ear chamber to expand as tympanic cavity surrounding auditory ossicles. *8,* Auditory (eustachian) tube. *9,* External ear canal. *10,* Aniage for the tympanic membrane.

The cartilage of the **third** pharyngeal arch is the precursor for the greater horn of the hyoid bone and part of the body (Fig. 13–7). The single muscle that develops from the third arch branchiomeric mesenchyme is the stylopharyngeus. The specific cranial nerve entering the third arch is the **glossopharyngeal**. It, therefore, supplies the muscle that develops from this arch. The cartilages in the remainder of the arches form into the thyroid, cricoid, and arytenoid components of the larynx. From fourth arch branchiomeric mesenchyme, the cricothyroid and pharyngeal constrictor muscles are formed. The specific nerve of the fourth pharyngeal arch is the superior laryngeal branch of the **vagus**. The intrinsic laryngeal muscles develop from the sixth arch and are innervated by that arch's resident nerve, which is the recurrent laryngeal branch of the vagus.

In each second pharyngeal pouch, the lining endoderm and underlying mesenchyme proliferate to form the paired **palatine tonsils**. From the lining of the third pouch develops **parathyroid III** (so called because of its third arch origin). This will form the "inferior" parathyroid because it later descends to a level below parathyroid IV. The thymus also develops from the lining of the third pharyngeal arch. Parathyroid IV (the "superior" parathyroid) develops from the fourth pouch.

In the floor of the pharynx, the first (mandibular) arches rapidly give rise to growing **lingual swellings** (Fig. 13–11). A smaller midline swelling, the **tuberculum impar**, is also present, and these three structures develop into the mucosal covering for the anterior two thirds, or body, of the tongue. Since the mandibular nerve supplies first arch tissue, it therefore provides the sensory (tactile) innervation for the mucosa of the body of the tongue. The chorda tympani, which is a branch of VII that diverges from the second to the first arch by crossing through the branchial (tympanic) membrane to join the mandibular nerve (lingual branch), provides gustatory innervation for the tongue's mucosa.

At the root of the midventral parts of the second, third, and fourth pharyngeal arches, another prominent swelling occurs, the **copula**. This general region develops into the posterior third (root) of the tongue. The cranial nerves supplying the third and fourth arches are the glossopharyngeal and vagus, and these are thus the sensory nerves that innervate the mucosa of the root of the tongue. The core of the tongue is occupied by its "intrinsic" muscles. These originate from a more caudal region (probably from occipital somatic mesoderm) and grow into the expanding mucosal covering for the tongue being formed by the floor of the pharynx (described above). The motor innervation to these muscles is thus provided by the paired hypoglossal (XII) nerves. They are carried along with the intrinsic muscles as they migrate anteriorly into the formative body of the tongue.

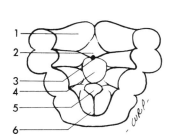 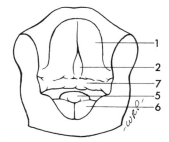

FIGURE 13–11. Developing tongue at 6 and 8 weeks. *1,* Lateral lingual swelling. *2,* Tuberculum impar. *3,* Foramen caecum. *4,* Copula. *5,* Epiglottis. *6,* Arytenoid swellings. *7,* Root of tongue.

Anatomically, the body of the tongue is separated from the root by a V-shaped sulcus (the **sulcus terminalis**). This marks the approximate line between the derivatives of first arch origin and those from the arches behind the first arch. At the midline in this developing groove, between the tuberculum impar and the copula, the thyroid primordium develops as an epithelial diverticulum into the pharyngeal floor (Fig. 13–12). It then separates from the mucosal lining and migrates caudally. The point of invagination, however, remains as a permanent pit termed the **foramen caecum** (Fig. 13–11). It is located at the apex of the V and is a landmark that identifies the adult position of the embryonic boundary between the first and second arches. As for most glandular tissues, the thyroid is thus of epithelial origin; and because the primordium develops from the pharyngeal lining, it is of endodermal derivation.

By the time an embryo is about 5 weeks old, the first pharyngeal arch has formed recognizable **maxillary** and **mandibular swellings**. Just above the stomodeum, the paired, laterally located **nasal placodes** have already differentiated by thickenings of the surface ectoderm. Horseshoe-like ridges (**nasal swellings**) have developed around them to form deepening **nasal pits**. The floor of each pit is termed the oronasal membrane, but it is a transient structure that soon breaks through, thus opening the nasal pits directly into the oral cavity. At the same time, the semicircular nasal swellings continue to enlarge. Each swelling is composed of a lateral and medial limb. The expanding **medial** limbs merge at the midline to form the primordium that will differentiate into the middle part of the nose, the philtrum (cupid's bow) of the lip, the "incisor" part of the maxilla (premaxilla), and the small primary palate. (See Figs. 13–1 and 13–2.)

The rapidly growing **lateral** limbs of each nasal swelling form the alae of the nose (Figs. 13–8 and 13–9. While these changes occur, the maxillary swellings are also enlarging, and they subsequently merge with the medial limbs of the nasal swellings. The furrow between them (not a complete cleft in normal development) disappears, and a closed, U-shaped arch is thereby formed. The medial limbs develop into the middle span of both the maxillary arch and the upper lip as mentioned above. The cuspid, premolar, molar, and lateral lip parts of the upper arch develop from the paired maxillary processes. (See Brin et al., 1990, for an evaluation of prenatal nasal and cuspid relationships.) **These** are all some of the lines of merger that can be involved in cleft lip and jaw. Sometimes, developmental variations are encountered in which the blastema of a tooth is caught on the "wrong" side of a cleft; this always causes excitement because that is not the way it is supposed to be.

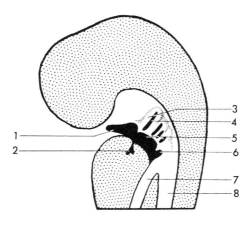

FIGURE 13–12. Body of tongue (lateral lingual swellings and tuberculum impar). *2*, Thyroid diverticulum. *3*, Mandibular arch. *4*, Pouch between first and second arches. *5*, Root of tongue (copula). *6*, Arytenoid swellings. *7*, Trachea. *8*, Esophagus.

An oblique groove is present between the maxillary swelling and the lateral limb of the nasal swelling (Fig. 13–8). This is the **nasolacrimal groove**, which will soon close, but the line of merger establishes a developmental pathway for the later formation of the nasolacrimal duct. If this merger fails, a permanent facial cleft or fissure results.

The superficial tissues in lateral areas of the maxillary process fuse with the mandibular process to form the cheek. **Epithelial pearls** often occur along such lines of mucosal and cutaneous fusion. These are small islands of epithelial cells that were "programmed" to form, but were caught up in the fusion process. **Fordyce's spots**, which are remnants of cutaneous sebaceous glands, can similarly be found in the adult buccal mucosa, for the same reason, along lines of fusion.

The growing right and left mandibular swellings join at the midline to form the lower jaw and lip. A cartilaginous interface forms at this junction.[‡]

The **frontal prominence** forms the forehead and a vertical zone of developing tissue between the merging right and left medial nasal swellings. Here, the midline **nasal septum** is formed, which was historically believed by some to function as a pacemaker in later fetal development when its core becomes cartilaginous (see Chapter 5).

To date, these multiple, regional facial changes are all occurring at about the same time and have proceeded **rapidly** from about the fourth to the sixth week of embryonic development. The paired **palatal shelves** are now forming from each side of the maxillary arch (Figs. 13–13 and 13–14). The oral cavity is still relatively small, however, and the sizable tongue remains interposed between the right and left shelves. The early shelves necessarily enlarge downward in an obliquely vertical manner because of this. However, the inferior expansion of the whole lower part of the face carries the tongue downward. The oral cavity increases greatly in size. The paired nasal chambers are still continuous with the oral cavity. (Right and left nasal cavities are present because the nasal septum, developing inferiorly from the frontal prominence, has sustained the original paired nature of the nasal primordia). The oral and nasal cavities at this stage are separated from each other only in the anterior-most region by the tiny, unpaired **primary palate** (median palatine process). The latter was formed by the fusion of the nasomedial ("premaxillary") processes. The whole lower part of the developing face, including the tongue and the floor of the oral cavity, now becomes displaced inferiorly to a greater extent than the enlarging palatal shelves are descending, so that the newly formed shelves of the maxilla are free to expand **medially** as well. They come together and soon fuse along the midline (the palatal raphe). The shelves "swing upward" in order to contact each other, but some of this apparent upward rotation is produced by differential growth. The shelves are growing and, especially, are becoming displaced inferiorly. By differential growth, the shelves expand downward as well as toward each other, but the **entire** nasal chamber on each side also expands laterally and inferiorly. Some of this apparent "upward swing" is relative and is a consequence of actual inferomedial growth. This is a process in which the different parts in the two nasal chambers and the oral cavity all grow at

---

[‡]Although a limited amount of endochondral ossification will later occur here, the two halves of the mandible fuse completely after birth, unlike the permanently separate lower jaw halves of nonprimate mammals. Except in the "secondary cartilage" of the mandibular condyle (and to a much lesser extent in the mandibular symphysis and a small cartilage on the coronoid process), the greater part of the mandibular ossification is by the intermembranous mechanism. Meckel's cartilage does not participate in the endochondral ossification process (except for random spots here and there) and disappears except for its contribution to the ear ossicles and ligaments. The maxilla is entirely of intramembranous origin.

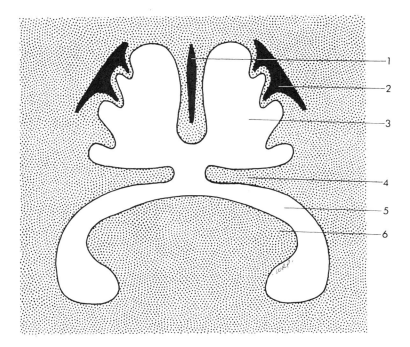

FIGURE 13–13. Frontal section through the oronasal region in a 7¹/₂-week embryo. *1*, Cartilage of the nasal septum. *2*, Cartilage of the nasal conchae. *3*, Nasal chamber. *4*, Palatal shelf. *5*, Oral cavity. *6*, Tongue. (Adapted from Langman, J.: *Medical Embryology*. Baltimore, Williams & Wilkins, 1969, with permission.)

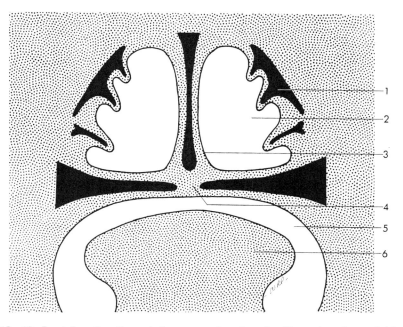

FIGURE 13–14. Frontal section through the oronasal region of a 10-week embryo. *1*, Nasal conchae. *2*, Nasal chamber. *3*, Nasal septum. *4*, Palatal shelves, fused at midline and fused with nasal septum. The intramembranous bone of the palatal shelves (from the maxilla) is beginning to form. *5*, Oral cavity. *6*, Tongue. (Adapted from Langman, J.: *Medical Embryology*, Baltimore, Williams & Wilkins, 1969, with permission.)

differential rates and to different extents as the whole midfacial region rapidly increases in size. While the schematic illustrations in Figures 13–13 and 13–14 are shown here as the same in size, in reality, a considerable enlargement is occurring.

The merger of the right and left palatal shelves forms the **secondary palate**. Bone tissue soon appears within it. This part of the palate is a direct extension of the maxilla from which it develops. The original primary palate, formed from the nasomedial (premaxillary) processes, is retained as a small median, unpaired, triangular segment of the palatal complex in the anterior region just ahead of the incisive foramen, a landmark that identifies the midline boundary between the primary and secondary parts of the palate (Fig. 13–15). The separate palatine bones and their posterior contribution to the palatal complex do not develop until somewhat later. In the meantime, the nasal septum has merged with the superior surface of the palate. The two nasal chambers are now completely compartmented, and both have been closed off from the oral cavity along the length of the palate (Figs. 13–14 and 13–16).

REMODELING IN THE FETAL FACE

The process of "remodeling," involving differential, regional "fields" of periosteal and endosteal resorptive and depository surfaces, first begins in the fetus at about 10 weeks in two principal locations: on lining surfaces of the bone around tooth buds and on the endocranial surface of the frontal bone. The major remodeling throughout the remainder of the early facial skeleton begins at about 14 weeks. Before this time the bones enlarge in all directions from their respective ossification centers. Remodeling, as a process that accompanies growth, starts when the definitive form of each of the individual bones of the face and cranium is attained (Fig. 13–17). As the officiation centers appear and begin to grow (Fig. 13–18), the **re-**

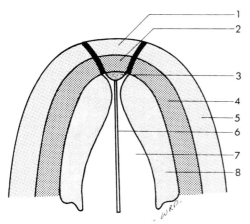

FIGURE 13–15. Oral view of the palatal shelves in a 7½-week embryo. *1,* Philtrum of upper lip. *2,* "Premaxillary" segment from medial nasal process. *3,* Primary palate. *4,* Upper arch (part derived from maxillary swelling. *5,* Cheek. *6,* Nasal septum. *7,* Open oral and nasal cavities. *8,* Palatal shelves. In this stage, the philtrum and premaxillary segment have already merged with the maxillary swellings.

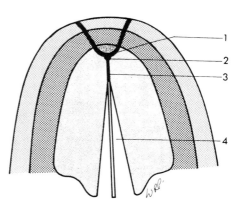

FIGURE 13–16. Oral view of palate showing beginning of fusion. *1,* Merger of midline plrimary palate with bilateral secondary palatal shelves. *2,* Incisive foramen. *3,* Palatal raphe (midline fusion). *4,* Open nasal and oral chambers.

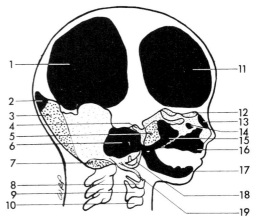

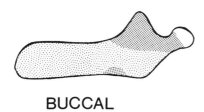

BUCCAL

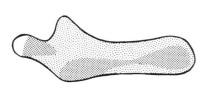

LINGUAL

FIGURE 13-17. Mandible in the last trimester of fetal development. Dark stippling represents resorptive fields, and light stippling indicates depository fields.

FIGURE 13-18. Human skull at about 3 months. Intramembranous bones are shown in black. Cartilage is represented by light stippling, and bones developing by endochondral ossification are indicated by darker stippling. Approximate time of appearance for each bone is indicated in parenthesis. *1*, Parietal bone (10 weeks). *2*, Interparietal bone (8 weeks). *3*, Supraoccipital (8 weeks). *4*, Dorsum sellae (still cartilaginous). *5*, Temporal wing of sphenoid (2 to 3 months; the basisphenoid appears at 12 to 13 weeks, orbitosphenoid of 12 weeks and presphenoid at 5 months). *6*, Squamous part of temporal bone (2 to 3 months). *7*, Basioccipital (2 to 3 months). *8*, Hyoid (still cartilaginous). *9*, Thyroid (still cartilaginous). *10*, Cricoid (still cartilaginous). *11*, Frontal bone (7½ weeks). *12*, Crista galli, still cartilaginous (inferiorly, the middle concha begins ossification at 16 weeks, the superior and inferior conchae at 18 weeks, the perpendicular plate of ethmoid begins ossification during the first postnatal year, the cribriform plate during the second postnatal year, the vomer at 8 total weeks). *13*, Nasal bone (8 weeks). *14*, Lacrimal bone (8½ weeks). *15*, Malar (8 weeks). *16*, Maxilla (end of 6th week; premaxilla, 7 weeks). *17*, Mandible (6 to 8 weeks). *18*, Tympanic ring (begins at 9 weeks, with complete ring at 12 weeks); petrous bone, (5 to 6 months). *19*, Styloid process, (still cartilaginous). (Modified from Patten, B. M.: *Human Embryology*, 3rd Ed. New York, McGraw-Hill, 1968, with permission.)

modeling process also begins and serves to progressively shape the individual bones as it simultaneously enlarges them.

Nasomaxillary Complex

The anterior part of the maxilla in both the fetus and the child is depository on lingual surfaces and resorptive on nasal lining surfaces. A major difference exists, however, on the anterior-most (labial) surface. Here it is depository in the fetus, but characteristically becomes resorptive after the first few years following birth when definitive arch length has been attained. During the fetal period, the exterior surface of the entire maxilla, including its anterior part,[§] remains depository to provide for increasing arch length in conjunction with the development of the tooth buds and their subsequent enlargement. Resorption occurs on the alveolar lining surfaces surrounding each of the tooth buds. The fetal maxillary arch thus lengthens horizontally in both posterior **and** anterior directions, in contrast to the largely posterior mode of elongation in the later periods of childhood development. In the postnatal face, after the primary teeth have

---

[§]An old game among facial researchers is arguing whether or not a premaxilla actually exists as a separate bone in man and how many ontogenic ossification centers are involved. Phylogenically, there is no question.

erupted and are being shed to make way for the permanent arch, the anterior (labial) surface of the maxillary arch begins to become resorptive (Kurihara and Enlow, 1980a). This is part of the growth and remodeling process that continues to produce the **downward** growth movement of the maxillary arch and palate.

The posterior and infraorbital surfaces of the maxilla proper are depository in both prenatal and postnatal life. The process of posterior deposition on the maxillary tuberosity progressively increases the maxilla in horizontal length. Deposition on the orbital floor in the fetal skull keeps it in a constant positional relationship with the eyeball, just as in the growing child. The eyeball enlarges in volume at a decreasing rate after the fourth to fifth fetal months. Its volume increases by over 100 per cent before the fifth month, by 50 per cent during the sixth and seventh months, and only by 23 to 30 per cent in the eighth and ninth months. Remodeling of the orbital floor takes place because the entire maxilla, including the orbit, is displaced in a progressively inferior direction in relation to continuing new bone growth at the frontomaxillary suture. At the same time, deposition on the orbital floor serves to carry it superiorly, thereby maintaining it in a constant position relative to the eyeball. The infraorbital canal is also compensating by resorption superior to and deposition inferior to the infraorbital nerve. This maintains a constant relationship between the nerve and the orbital floor, along which the infraorbital nerve passes before entering the infraorbital canal.

The external surface of the frontal process of the maxilla is depository during both prenatal and postnatal facial development. The contralateral nasal side is mostly depository, with some resorption at older fetal ages, but it is entirely resorptive postnatally. This area in the rapidly growing young child is characterized by a massive lateral expansion of the lateral nasal walls, including the ethmoidal plates and sinuses. The latter part of fetal life appears to be a transitory period in which these surfaces are just beginning a major lateral expansive movement.

In both the fetal and postnatal periods, the nasal side of the palate (including the palatine bone) is resorptive except along the midline, and the oral surface is depository. This provides for an inferior remodeling relocation of the palate and a vertical enlargement of the nasal chambers and also, significantly, provides a key means that sustains functional alignment of the palate as the entire maxilla undergoes variable displacement rotations.

The mucosal surface of each vertical plate of the palatine bone is resorptive, and the opposite surface on the lateral nasal wall is depository in both the prenatal and postnatal periods. This provides for the bilateral expansion of this part of the nasal chamber in width.

The Mandible

The beginning fetal mandible, as in the earliest growth stages of the other bones of the skull, initially has outside surfaces that are entirely depository in character. At about 10 weeks, however, resorption begins around the rapidly expanding tooth buds and is present thereafter. By 13 weeks, distinct resorptive fields are becoming established on the buccal side of the coronoid process, on the lingual side of the ramus, and on the lingual side of the posterior part of the corpus. The anterior edge of the ramus is already resorptive, and the posterior border is depository. In some specimens, however, the anterior margin along the tip of the coronoid process shows deposition, suggesting a "rotation" to a more upright position (see Chapter 4). By 26 weeks, the basic growth and remodeling pattern that continues on into postnatal development is seen except, notably, in the incisor region (Fig. 13–17). In the fetal and early postnatal mandible, the entire labial side of the anterior part of the corpus is still depository. As in the fetal and young postnatal maxilla, the fetal mandibular corpus grows and lengthens **mesially** as well as distally in conjunction with the establishment of the primary dentition. The lingual side of the fetal corpus in the incisor region is resorptive after about the fifteenth week in most (but not all) mandibles. This contributes to a forward remodeling movement of the entire incisor region of the corpus. Subsequent to the deciduous dentition period of childhood growth, however, the alveolar bone on the labial side in the forward part of the arch undergoes a reversal to become **resorptive**, and the opposite lingual side becomes uniformly depository. This change occurs in conjunction with the unique lingual direction of incisor movement in the child's mandible. From this time, the chin begins to take on a progressively more prominent form; the mental protuberance continues to remodel anteriorly, while the alveolar bone above it remodels posteriorly until the lower permanent incisors reach their definitive positions. (See Kurihara and Enlow, 1980a, for more details.)

A DEVELOPMENTAL TIMETABLE

A "priority plan" exists during the prenatal growth and development of the face and the body in general. Some specific organs and anatomic parts are given priority status in earlier timing and/or growth rate; some other parts receive partially deferred attention. This is determined, in general, by the urgency of a given part's functional role in the early physiologic relationships of the developing fetus. Certain developing anatomic components, such as the cardiovascular system and many parts of the nervous system, are essential to the maturation of all other parts and to fetal life itself. Components such as the lungs and the nasal and oral parts of the face and the urogenital and digestive systems are essentially nonfunctional during the fetal period. Their respective roles are carried out by placental interchanges. Although their prenatal maturation is incomplete, these growth-delayed parts must nonetheless achieve readiness for immediate and full newborn-level function at the instant of birth. This is "prospective developmental differentiation." That is, structure develops even though function has yet to exert its ontogenic influence on structural design and differentiation. This is an extension, not an exception, of the "structure and function interplay" principle of biology, with the phylogeny of function establishing a provisional developmental program. Airway size must be prepared and adequate to accommodate newborn lung size, which, in turn, must be sufficient to meet the functional needs for the size of the body at the time. Neonatal oral functions must also be ready to respond, virtually instantaneously, upon birth. Thereafter, as described throughout earlier chapters, differential extents and rates of developmental maturation occur among the multitude of different body (and facial) regions and parts. The neonatal brain, calvaria, basicranium, and eyes are relatively large in comparison with the proportionately much shorter face. However, as general body size progressively increases, the lungs enlarge to match, and the nasal part of the face (not just the external nose) correspondingly begins to increase significantly in height and length. The dentition begins to emerge, chewing begins to replace suckling, neural reflexes change, swallowing patterns change, and the oral part of the face, with its rapidly enlarging masticatory muscles and growing and developing jaw bones, keeps pace. All of the multitude of regional parts proceed developmentally within a general field of facial growth, which has a perimeter prescribed by the precocious basicranial template.

14

Maturation of the Orofacial Neuromusculature

ROBERT E. MOYERS, D.D.S., Ph.D. *and* DAVID S. CARLSON, Ph.D.

PRENATAL MATURATION

During prenatal life the human neuromuscular system matures unevenly. It is not accidental that the orofacial region matures (in the neurophysiologic sense) ahead of limb regions, because the mouth is the primary site of respiration, nursing, and protection of the oropharyngeal airway. In the human fetus, by about the eighth week, generalized uniform reflex movements of the entire body can be elicited by tactile stimulation. A few spontaneous movements, in response to as yet unidentified stimuli, have been observed as early as $9\frac{1}{2}$ weeks. Localized specific and more peripheral responses can be produced before 11 weeks. At this time, stimulation of the nose-mouth region causes lateral body flexion. By 14 weeks, the movements have become much more individualized, and very delicate activities can be executed. When the mouth area is stimulated, general bodily movements no longer are seen; instead, facial and orbicular muscle responses are produced. Stimulating the lower lip, for example, causes the tongue to move. Stimulation of the upper lip causes the mouth to close and, often, deglutition to occur.

Respiratory movements of the chest and abdomen are first seen at about 16 weeks. The gag reflex has been demonstrated in the human fetus at about $18\frac{1}{2}$ weeks (menstrual age). By 25 weeks, respiration is shallow but may support life for a few hours if established.

Stimulation of the mouth at 29 weeks has elicited suckling, although complete suckling and swallowing are not thought to be developed until at least 32 weeks.

Davenport Hooker and Tryphena Humphrey have shown us that there is an orderly, sequential staging of events in prenatal orofacial neuromuscular maturation—a staging seen throughout the body, but which is much more advanced in the oropharyngeal region. All this has to be established by the time of birth in order for the child to survive (Humphrey, 1970).

NEONATAL ORAL FUNCTIONS

At birth, tactile acuity is much more highly developed in the lips and mouth than it is in the fingers. The infant carries objects to his mouth to aid in the perception of size and texture; later they go into the mouth as a part of teething. The neonate slobbers, drools, chews toes, sucks thumbs, and discovers that gurgling sounds can be made with the mouth.

Freudians consider all of this oral eroticism, as they do adult smoking; but in the infant surely it is also explanatory and exercises the most sensitive perceptual system in the body at that time. Oral functions in the neonate are guided primarily by local tactile stimuli, particularly those in the lips and front part of the tongue.

The tongue at this age does not guide itself; rather, it follows superficial sensation. The posture of the neonate's tongue is between the gum pads, and it is often far enough forward to rest between the lips, where it can perform its role of sensory guidance more easily. The young infant, to a great extent, interprets the world with the mouth, and the integration of oral activities is therefore by sensory mechanisms.

If you touch a young child's lips or tongue and have him follow your finger, both the head and body turn. A little bit later the head turns separately from the body, and still later the mandible is moved without moving the head. It is only last of all that the neonate can follow with the tongue, while not moving the mandible. These stages appear in a natural sequence, just as teeth erupt on a kind of schedule.

The infant uses the mouth for many purposes. The perceptual functions of the mouth and face are combined with the sensory functions of taste, smell, and jaw position. The neonate's primary relationship to its environment is by means of the mouth, pharynx, and larynx. Here a high concentration of readily available receptors becomes stimulated and modulates the already matured brain stem coordinations that regulate respiration and nursing and determine head and neck positions during breathing and feeding.

The sensitivity of the tongue and lips is perhaps greater than that of any other body area. The sensory guidance for oral functioning, including jaw movements, is from a remarkably large area. These sensory inputs are compounded by many dual contacting surfaces, such as the tongue and lips, the soft palate and posterior pharyngeal wall, and the compartments of the temporomandibular articulation. A great array of sensory signals is required for the integration, coordination, and interpretation of this complex system.

INFANTILE SUCKLING AND SWALLOWING

The effectiveness of oral motor activities is a good indication of the neurologic maturation of premature infants. It has been found that a child will follow the same patterns in certain oral reflex movements years after initial learning. For example, a study was made of children whose records had been kept from infancy. As long as 9 years after weaning, if given a bottle from which to suckle, they producing the same suckling, swallowing, and respiratory rhythms they had when infants. If they swallowed in a suckle-suckle-swallow type of pattern (i.e., two suckles for one swallow, two-for-one), this same rhythm appeared years later. It may be a three-for-one or even a four-for-one ratio, but the pattern is maintained. Such primitive reflexes are difficult for us to change. How foolish it is for us, with our present ignorance about conditioning such basic mechanisms, to try and alter some of these reflexes. We must spend more time with those problems that we have at least a theoretical chance to condition.

Rhythmic elevation and lowering of the jaw provide sequential changes in positions of the tongue in coordination with its suckling contractions.

The activities of suckling are closely related temporally to the motor functions of positional maintenance of the airway.

Electromyographic studies in our own laboratory have confirmed visual observations reported in England by a number of people, revealing that while the mandibular movements are carried out by the muscles of mastication, the mandible is primarily stabilized during the actual act of infantile swallowing by concomitant contractions of the tongue and the facial (rather than masticatory) muscles (Moyers, 1964). At the actual time of the infantile swallow, the tongue lies between the gum pads and in close approximation with the lingual surface of the lips. Thus, the infantile swallow is neuromuscularly a different mechanism from the mature swallow.

Characteristic features of the infantile swallow are that (1) the jaws are apart, with the tongue between the gum pads; (2) the mandible is stabilized primarily by contractions of the muscles of the seventh cranial nerve and the interposed tongue; and (3) swallowing is guided, and to a great extent controlled, by sensory interchange between the lips and the tongue.

Maintenance of the Airway

The oral-jaw musculature is responsible for the vital positional relationships that maintain the oral pharyngeal airway. While the infant is resting, a rather uniform diameter for the airway is provided by (1) maintaining the mandible anteroposteriorly and (2) stabilizing the tongue and posterior pharyngeal wall relationships.

The axial musculature around the vertebrae is also involved. These primitive neonatal protective mechanisms provide the motor background upon which, with growth, all the postural mechanisms of the head and neck region are developed. Physiologic maintenance of the airway is of vital, continuing importance from the first day throughout life.

This little neonate who cannot focus his eyes, who cannot make a purposeful movement of his limbs, who cannot hold his head upright, who has absolutely no control of the lower end of his gastrointestinal tract has absolutely exquisite control of some functions in the orofacial regions. Why? Such control is necessary for survival.

Infant Cry

When the aroused baby is crying, the oral region is unresponsive to local stimulation. The mouth is held wide open, while the tongue is separated from the lower lip and from the palate. The steady stabilization of the size of the pharyngeal airway is given up during crying, and there are irregular, varying constrictions during expiration of the cry and large, reciprocal expansions during the alternating inspirations.

Gagging

Gagging, the reflex refusal to swallow or accept foreign objects in the throat, is an exaggeration of the protective reflexes guarding the airway and alimentary tract. The gag reflex is present at birth, but it changes as the child grows older in order to accommodate visual, acoustic, olfactory, and psychic stimuli that are remembered and thus condition it.

EARLY POSTNATAL DEVELOPMENT OF ORAL NEUROMUSCULAR FUNCTIONS

Mastication

The interaction between the rapidly and differentially growing craniofacial skeleton and the maturing neuromuscular system brings about sequentially progressive modifications of the elementary oral functions seen in the neonate (Moyers, 1964, 1969, 1988). Mandibular growth, downward and forward, is greater during this time than midfacial growth and is associated with a greater separation of the thyroid bone and thyroid cartilage from the cranial base and mandible.

Maturation of the musculature and delineation of the temporomandibular joint help provide a more stable mandible. Although mandibular growth carries the tongue away from the palate and helps provide differential enlargement of the pharynx, patency of the airway is maintained —a most important point.

The soft palate and the tongue are commonly held in apposition, but as the tongue is no longer lowered by mandibular growth, its functional relationship with the lips is altered, an alteration aided by the vertical development of the alveolar process. So the morphologic relationship of the tongue and lips is strained. At rest now, the tongue is no longer in generalized apposition with the lips, buccal wall, and soft palate. The lips elongate and become more selectively mobile; the tongue develops discrete movements that are separate from lip and mandibular movements. The labial valve mechanism is constantly maintained during rest and feeding so that food is not lost.

The development of speech and mastication as well as of facial expression requires a furthering of the independent mobility of the separate parts. In the neonate, however, the lips tightly surround a plunger-like tongue, moving in synchrony with gross mandibular movements. Speech, facial expression, and mastication require the development of new motor patterns as well as greater autonomy of the motor elements. Not all the developmental aspects of these functions are known. But mastication certainly does not gradually develop from the infantile nursing. Rather, it seems that the maturation of the central nervous system permits completely new functions to develop. These functions are triggered to an important extent by the eruption of the teeth.

One of the most important factors in the maturation of mastication is the sensory aspect of newly arriving teeth. The muscles controlling mandibular position are cued by the first occlusal contacts of the antagonistic incisors. Serial electromyographic studies at frequent intervals during the arrival of the incisors have demonstrated conclusively that the very instant the maxillary and mandibular incisors accidentally touch one another, the jaw musculature begins to learn to function in accommodation to the arrival of the teeth (Moyers, 1964).

Thus, since the incisors arrive first, the closure pattern becomes more precise anteroposteriorly before it does mediolaterally. All occlusal functions are learned in stages. The central nervous system and the orofacial and jaw musculature mature concomitantly, and usually synchronously, with the development of the jaws and dentition.

The earliest chewing movements are irregular and poorly coordinated, like those during the early stages of the learning of any motor skills. As the primary dentition is completed, the chewing cycle becomes more stabilized, using more efficiently the individual's pattern of occlusal intercuspation. In the very young child, sensory guidance for masticatory movement is provided by the receptors in the temporomandibular articulation, the periodontal membrane, the tongue, and the oral mucosa and muscles; of these it seems by far that the most important are those of the temporomandibular articulations, and next those of the periodontal membrane. Cuspal height, cuspal angle, and incisal guidance (which is usually minimal in the primary dentition) play a role in the establishment of chewing patterns in the infant. However, condylar guidance is not important at this age, since the eminentia articularis is ill-defined and the temporal fossae are shallow. Rather, it may be supposed that the bone of the eminentia articularis forms where temporomandibular function permits (or causes) it to develop. In a similar fashion, the plane of occlusion is established by the growth of the alveolar process, during eruption of the teeth, to heights permitted by the configuration and functioning of the neuromusculature.

The individual's movements during the chewing cycle are a developed, integrated pattern of many functional elements. In the young child, at the time of completion of the primary dentition, masticatory relationships are nearly ideal, since all three systems (bone, teeth, and muscle) still show the adaptability characteristic of development. Cusp height and overbite in the primary dentition are more shallow, bone growth more rapid and adaptive, and neuromuscular learning more easily cued because pathways and patterns of activity are not yet well established. Adaptations to masticatory change are much more difficult in later years, as every dentist knows.

Facial Expression

In a not dissimilar way, most subtle facial expressions are learned, largely by imitation, so we think, and begin about the time the primitive uses of the seventh nerve musculature for infantile swallowing are abandoned. Those of us who are parents imagine all sorts of facial expressions in the young neonate. Actually, observing the infant objectively, we must admit that the expression is often rather blank. The reason is that the facial muscles are busy being used for the massive efforts of mandibular stabilization necessary during infantile swallowing. Eventually the mandible becomes controlled and stabilized more by the muscles of mastication, particularly during unconscious reflex swallowing, and the delicate muscles of the seventh cranial nerve become truly "muscles of facial expression."

Although many facial expressions are learned through imitation, some facial responses are not learned and can be traced back to reflexes of earlier primates. Similar facial displays have evolved in the four lines of modern primates in which monkey-like forms have developed. Comparative studies have been made revealing similar reflex expressions of protective anger, for example, in various primates—the same primitive expressions you have seen on your best friend.

Speech

Purposeful speech is different from the reflex infant cry. Infant crying is associated with irregular tongue and mandibular positions related to sporadic inspirations and expirations. Speech, on the other hand, is performed on a background of stabilized and learned positions of the mandible, pharynx, and tongue. The infant cry is usually a simple displacement of parts, accompanied by a single explosive emission, whereas speech can only be carried out by polyphasic and sequential motor activities synchronized closely with breathing. Speech is regular; the infant cry is sporadic. Speech requires complicated, sophisticated, varying sensory conditioning elements during learning; the infant cry is primitive and not learned.

Speech consists of four parts: (1) language—the knowledge of words used in communicating ideas; (2) voice—sound produced by air passing between the vibrating vocal cords of the larynx; (3) articulation—the movement of the speech organs used in producing a sound, (i.e., the lips, tongue, teeth, mandible, palate, and so forth); and (4) rhythm—variations of quality, length, timing, and stress of a sound, word, phrase, or sentence. If there is no impairment of hearing, sight, or oral sensation, the child will learn to speak from the speech that is heard. Speech defects are a loss or disturbance of language, voice, articulation, and rhythm or combinations of such losses and disturbances.

Mature Swallow

During the latter half of the first year of life, several maturational events usually occur that alter markedly the orofacial musculature's functioning. The arrival of the incisors cues the more precise opening and closing movements of the mandible, compels a more retracted tongue posture, and initiates the learning of the mastication. As soon as bilateral posterior occlusion is established (usually with the eruption of the first primary molars), true chewing motions are seen to start, and the learning of the mature swallow begins. Gradually, the fifth cranial nerve muscles assume the role of muscular stabilization during swallowing, and the muscles of facial expression abandon the crude infantile function of suckling and the infantile swallow and then begin to learn the more delicate and complicated functions of speech and facial expressions. The transition from infantile to mature swallowing takes place over several months, aided by maturation of neuromuscular elements, the appearance of upright head posture, and hence a change in the direction of gravitational forces on the mandible, the instinctive desire to chew, the necessary ability to handle textured food, dentitional development, and so forth. Many children achieve features of the mature swallow at 12 to 15 months, but there is a great variability. Characteristic features of the mature swallow are as follows: (1) the teeth are together (although they may be apart with a liquid bolus); (2) the mandible is stabilized by contractions of the fifth cranial nerve muscles; (3) the tongue tip is held against the palate above and behind the incisors; and (4) minimal contractions of the lips are seen during swallowing.

Neural Regulation of Jaw Positions

Jaw position, like a number of other automatic-somatic activities, normally is largely reflexively controlled, even though it can be altered voluntarily. A surprising number of jaw functions are carried out at the subconscious level, even though conscious control is possible and sometimes necessary. Receptors in the temporomandibular capsule area are far more important than previously thought.

Since more research on the neurophysiologic regulation of jaw position and function has been done on the adult, there has been a tendency to transfer prosthodontically oriented concepts, based on sound adult clinical practice, to children. Our knowledge about the developmental aspects of orofacial and jaw neurophysiology is incomplete at this time, although much research is under way. We must remember that many of our attitudes are victims of our experience with degenerating occlusions in adults, and the critical clinical factors that apply under those circumstances may not be present in the child or may have different relative significance during development.

Unconditioned jaw positions and functions include mandibular posture for the maintenance of the airway and unconscious or reflex swallowing. The neural mechanisms that determine mandibular posture are important to the dentist, because mandibular posture (sometimes in dentistry called the rest position) is a determinant of the vertical dimension of the face. In the opinion of many, the position of the mandible during unconscious swallowing is an important factor in occlusal homeostasis, because every time a person swallows unconsciously, the occlusal relationship is stabilized or, because of tooth interferences, shifts interfering teeth by lower jaw movement until a stable occlusal relationship finally is obtained.

Conditioned jaw positions and functions include all those of mastication, the mature swallow, and speech and most of facial expression.

OCCLUSAL HOMEOSTASIS

Occlusal stability at any moment is the result of the sum of all forces acting against the teeth. Some of these forces have been measured in research, but it is not yet possible to describe precisely in summation all the forces and counterforces that produce occlusal homeostasis. Occlusal homeostasis is dependent upon elaborate and sophisticated sensory feedback mechanisms from the periodontal membrane, temporomandibular joint, and other parts of the masticatory system. Such sensory feedback serves as a regulating mechanism helping to determine the strength and nature of muscle contractions. Each individual tooth is positioned between contracting sets of muscles. It is also in contact with adjacent teeth and in occlusion with the teeth of the opposite arch. A number of physiologic forces determine the tooth's position occlusally, including eruption, the occlusal force during swallowing, the forces of mastication, occlusal wear of the crown of the tooth, and so forth. Occlusal interferences in or near the unconscious swallowing position of the mandible tend to diminish reflexively the force of muscle contractions during swallowing. Because reflex swallowing occurs so frequently, it plays an important role in occlusal homeostasis. Other factors involved in occlusal homeostasis include the natural mesial drifting tendencies of the teeth, the anterior component of force, the growth of bones of the craniofacial complex, and alveolar bone growth and remodeling. It is now believed that the neuromuscular mechanisms and bone growth factors are far more important in the nature of occlusal relations than are the oft-mentioned factors of cuspal inclination, cusp height, condylar guidance, and so on. The occlusal relationships are now generally held to be nowhere near as stable as depicted in some dental textbooks, if for no other reason than that occlusal adaptations must occur constantly to accommodate, in their way, changes in the neuromusculature and the craniofacial skeleton. Occlusal homeostasis is achieved and maintained in a complex system of responses and adaptations in several tissue systems.

EFFECT OF NEUROMUSCULAR FUNCTION ON
FACIAL GROWTH

From the earliest periods of embryonic growth, an intimate functional relationship exists between muscles and the bones to which they are attached. Obviously, as the bones grow, the muscles must also change their size. Therefore, a relationship exists between the overall growth of any bone and the muscles attached to that bone; and adjustments between muscle and bone are a normal part of growth and development. During growth, muscles also must migrate to occupy relatively different positions with time. As the skeleton grows, there is a constant adjustment of the attachment relationships between muscle and skeleton.

Functional use and disuse determine to some extent the thickness of the cortical plate of limb bones. However, the relationship of muscle function and bone form and growth in the craniofacial skeleton is much more difficult to assess. Certain parts of some of the facial bones are very dependent on function—for example, the alveolar process around the roots of the teeth and the coronoid process to which the temporal muscle is attached. In a more general way, the conformation of the bone and the craniofacial relationships are determined by such factors as mouth breathing, excessive masticatory function, and so forth. In the case of the calvaria, cranial base, and nasomaxillary complex, functional features other than those of muscle apparently play an important role in development and growth—namely, the growth of the brain, the eyeballs, cartilage growth, and so on.

The mandible, with its important condylar cartilage, holds a special interest for dentists, particularly orthodontists. Although there is general agreement that variations in muscle function affect markedly the areas of muscle attachment and that the development and use of the dentition affect the alveolar process, there is some dispute over whether or not muscle function can have a more general effect on the size and form of the mandible. The point is a very important one for orthodontists treating Class II malocclusions in children who are still growing.

Although the evidence is still not complete, most workers now believe that function plays a more dominant role in the determination of mandibular size and conformation than was previously thought. For example, extensive experimental research has shown that the masseter and lateral pterygoid muscles may play a major role in the growth of the mandibular condylar cartilage. It remains unclear, however, whether this effect is a direct one, or whether muscle function influences condylar growth simply by alteration of the biomechanical environment.

EFFECTS OF ORTHODONTIC TREATMENT ON THE MUSCULATURE

It is known that severe malocclusion is often associated with pathologic changes in the temporomandibular articulations, which in turn impair the sensory receptors within the joints, causing such orthodontic patients to have a less precise ability to determine mandibular position than persons who have normal occlusion. After malocclusions have been treated orthodontically, there is a significant change in the range of mandibular movements and an improvement in the precision of the determination of mandibular positions. Occlusal equilibration on treated orthodontic patients has been shown to change significantly teeth-apart swallowing to teeth-together swallowing (Moyers, 1988). Thus, orthodontic treatment including occlusal equilibration conditions swallowing reflexes, which in turn help stabilize the orthodontic occlusal result. Occlusal disharmonies, at the end of orthodontic treatment, have been shown to be disruptive to the stability of treated orthodontic occlusions and thus an important cause of relapse in treated malocclusions. Other adaptive muscular changes following orthodontic therapy may include an altered lip posture, tongue posture, mandibular posture, chewing stroke, and method of breathing.

15

Cephalometrics

B. HOLLY BROADBENT, Jr., D.D.S.

Cephalometric radiography, or "cephalometrics" as it is more frequently called, is a technique employing oriented radiographs for the purpose of making head measurements. It has found wide use in growth research and in orthodontic diagnosis and treatment evaluation. The principles of cephalometrics are patterned closely after the science of craniometry, which has long been used in anthropology in the quantitative study of the skull.

Craniometry was initially applied in measuring dried skulls. Standard landmarks and measurements were developed, and much useful information was obtained. The technique, however, had the obvious shortcoming of being a one-time-only evaluation of a static subject. Serial study of growth changes was obviously not possible. When the technique was transferred to living subjects for growth measurement, accuracy was lost because landmarks were obscured, the soft tissue was of varying thickness, and there was no access to deeper structures.

In 1931 the first comprehensive publication on the basic technique of cephalometric radiography was introduced by Dr. B. Holly Broadbent, Sr. From the early 1920s, Broadbent had been associated with Dr. T. Wingate Todd of the anatomy department of Western Reserve University of Cleveland, Ohio. Todd had been brought from Manchester, England, to head the Brush Inquiry, a study conceived and financed by the famous inventor Charles F. Brush, who was interested in "normal" human development. The Brush Inquiry included, among a very comprehensive group of tests, the concept of the study of the skeletal development of youngsters through serial or longitudinal radiographs of developing epiphyses throughout the entire body.

At that time there was no method for accurately positioning the child's head so that cephalometric radiographs could be compared in a serial study. Dr. Broadbent, through his association with Todd, and with the assistance of an excellent machinist and arduous experimentation, transformed the Todd craniostat into the first cephalometer (Fig. 15–1) in 1925. Thus, cephalometric radiography became a means for producing serial lateral and frontal cephalograms, with the subject in a fixed and reproducible position.

Concurrent with the Brush Inquiry, but as an autonomous research product, the Bolton Study was initiated and supported through the interest of Mrs. Frances P. Bolton and her son Charles. This study investigated the craniofacial and dental development of the Brush Inquiry group as

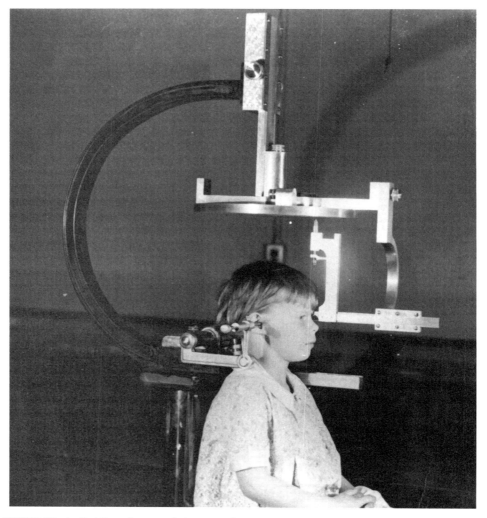

FIGURE 15–1. First Broadbent cephalometer, designed to hold the living head in a manner similar to that used by the radiographic craniometer. (From Broadbent, B. H., Sr., B. H. Broadbent, Jr., and W. Golden: *Bolton Standards of Dentofacial Developmental Growth.* St. Louis, C. V. Mosby, 1975, with permission.)

well as others brought in by interested clinicians. The Broadbent-Bolton cephalometer was used in collecting cephalometric records, many of them comprehensive longitudinal studies, on over 5000 children. The Brush Inquiry and Bolton Study records and data are housed at Case Western Reserve University in Cleveland as the Bolton-Brush Growth Study Center.

Simply stated, cephalometrics involves making measurements from lateral and frontal head radiographs taken with the head held in a fixed position in a cephalometer (Fig. 15–2). The head is held in this position by means of ear rods, which are aligned on the central axis of radiation from the x-ray tube. Thus, for a profile view, the sagittal plane of the head is at right angles to the direction of the x-rays, the film cassette placed as close as possible to the left side of the face. For a frontal or posteroanterior (PA) view, the frontal plane of the head is perpendicular to the x-ray beam, the film cassette placed as close as possible to the face. A standard distance

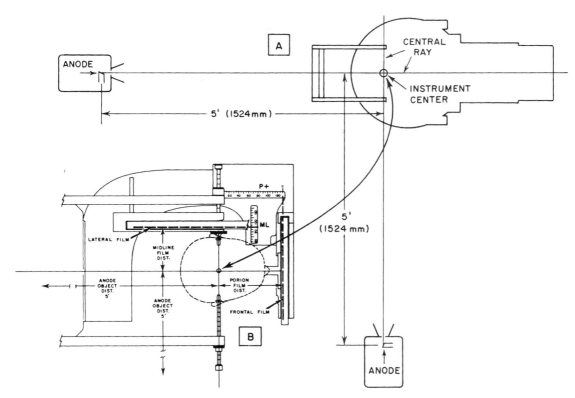

FIGURE 15–2. Bolton cephalometric floor plan. *A,* Relation of the anodes, the central rays, and the instrument center. *B,* Relation of the instrument center to the lateral and frontal films and the ML (midline-lateral film distance) and P+ (porion film distance) scales. (From Broadbent, B. H., Sr., B. H. Broadbent, Jr., and W. Golden: *Bolton Standards of Dentofacial Developmental Growth.* St. Louis, C. V. Mosby, 1975, with permission.)

of 60 inches from the source of radiation to the midsagittal plane or to the porionic axis is maintained. Vernier scales for measuring the film distances from the midsagittal plane or porionic axis for varying head sizes permit accurate correction for enlargement.

Standardization of the technique is necessary to minimize error when serial radiographs of the same individual are taken at different times and to permit universal use of cephalometric data obtained from many different sources. Possible errors in the technique include (1) a lack of perpendicularity of the x-ray beam to the subject's midsagittal plane and the film surface and (2) not placing the film in the closest approximation to the head and face for minimizing enlargement (Fig. 15–3).

Obviously, norms and standards developed from the Broadbent-Bolton technique, where the enlargement factor is minimized, may not be compatible with those derived from a fixed cassette relationship, which may vary from 12 to 18 cm distance from midsagittal plane to film surface, thus causing a disparity in the enlargement factor.

The safety features of the cephalometric technique include the use of the 90-kv peak to minimize softer x-rays, which are absorbed by the patient and are ineffective in contributing to the resulting picture. Additionally, the beam is filtered to remove as many of these softer x-rays as possible. The film is a double-emulsion film sandwiched in a cassette with compatible intensifying screens, which greatly reduce the radiation nec-

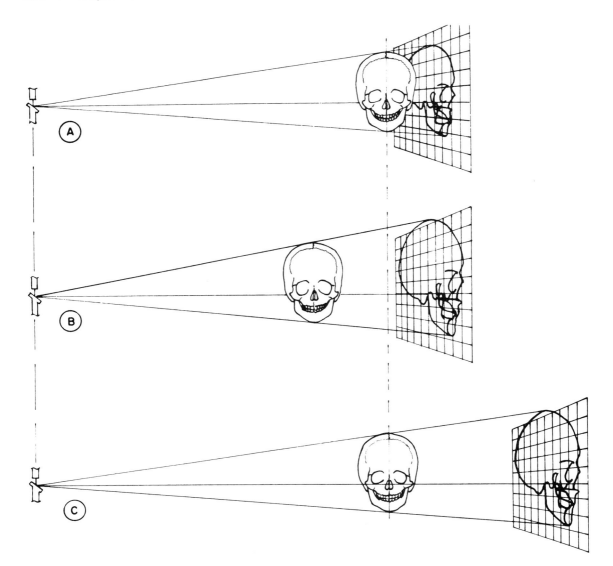

FIGURE 15–3. Enlargement of shadow. *A,* Skull distant from the anode and close to the film produces minimal enlargement and a sharp shadow. *B,* Skull situated closer to the anode and more distant from the film produces unnecessary enlargement and less sharpness of the shadow. *C,* Skull far from the anode and also distant from the film produces unnecessary enlargement and less sharpness of the shadow. (From Broadbent, B. H., Sr., B. H. Broadbent, Jr., and W. Golden: *Bolton Standards of Dentofacial Developmental Growth.* St. Louis, C. V. Mosby, 1975, with permission.)

essary for a satisfactory radiograph. Patient and operating personnel protection is, of course, a prime consideration.

ORIENTATION

In the Broadbent technique, as was noted in the diagrammatic representation of the head holder, a recording of the distance of the lateral film from the midsagittal plane and also the distance of the frontal film surface from the porionic axis allows for direct orientation of the frontal to the lateral for transfer of right and left structures, peripheral to the midline, from the lateral x-ray to the frontal, and the reverse (Fig. 15–4). This orientation is of significant assistance, not only in discerning right and left structures, but also where correction might be necessary for a frontal radiograph in which the head has been tilted down or up from Frankfort relation.

Most contemporary cephalometers used in orthodontic offices incorporate the basic elements of roentgenographic cephalometry but utilize only one x-ray source, with the associated ability to rotate the head holder 90 degrees to take a complimentary frontal view. The wall-mounted arrangement (Fig. 15–5) allows for conservation of space and is very utilitarian, because the x-ray tube may also be used for periapical radiographs. Cephalometers that have provision for taking panoramic radiographs are also available for clinical use.

TRACING THE X-RAYS

Because of the need for measuring angles, planes, and linear dimensions on the radiographs, as well as comparing morphologic features, the historic technique of tracing the x-rays on 0.003 matte acetate paper is widely used so that the tracings of serial records may be superimposed and viewed on a transilluminated screen. The Broadbent-Bolton technique is that of averaging right and left structures in order to produce a tracing that represents these structures as they might be projected on the mid-sagittal plane. Figure 15–6 indicates the tracing technique of drawing between points of the right and left structures, rather than just between lines, in order to make an accurate average of the two images.

Figure 15–7 is a diagram of comprehensive lateral and frontal tracings and also includes many of the landmarks used in the cephalometric analy-

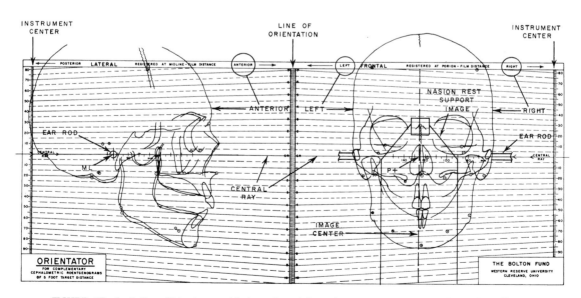

FIGURE 15–4. Bolton Orientator with lateral and frontal tracing in position. (From Broadbent, B. H., Sr., B. H. Broadbent, and W. Golden: *Bolton Standards of Dentofacial Developmental Growth.* St. Louis, C. V. Mosby, 1975, with permission.)

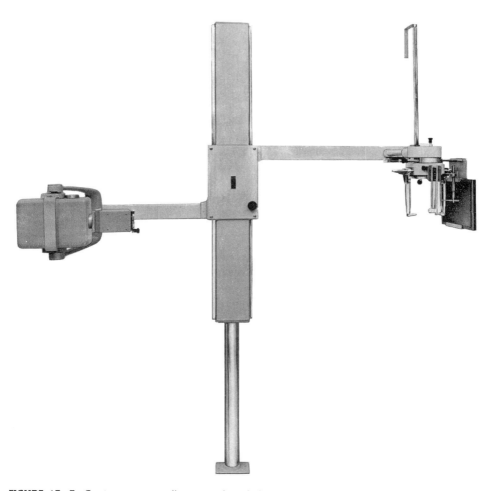

FIGURE 15–5. Contemporary wall-mounted cephalometer. (From the Bolton Study, Bolton-Brush Growth Study Center, Case Western Reserve University, Cleveland, Ohio, with permission.)

ses to be described. A glossary of definitions is included at the end of this chapter.

In making the tracing, of course, the individual investigator or diagnostician may elect to trace whatever features are of interest.

Although the lateral cephalogram is most routinely used in orthodontic practice today, a complementary frontal picture can be of inestimable value in understanding facial proportions (Fig. 15–8), asymmetries that may be present, and the positions of specific dental units such as the incisors, cuspids, and molar series.

Soft tissue structures are of significant importance to the cephalometrician in understanding the relationship of these structures to the skeletal elements as well as to the dentition. Diagnosis of an enlarged adenoid mass, turbinates, tongue and lip position and thickness, and so forth are of great value in the process of diagnosis, treatment planning, and prognosis.

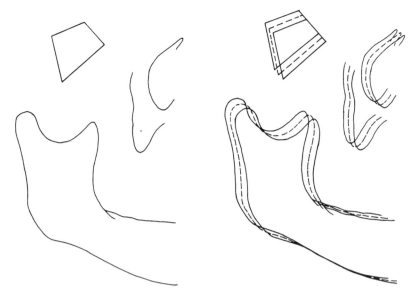

FIGURE 15–6. Averaging method. Note that the average (broken line) maintains the contours of the surfaces being averaged. The average depicts identical facets of right and left structures and not simply adjacent structures. (From Broadbent, B. H., Sr., B. H. Broadbent, Jr., and W. Golden: *Bolton Standards of Dentofacial Developmental Growth.* St. Louis, C. V. Mosby, 1975, with permission.)

NORMS, VARIABILITY, AND COMPARISON

Before entering into a description and discussion of the various cephalometric measurements, it seems appropriate to attempt to define a concept of how and for what purpose we are to use this technique.

It has already been stated that measurements made on oriented headfilms provide useful information in both research and clinical practice. In the research application three primary efforts have been made: first, the accumulation of data related to craniofacial growth changes; second, the establishment of statistical norms for numerous cranial and dentofacial dimensions; and third, the evaluation of response to various treatment procedures. All these approaches have taken into account the obvious variables of age, sex, and racial and ethnic background. In growth research much has been learned of the morphologic and dimensional patterns of skull growth. However, the information is limited to just those aspects: change in shape and size. Although it is true that changes in rate, direction, and pattern of growth have been recorded, the cephalometric technique does not locate the sites of growth or measure the contribution of growth sites. Realistically, the single film provides only a static evaluation of that individual's size and shape at that point in time. A subsequent film on the same individual permits an evaluation of size and shape changes that occurred in the interval between films but does not tell exactly where the growth occurred.

In addition, and not covered in this overview, is the importance of the individual's biologic age (skeletal age), because either delayed or accelerated development is of utmost importance when "normal" comparisons are made. In orthodontic clinical application, the common practice is to make any number of the prescribed measurements on the film and to compare these with established norms. When the word "normal" is used, the researcher and clinician alike may ask, "What is a normal face—or a normal

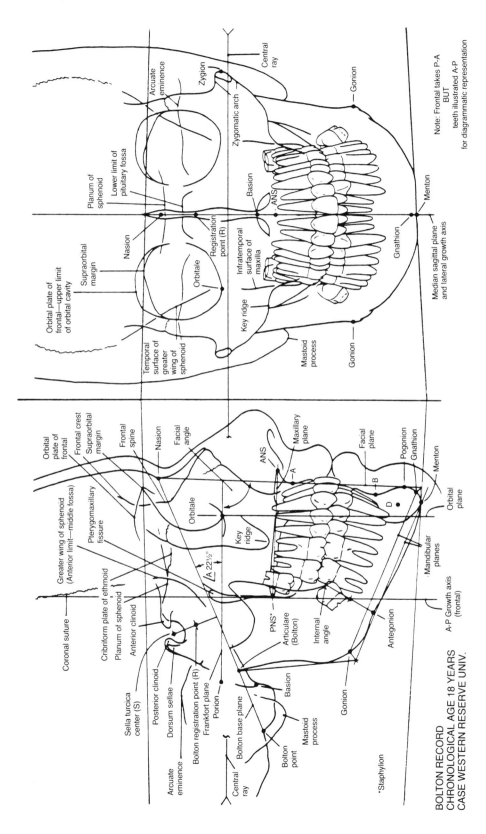

FIGURE 15–7. Lateral and posteroanterior tracings of an 18-year Bolton record. The structures, lines, and points that are frequently traced have been labeled. (From Broadbent, B. H., Sr., B. H. Broadbent, Jr., and W. Golden: *Bolton Standards of Dentofacial Developmental Growth.* St. Louis, C. V. Mosby, 1975, with permission.)

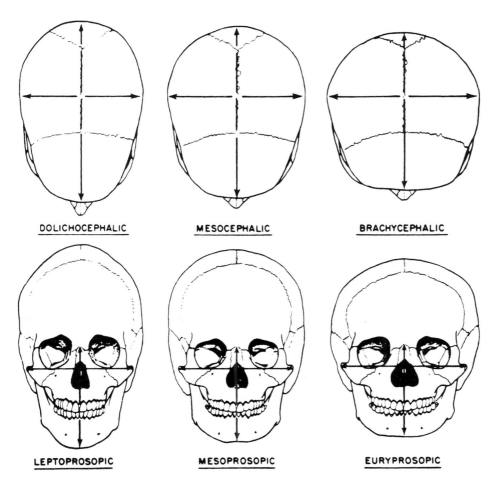

DOLICHOCEPHALIC   MESOCEPHALIC   BRACHYCEPHALIC

LEPTOPROSOPIC   MESOPROSOPIC   EURYPROSOPIC

FIGURE 15–8. Cephalic and facial indices. Three distinct facial types as related to the height, width, and depth of the skull. (From Broadbent, B. H., Sr., B. H. Broadbent, Jr., and W. Golden: *Bolton Standards of Dentofacial Developmental Growth.* St. Louis, C. V. Mosby, 1975, with permission.)

head?" or they may ask, "Normal with reference to what?" Many thousands of cephalometric headfilms have been traced and as many comparisons made in a massive effort to find this elusive "norm." But when we combine the obvious differences in age, sex, race, and environment and add to these the vicissitudes of biologic and genetic variation, it becomes evident that variation is indeed the name of the game.

Realistically, the clinician works with one patient at a time, and when he compares that individual's measurement with statistically derived norms, he is comparing his patient with a generalization drawn from a large group of individuals. Or he may be attempting to forecast the pattern of facial growth of a young patient by comparing his static measurements with those of a large group of similar individuals whose patterns of facial growth have been statistically evaluated. In the world of biology, where variability is still the rule, these efforts, although meeting with increased success, continue to entail a certain amount of hazard.

In practice, the orthodontist compares his patient's measurements with the norms and notes areas of deviation. These norms are calculated means or averages of many equivalent measurements. Along with the mean, a standard deviation (SD) is usually calculated. In clinical use, this SD might be called an acceptable range of variability. In other words, when there is variation within 1 SD, treatment by conventional orthodontic means should yield a good result. As the degree of deviation increases, the relative success of treatment decreases. This may appear to be an over-simplification, but essentially it means that, to some extent, the treatment is the victim of the individual pattern presented.

On the positive side, cephalometric-aided research has identified growth patterns and predictable responses to certain treatment procedures, either of which may assist the treatment planning process. The extent to which deviations from the norm influence the evaluation of the individual patient is a judgment made by the clinician, which he incorporates with all the other diagnostic information he has accumulated.

BOLTON STANDARDS

Many different types of overlay cephalometric appraisals have been conceived through the years, from grids to polygonal patterns, to various transparencies, and so forth. Each has made a contribution to our ever-increasing knowledge of "normal" dentofacial growth and development.

Probably the most comprehensive of these to date are the Bolton Standards of Dentofacial Development Growth. These standards are optimum serial facial patterns that include annual lateral transparencies from 1 to 18 years with coordinated frontal standards from 3 to 19 years for both males and females (Fig. 15–9).

Published by Broadbent, Broadbent, and Golden in 1975, they provide a comprehensive method of analysis, because the soft tissue profile as well as the skeletal elements of the cranium, face, and dentition are provided for morphologic comparison as well as cephalometric measurement.

Because there is no dichotomy of size differentiation between the male and female groups, an average of the two sexes is used as the "standard" for each age. There is, of course, the need to consider sexual dimorphism in the peripheral skeletal morphology (Fig. 15–10 and Table 15–1), but the basic difference in size takes place after puberty, with the males growing for a longer period and to a larger size, as a group, than the females (Fig. 15–11).

It must be recognized that in the averaging tracing technique employed for arriving at single annual "norms," the individual circumpubertal growth spurts of the subjects, which occur at differing ages, are blended out. The Bolton Standards may be superimposed over the cephalogram directly, or, for greater ease of interpretation, over the traditional tracing of the radiograph.

There is no set method of superpositioning, and the diagnostician is free to use whatever landmarks suit the case at hand. Usually, the four basic areas of morphology—cranial base, skeletal maxillary base, mandibular base, and soft tissue—are compared with appropriate chronologic standards; and then specific relationships of these bases and the dentition are assessed (Fig. 15–12).

An example of the use of the standards in analyzing the lateral cephalogram of a 10-year-old Angle Class II, Division I female is shown in Figure 15–13. The superpositioning is arbitrarily done in this instance on the Bolton plane at nasion.

The frontal example is that of a case with a significant mandibular asymmetry. The frontal standard is superimposed on a "best fit" basis on the orbits and upper face to most clearly show the lower face deviations (Figure 15–14).

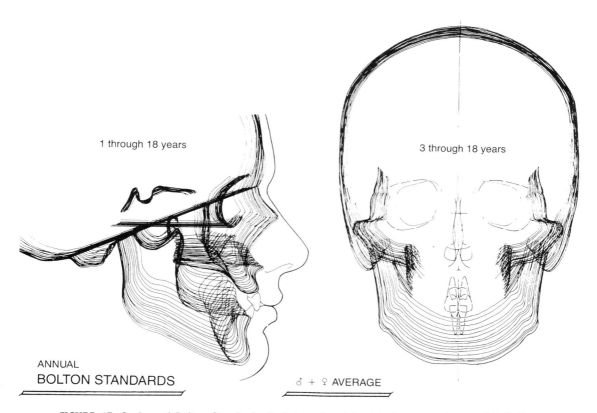

FIGURE 15–9. Annual Bolton Standards. Both lateral and frontal views superimposed in Bolton relation. (From Broadbent, B. H., Sr., B. H. Broadbent, Jr., and W. Golden: *Bolton Standards of Dentofacial Developmental Growth.* St. Louis, C. V. Mosby, 1975, with permission.)

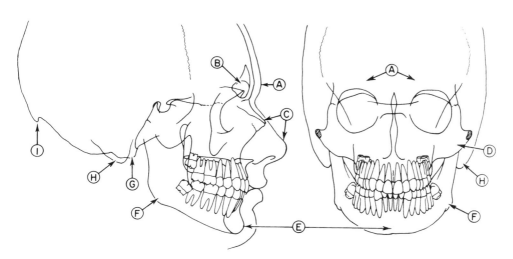

FIGURE 15–10. Sexual dimorphism in craniofacial development. The diagram indicates the basic areas of differentiation that occur between males and females in the adolescent years. (From Broadbent, B. H., Sr., B. H. Broadbent, Jr., and W. Golden: *Bolton Standards of Dentofacial Developmental Growth.* St. Louis, C. V. Mosby, 1975, with permission.)

TABLE 15–1. SEXUAL DIMORPHISM IN CRANIOFACIAL PATTERNS: THREE AREAS OF COMPARISON OF MALES AND FEMALES THAT INDICATE THEIR DISSIMILARITIES*

	Females	Males
Circumpubertal growth spurt	10 to 12 years	12 to 14 years
Mature size	Growth plateaus at approximately 14 years Moderate increase to 16 years	Active to approximately 18 years
Physical characteristics (differences develop in middle to late adolescence)		
Supraorbital ridges (A)	Virtually absent	Well developed
Frontal sinuses (B)	Small	Large
Nose (C)	Moderate	More massive
Zygomatic prominences (cheekbones) (D)	Small	Large
Mandibular symphysis (pogonion) (E)	Rounded	Prominent
External mandibular angle (gonion) (F)	Rounded	Prominent lipping
Occipital condyles (G)	Small	Large
Mastoid processes (H)	Small and delicate	Large
Occipital protruberance (inion) (I)	Insignificant	Prominent

*These dissimilarities are not significantly related to skeletal balance or malocclusion.
From Broadbent, B. H., Sr., B. H. Broadbent, Jr., and W. Golden: *Bolton Standards of Dentofacial Developmental Growth*. St. Louis, C. V. Mosby, 1975, with permission.

It goes almost without saying that standards of the Broadbent-Bolton Standards can only be used, with accuracy, in analyzing cephalograms taken by a similar (i.e., minimal enlargement) technique.

SUMMARY

This discussion of cephalometrics has been admittedly a very brief overview of the technique and principles used in this form of craniofacial evaluation. The technique of acquiring headfilms and tracing and measuring them is straightforward and has demonstrated good accuracy. Over the past 60-odd years, various measurements and systems of analysis have been developed and currently are widely used, especially in the orthodontic field. Cephalometric research and its clinical application have centered on facial pattern evaluation, growth prediction, and treatment evaluation, all of which are external morphologic appraisals. The widespread clinical interest in cephalometrics has undoubtedly resulted in the development of measurements and analyses that help the clinician evaluate areas of primary interest, with emphasis on locating and quantifying external positional deviation, rather than pinpointing sites of growth change or treatment response. The immediate concern of the clinician was, "What is the problem? Where is it? How severe is it? What can I do to correct it?" Cephalometrics has helped answer these questions, but it has not added

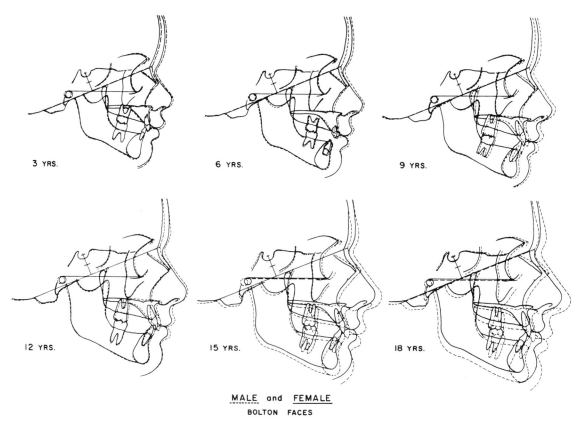

FIGURE 15–11. Average male and female Bolton faces superimposed in Bolton relation. The similar morphologic pattern is demonstrated with the first significant change in size occurring between 12 and 15 years at approximately 14 years. (From Broadbent, B. H., Sr., B. H. Broadbent, Jr., and W. Golden: *Bolton Standards of Dentofacial Developmental Growth*. St. Louis, C. V. Mosby, 1975, with permission.)

significantly to an understanding of the true nature of the deviation, how it got that way, and by what mechanism it will respond to treatment.

In defense of cephalometrics, it must be stated that many of the landmarks and lines were carry-overs from preradiographic craniometric techniques, and although they bore little relationship to sites of growth and/or treatment change, they were easy to locate and lent themselves well to the kind of geometric evaluation in current use.

Deviation was recognized by comparison of patient measurements with statistically derived means obtained by study of selected population samples. Perhaps it is an overstatement to say that this procedure appears to have the potential error of not recognizing biologic variability, and there is an implication of trying to make everybody look alike.

More recently, growth and development research has shifted emphasis to a more complete understanding of individual patterns of growth change and of what is happening in this complex anatomic area to cause these patterns to develop. The principal author of this text, as a counterpoint to the system and philosophy of analysis just described, visualizes use of the cephalometric principle and technique for a quite different purpose. Although the cephalometric study to be described by Enlow in subsequent pages may not be designed for routine clinical use, an understanding of it

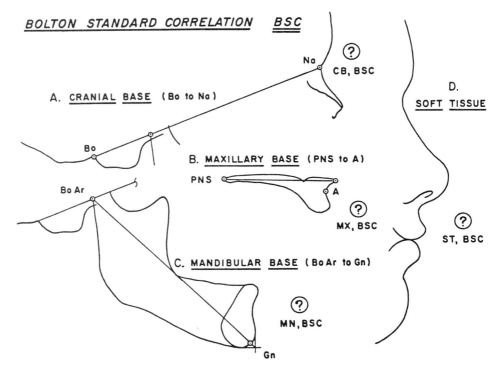

FIGURE 15–12. Bolton Standard Correlation (BSC). Diagrammatic representation of the landmarks employed when the composite standards are used for assigning Bolton Standard age levels to the three skeletal components of the craniofacial complex. (From Broadbent, B. H., Sr., B. H. Broadbent, Jr., and W. Golden: *Bolton Standards of Dentofacial Developmental Growth.* St. Louis, C. V. Mosby, 1975, with permission.)

may help to close the "gap" between the questions, "What is the problem?" and, "How did it get that way?"

COUNTERPART ANALYSIS (OF ENLOW)

This is a method in which the various facial and cranial parts are compared with each other to see, simply, how they fit. The individual is measured against himself, rather than compared with population standards and norms. Most conventional methods of analysis and cephalometric growth studies are intended essentially to determine **what** a particular growth or form pattern is. This procedure was developed to explain **how** such a pattern was produced in any given person. The ANB angle, for example, tells one the nature of the positional relationship between the anterior part of the upper and lower arches and provides an index with which one can gauge the extent of malocclusions. The counterpart procedure is intended to account for the composite of the anatomic and morphogenetic factors that **produced** the particular ANB angle (and other measurements) found in a given person.

Most conventional cephalometric planes and angles are not intended to coincide with or indicate actual sites and fields of growth and remodeling, and they are thus not appropriate for the essentially anatomic purposes just described. Because most standard planes and angles do not represent the patterns and distribution of growth fields, comparisons of the individ-

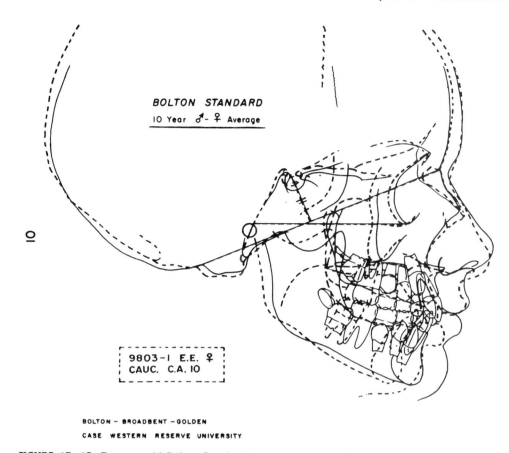

FIGURE 15–13. Ten-year-old Bolton Standard (superimposed on the Bolton plane at nasion) to indicate the structural variables in a typical Class II, Division 1 case. (From the Bolton Study, Bolton-Brush Growth Study Center, Case Western Reserve University, Cleveland, Ohio, with permission.)

ual with population standards are required; there is usually no other basis for interpretation, owing to the nature of the planes themselves. However, if planes are constructed so that the activities of the growth and remodeling fields are in fact directly represented, a built-in and morphologically natural set of "standards" is identifiable that allows meaningful evaluation of overall craniofacial form and pattern without population comparisons.

The analysis is based on the **counterpart principle**. This is the actual design basis upon which the face is constructed and which underlies the plan of its intrinsic growth process. The counterpart concept was described in Chapters 3, 9, and 10, and it was used as the working basis for explaining how the face grows. The counterpart analysis is, in effect, the same. It shows **where** imbalances exist, **how much** is involved, and what the **effects** are.

In Figures 15–15 and 15–16 construction lines have been drawn on a headfilm tracing to represent several key fields and sites of growth. These include the maxillary tuberosity, the mandibular condyle (using articulare for convenience, rather than condylion), the ramus-corpus junction, the posterior border of the ramus, the anterior surfaces of both the maxillary and mandibular bony arches, the occlusal plane, and the junction between the middle and anterior cranial fossae (the anterior-most extent of the great wings of the sphenoid where they cross the cranial floor). Other

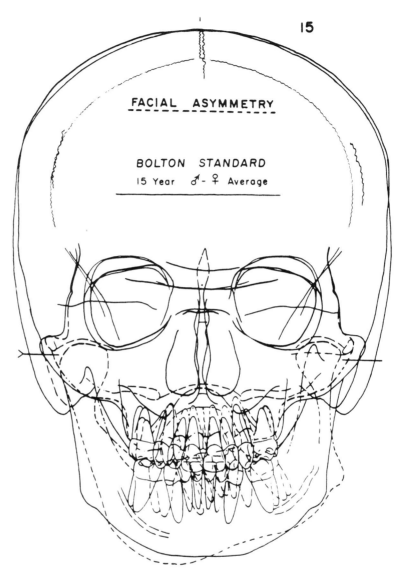

FIGURE 15–14. Fifteen-year-old frontal Bolton Standard (superimposed on the midsagittal plane and orbits) to indicate facial asymmetry in a typical case. (From the Bolton Study, Bolton-Brush Growth Study Center, Case Western Reserve University, Cleveland, Ohio, with permission.)

planes may be added to represent other major growth areas, if desired, such as the zygomatic arch, the palate, the olfactory plane, and the anterior-vertical plane of the midface.

Note that the **PM** vertical plane is represented. This is the important boundary that separates the anterior cranial fossa and nasomaxillary complex from the middle cranial fossa and pharynx. The ramus relates to the latter and the corpus to the former (see page 160).

Two basic factors are important in evaluating the role of any bone or part of a bone in a composite assembly of several different bones. The first

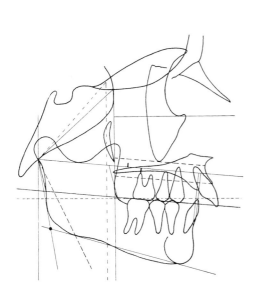

FIGURE 15–15. Headfilm tracing of a Class II patient. Construction lines have been added for the counterpart analysis. (From Enlow, D. H., T. Kuroda, and A. B. Lewis: The morphological and morphogenetic basis for craniofacial form and pattern. Angle Orthod., 41:161, 1971, with permission.)

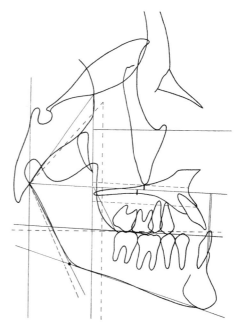

FIGURE 15–16. Headfilm tracing of a Class III patient. Compare with Figure 15–15. (From Enlow, D. H., T. Kuroda, and A. B. Lewis. The morphological and morphogenetic basis for craniofacial form and pattern. Angle Orthod., 41:161,1971, with permission.)

is the bone's **size** (horizontal and vertical), and the second is its **alignment** (rotational position). In this analysis, both must be considered. The reason is that the nature of the alignment of any bone affects the **expression** of its various dimensions, as explained in Chapters 3 and 10. The determination of a bone's dimension alone is not enough (and can be misleading); its alignment must also be known for one to see just how this factor affects its actual dimensions. In the counterpart analysis, both are determined for all the various bony parts and counterparts.

The rationale, in brief, is that the vertical and/or horizontal size of one given part is compared with that of its specific counterpart(s). If they exactly match, or nearly so, a dimensional "balance" exists between them. If one or the other is long or short, however, the resulting imbalance can cause either **protrusion** or **retrusion** of the part of the face involved and thereby affect the profile, either directly or indirectly. The various parts and counterparts are then checked for their alignment to see if each, independently, has a protrusive or a retrusive effect, regardless of the nature of the dimensions. Then all the regional part-counterpart relationships are added up to see how the sum of all underlies the face of any given individual. This may be done on a single headfilm tracing at any age, or serial headfilms can be used for determining the progressive effects of age changes or of treatment results.

Figure 15–15 shows a Class II individual in whom major variations and imbalances are present for the different horizontal and vertical dimensions and for the alignment relationships (compare with the Class III individual described in the next paragraph). Note that (1) the mandibular corpus is short **relative** to its counterpart, the maxillary bony arch (both skeletally and dentally in this individual); (2) the corpus is aligned (rotated) upward (i.e, the "gonial angle" is more closed); (3) the middle cranial fossa is aligned obliquely more forward (the dashed lines represent "neutral" alignment positions); (4) the ramus is aligned more backward; and (5) the nasomaxillary complex is vertically long (resulting in a downward and backward ramus rotation). **All** these features are either mandibular retrusive or maxillary protrusive, and they have combined to produce the multifactorial basis for a Class II malocclusion and retrognathic profile. Note, however, that the horizontal breadth of the ramus **exceeds** its counterpart, the horizontal (not oblique) dimension of the middle cranial fossa. This is a compensatory feature that has partially offset the aggregate effects produced by other features and thereby reduced the severity of the malocclusion. If desired, the actual amounts of each and all of these effects can be measured.

Figure 15–16 shows an individual in whom the dimensions and alignments combine to produce the composite, multifactorial basis for a Class III malocclusion. Note that (1) the dental **and** skeletal dimensions of the mandibular corpus in this individual exceed maxillary arch length; (2) the corpus is aligned (rotated) markedly downward; (3) the middle cranial fossa is aligned backward; and (4) the ramus is aligned forward. These relationships are all mandibular protrusive or maxillary retrusive, and they combine to produce the prognathic face and Class III malocclusion. The horizontal breadth of the ramus, however, is less than that of its counterpart, the middle cranial fossa. This is a compensatory feature that, in this particular individual, has partially offset the composite effects of the other relationships and thereby reduced the extent of the malocclusion.

For a more detailed description of the construction lines used, how to determine the actual dimensions, and how to establish the "neutral" alignment planes for any given individual, see Enlow et al. (1971a).

The "counterpart analysis" is not intended as a routine clinical tool for everyday office use in diagnosis and treatment planning. It is not needed for this, because the rationale for treatment procedures, at least today, is not usually based on corrections of the actual underlying causes of malocclusions and other kinds of facial and cranial dysplasias. The counterpart analysis is useful, however, in determining what treatment has done in terms of the specific anatomic and developmental changes that have been brought about, more so than most types of analyses, because the others deal more with correlative geometry than with morphologic and morphogenetic relationships. Actually, the immediate payoff for the counterpart analysis has already been largely achieved. It has pointed out more clearly the multifactorial basis for malocclusions and just what some of the specific anatomic and developmental factors are. It has shown how a number of compensatory features participate. It has explained how and why population groups have either Class II or Class III tendencies. Except for such specific types of research studies, however, the counterpart analysis is inappropriate as a routine clinical method. When the intrinsic control processes of facial growth become better understood, when the control processes themselves can be controlled, and when treatment procedures can **then** become based on the real causative factors that underlie structural imbalances, then cephalometric analyses utilizing genuine anatomic and developmental relationships will become increasingly more relevant. The counterpart analysis itself, of course, is far from complete and is only a beginning, but it is a concept. It is also very useful in understanding the rationale for the basic plan of normal facial construction as well as malocclusions and in explaining and teaching this complex subject to students in a way that is relatively easy to understand.

COMPUTERIZED CEPHALOMETRICS AND VIDEOIMAGING

Rapid changes in the field of computer science have led to an increase in the use of computers to analyze and/or store cephalometric radiographs. Two methods of analysis are currently in use. The first, and by far the most common, is to connect an x-y coordinate recording device to the computer. The cephalometric radiograph or tracing is placed on the recording tablet and a pointer is used to locate each cephalometric landmark. Once the landmark is located, the operator depresses a button on the pointer and the x and y coordinates of the landmark are recorded in a computer file. This method has been successfully implemented by a number of commercial manufacturers. Users can store the x-y coordinates of landmarks and automatically measure and record linear and angular distances between and among them. All of the software programs will produce the measurements needed to construct the conventional cephalometric analyses. Most software programs also record the means and standard deviations for each measurement and highlight measures that are greater than one or two standard deviations from the mean. Because of their ease of use, these new methods will probably replace the traditional means of pencil and tracing paper analysis of cephalometric radiographs within the next few years.

More recently computers have been used to store video images of the face. These video images can be used in much the same way as 35 mm slides or photographs have been used in the past. In addition, the video images can be linked to the x-y coordinate data derived from the cephalometric radiograph. Linking these two data formats together allows the practitioner to simulate treatment changes on the cephalometric tracing and perform similar modifications on the video image of the face. This combined radiographic and photographic display is being used by practitioners to communicate with patients regarding the potential facial changes that can be achieved with orthodontics alone or in combination with orthognathic surgery.

Another potential use of the computer in clinical orthodontics is to store the actual radiographic image instead of just the x-y coordinates of the anatomic landmarks. This type of digital record has many advantages over storing landmark data. For example, image contrast and brightness can be modified over the whole radiograph or selectively in a small region. To bring out details in the image, one may have higher contrast in the lighter areas of the image, and less contrast in the darker areas. In addition, various structures can have their edges enhanced, thereby improving their visibility. Edge enhancement, like contrast and brightness, can also be selectively applied to either darker or lighter areas or to the entire image. The net result of computerized digital imaging is that one can consistently acquire images of uniform density and selectively enhance any particular structure within the image. In particular, this means that soft tissue will be more easily visualized on digital films than conventional films. Digital images can also be stored, copied, and transmitted without loss of quality or distortion. This would be particularly useful when multiple healthcare providers need access to a patient's radiographic record.

Although digital images have many advantages, this new technology presents a new set of practical, legal, and theoretical problems that need to be addressed. For example, when a film is scanned, whether by video camera or flatbed scanner, the information content of the image must be preserved. The two major parameters which affect the quality of the scanned images are: (1) the spatial resolution, and (2) the gray scale resolution. Traditionally, resolution refers to the quality of an image in terms of the fidelity of the finest details in the content of the image. Thus, the spatial resolution refers to the image quality in terms of the spatial detail. When the spatial resolution is poor, two adjacent spatial features may be blurred together so that they appear as a single feature rather than two separate features. This classical definition of resolution is obviously dependent on the image content, and on the importance of small features as carriers of image information. In digital images, an image-independent and display-independent specification is simply the number of pixels (short for picture elements) in the horizontal and vertical directions. While this is not the only determinant of spatial resolution (in terms of resolving the details in an image), it has become a standard measure.

In terms of cephalometric radiographs, what is the significance of the spatial and gray scale resolutions? Suppose we wish to locate a single landmark, as is necessary to make certain distance measurements. If the spatial resolution were too low (i.e., insufficient number of horizontal and vertical pixels in a digital image), then the image would appear to be blurred. The blurring may completely obscure a landmark, and measurement would be impossible. Less severe blurring would make the landmark less "sharp," larger, and merged with neighboring features, thus introducing ambiguity and error in the measurement of the location of the landmark. In addition to errors introduced by insufficient spatial resolution, the information content of a cephalometric radiograph can be obscured or lost if too few shades of gray are available to represent each pixel. A digital image scanned by a video camera may have 256 gray scale levels. Many texts and sales persons state that 64 gray levels are sufficient for human viewing. However, a simple experiment can show that we easily see a difference of one in 256 gray levels. Thus, the requirement is highly dependent on the image content and the actual measurement made on the image. In terms of the cephalometric radiograph scan, if a landmark feature is in an image region with relatively slow and perhaps subtle changes in gray scale, then too few gray levels may obscure the landmark or change its apparent location. Work done in the Bolton-Brush Growth Study Center at Case Western Reserve University has shown that a spatial resolution of 1500 by 1000 pixels and a gray scale dynamic range of 12 bits preserve all of the information contained on silver halide cephalometric radiographs. Systems that meet these requirements should be available in the near future allowing practitioners and patients to benefit from digital radiographs.

GLOSSARY OF TERMS

The terms to be defined are primarily related to landmarks used in roentgenographic cephalometry. The definitions used are those most commonly found in the craniometric and orthodontic literature.

A: See Subspinale

Antegonion: The highest point of the notch or concavity of the lower border of the ramus where it joins the body of the mandible.

ANS, Anterior nasal spine: A sharp median process formed by the forward prolongation of the two maxillae at the lower margin of the anterior aperture of the nose.

Anteroposterior (AP) or frontal growth axis of the head and face: A transverse zone delineated by a plane through the coronal suture above, passing down through the pterygomaxillary fissure near the posterior termination of the hard palate along the anterior border of the ascending rami, and through the junction of the horizontal and vertical components of the mandible. It marks the division of the anterior from the posterior component of craniofacial developmental growth when lateral tracings are oriented in Bolton relation.

Ar, Articulare: Bjork—The intersection of the image of the posterior border of the ramus with the base of the occipital bone. Bolton—The point of intersection, in lateral aspect, of the posterior border of the condyle of the mandible with the Bolton plane.

B: See Supramentale.

Ba, Basion: The point where the median sagittal plane of the skull intersects the lowest point on the anterior margin of the foramen magnum.

Bolton plane: A line joining the Bolton point and nasion on the lateral cephalogram.

Bo, Bolton point: A point in space about the center of the foramen magnum that is located on the lateral cephalogram by the highest point in the profile image of the postcondylare notches of the occipital bone.

BSC, Bolton standard correlation:

  CB, Bolton cranial base: A line from Bolton articulare to nasion.

  MX, Bolton maxillary base: A line from PNS to ANS.

  MN, Bolton mandibular base: A line from Bolton articulare to gnathion.

Bregma: The point on the skull corresponding to the junction of the coronal and sagittal sutures.

Cephalogram or Radiograph: A generally accepted term describing a standardized roentgenographic (x-ray) picture of the head.

Cephalometer (roentgenographic cephalometer): In craniometry, an instrument for measuring the head. A cephalometer (device for holding the head) combined with roentgenographic equipment for the production of standardized complementary lateral and frontal radiographs used for measuring developmental growth of the dentition, face, and head.

Cd, Condylion: The most superior point on the head of the condyle.

Convexity, angle of: The angle formed by a line nasion to A and a projection of a line pogonion to A.

Coronal suture: The transverse union of the frontal with the parietal bones.

Craniostat: A device for holding the head for craniometric study.

Dacryon: A point on the inner wall of the orbit at the junction of the frontal and lacrimal bones and maxilla.

Facial angle: The angle formed by the junction of a line connecting nasion and pogonion, FP (facial plane), with the horizontal plane of the head, FH (Frankfort plane).

Facial height:

  Total: The distance between nasion and gnathion when projected on a frontal plane.

  Lower face: The distance between ANS and gnathion when projected on a frontal plane.

  Upper face: The distance between ANS and nasion when projected on a frontal plane.

FP, Facial plane: The line connecting nasion and pogonion on the lateral cephalogram.

FH, Frankfort horizontal plane: A horizontal plane determined by the two poria and left orbitale. It approximates closely the position in which the head is carried during life and is established on the lateral cephalogram by a line joining orbitale with porion as indicated by the top of the ear rod.

FMA angle: The angle formed by the mandibular plane and the Frankfort horizontal plane.

Foramen rotundum: A round opening in the greater wing of the sphenoid bone for the passage of the superior division of the fifth nerve.

FOP, Functional occlusal plane: A horizontal line from the posterior-most occlusal contact of the last fully erupted maxillomandibular molars extending anteriorly to the anterior-most occlusal contact of the fully erupted premolars.

Frontotemporale: A point near the root of the zygomatic process of the frontal bone at the anterior-most point along the curvature of the temporal line.

Gl, Glabella: The most anterior point on the frontal bone.

Gn, Gnathion: The lowest, most anterior midline point on the symphysis of the mandible.

Go, Gonion: The external angle of the mandible, located on the later cephalogram by bisecting the angle formed by tangents to the posterior border of the ramus and the inferior border of the mandible.

Ii, Incisor inferius: The tip of the crown of the most anterior mandibular central incisor.

Is, Incisor superius: The tip of the crown of the most anterior maxillary central incisor.

Id, Infradentale: The most anterior point of the tip of the alveolar process between the mandibular central incisors.

I, Inion: The apex of the external occipital protuberance.

Interincisal angle: The angle formed by the long axis of the lower incisor and the long axis of the upper incisor.

Internal angle of the mandible: Located on the lateral cephalogram by bisecting the angle formed by tangents to the anterior border of the ramus and the superior border (alveolar crests) of the mandible. Note: A line joining the internal angle and the antegonion marks the junction of the ramus with the body of the mandible.

Key ridge: The prominent ridge, formed by the malar process, which divides the canine fossa from the infratemporal fossa on the lateral surface of the maxillary bone.

Lateral growth axis: The division between the right and left lateral components of growth (see median sagittal plane).

MP, Mandibular planes: Variations of definitions include:
A tangent to the lower border of the mandible.
A line joining gonion and gnathion.
A line joining gonion and menton.
A line from menton tangent to the posteroinferior border of the mandible.

Maxillary plane: See Palatal plane.

Median sagittal plane: See Lateral growth axis. The anteroposterior median plane of the cranium and face.

Me, Menton: The most inferior point on the symphysis of the mandible in the median plane. Seen on the lateral cephalogram as the most inferior point on the symphyseal outline.

N, Na, Nasion: The craniometric point where the midsagittal plane intersects the most anterior point of the nasofrontal suture. (The anterior termination of the Bolton plane.)

Normal face: By normal face, we do not mean a face of certain dimensions or particular form (features), but a well-grown face, harmoniously developed, skeletally and dentally, and consistent in developmental progress with its years (Bolton).

O point: Center for convergence area of horizontal planes used in Sassouni's analysis.

Occ, Occlusal plane: A line passing through one-half of the cusp heights of the first permanent molars and one half of the overbite of the incisors.

Op, Opisthion: The most posterior point of the foramen magnum.

Orbital plane: The frontal (transverse) plane of the head passing through the left orbital point.

Or, Orbitale: In craniometry, the lowest point on the inferior margin of the orbit. The left orbital point is used in conjunction with the poria to orient the skull on the Frankfort horizontal plane.

Pal, Palatal plane, Maxillary plane: A line connecting the tip of the anterior nasal spine with the tip of the posterior nasal spine as recorded in the lateral cephalogram.

PM, Posterior maxillary plane: A vertical line from the averaged intersections of the great wings of the sphenoid and the anterior cranial floor, extending inferiorly to the averaged lower-most points of PTM.

Po, Pog, Pogonion: The most anterior point on the symphysis of the mandible in the median plane.

Points:

   A: See Subspinale.

   B: See Supramentale.

   D: The center of the cross section of the body of the symphysis. It is established by visual inspection.

   R: Bolton registration point. The center of the Bolton cranial base; a point midway on the perpendicular erected from the Bolton plane to the center of the sella turcica (S).

P, Porion: Anatomic porion is the outer upper margin of the external auditory canal; machine porion is the uppermost point on the outline of the ear rods of the cephalometer.

Porionic axis: A line drawn between the two poria.

PNS, Posterior nasal spine: A process formed by the united, projecting median ends of the posterior borders of the two palatine bones.

Pr, Prosthion: The most anterior point of the alveolar portion of the premaxilla, between the upper central incisors.

PTM, Pterygomaxillary fissure: In the lateral cephalogram, an inverted, elongated, teardrop shaped area formed by the divergence of the maxilla from the pterygoid process of the sphenoid. The posterior nasal spine and staphylion are generally located beneath the lower pointed end of this area.

Pt-vertical: A vertical line tangent to the posterior contour of PTM perpendicular to FH.

S, Sella turcica (Turkish saddle): The hypophyseal or pituitary fossa of the sphenoid bone lodging the pituitary body. The landmark S is the center of sella as seen in the lateral cephalogram and located by inspection.

SE, Sphenoethmoidal suture: The most superior point of the suture.

Si: The most inferior point on the lower contour of the sella turcica.

SN, Sella-nasion plane: The plane formed by connecting a line from sella to nasion.

Skeletal age: The maturational age of an individual as determined by the analysis of bone age indicated by the hand-wrist x-ray (biologic age).

SO, Spheno-occipital synchondrosis: The most superior point of the junction between the sphenoid and occipital bones.

Sp: The most posterior point on the posterior contour of the sella turcica.

Supraorbital plane: A line tangent to the anterior clinoid process and the most superior point on the roof of the orbit, as seen on the lateral cephalogram.

Sta, Staphylion: The point in the medial line (interpalatal suture) of the posterior part of the hard palate where it is crossed by a line drawn tangent to the curves of the posterior margins of the palate. (In the lateral cephalogram, the posterior curved margins of the hard palate frequently may be seen more clearly than the posterior nasal spine).

SOr, Supraorbitale: The uppermost point of the orbital ridge on the lateral cephalogram, it can be located at the junction of the roof of the orbit and the lateral contour of the orbital ridge.

Subspinale (Point A): That point in the median sagittal plane where the lower front edge of the anterior nasal spine meets the front wall of the maxillary alveolar process (Downs' point A).

Supramentale (Point B): The deepest midline point on the mandible between infradentale and pogonion (Downs' point B).

Te, Temporale: The intersection of the shadows of the ethmoid and the anterior wall of the infratemporal fossa.

Vertex: The most superior point on the cranial vault.

Y-axis: The line joining the sella turcica (S) center and gnathion.

Zygion: The point on the zygoma on either side, at the extremity of the bizygomatic diameter.

16

Bone and Cartilage

Cartilage provides three basic functions. It gives **flexible** support in appropriate anatomic places (the nasal tip, ear lobe, thoracic cage, tracheal rings); it is a **pressure-tolerant** tissue located in specific skeletal areas where direct pressure occurs (articular cartilage); and it functions as a **"growth cartilage"** in conjunction with certain enlarging bones (synchondrosis, condylar cartilage, epiphyseal plate). Cartilage is a nonvascular connective tissue and it is ordinarily noncalcified. Both vascularization and calcification, however, are involved as steps in the replacement process by bone tissue.

Several distinctive structural features relate to cartilage. First these are listed, and then the nature of their interrelationships is explained in terms of the various fundamental functions of cartilage.

Cartilage is a special type of connective tissue that has a stiff, firm, but **not hard** intercellular matrix. It provides rigid support, but it is so soft that it can be cut with a fingernail. This feature is based on the exceptionally high content of water-bound ground substance. The rich amount of chondroitin sulfate (Gr. *chondros*, cartilage) in the cartilage matrix is associated with a noncollagenous protein, and this combination has the special property of marked hydrophilia. This gives the turgid, firm character to the matrix. Cartilage thus develops in a variety of body locations where flexible (not brittle) support is appropriate. Cartilage has an enclosing vascular chondrogenic membrane, but it can have surfaces without one. Cartilage can grow appositionally and/or interstitially.

Because the matrix is noncalcified, the matrix is also able to be nonvascular. Nutrients and metabolic wastes diffuse directly through the soft matrix to and from cells. Thus, blood vessels are not required within cartilage as they usually are in bone, with its hard, impervious matrix.

Because the matrix is nonvascular, cartilage is pressure tolerant. There are no vessels near the surface to mash closed by compression, thereby allowing cartilage to operate metabolically because there are no pathways of supply to occlude. The water-bound, noncompressible matrix, furthermore, is not badly distorted by the force, and its turgid nature protects the cells within it from surface pressures.

Unlike bone, cartilage can function without a covering membrane because its nonvascular matrix is thus not dependent upon **surface** blood vessels in an enclosing **surface** membrane.

Because cartilage can function without a covering membrane, it is especially adaptable to sites involving pressure, as on long-bone articular surfaces and the surfaces of epiphyseal plates. If a soft connective tissue membrane were present, its vessels would be closed off by the compression, and the cells would be subject to anoxia as well as damage by the direct pressure itself. Furthermore, a delicate perichondrial membrane could not withstand abrasive articular movements. In conjunction with synovial secretions, however, the naked surface of the articular cartilage provides relatively frictionless movements while bearing great weight under severe pressure. (Note: The "secondary" cartilage of the mandibular condyle involves a specialized tissue system. Another tissue type having a characteristic capacity for pressure tolerance is dense non-vascular and relatively acellular collagenous connective tissue. The secondary condylar cartilage has a unique "capsule" composed of such tissue.)

Because cartilage has an interstitial as well as a membrane-dependent appositional mode of growth, it can thereby still grow in those pressure areas where an enclosing connective tissue membrane is absent. This includes articular surfaces, synchondroses, and epiphyseal plates. (Note again, the "secondary" nature of the condylar cartilage has a specialized system, as described in Chapter 4.)

Because ordinary cartilage matrix is not calcified, cell divisions can take place—which is not the case in bone—thus providing interstitial growth.

One can readily see how each and all of the above features interrelate and are directly interdependent. To perform the functions of a **growth cartilage** in endochondral sites of bone growth, no one of these features could work without all the others. Cartilage exists as a separate, special tissue type because of these special features, and its multiple functions could not be carried out by **any** of the other soft or hard tissues.

BONE

Bone provides the specialized feature of **hardness**. Because of this, it has several unique developmental characteristics. A bone, of course, cannot enlarge by interstitial growth because its cells are locked into a non-expandable matrix. It is thus dependent upon covering vascular membranes (periosteum and endosteum) providing the osteogenic capacity for an appositional system of growth. This is also why bone is necessarily a **traction** (tension) -adapted kind of tissue and why "bone" is said to be "pressure-sensitive."* The covering soft tissue membrane is sensitive to direct compression, because any undue amount would occlude its blood vessels, interfere with osteoblastic deposition of new bone, and cause avascular necrosis. Actually, it is the periosteal **membrane** and not the hard part of the bone itself that is pressure sensitive (see page 208). The mag-

---

*The whole subject of pressure and tension is greatly oversimplified in most routine descriptions, as it is also in the present discussion. The actual nature of the forces that act on a bone is quite complex and can seldom be designated purely as either tension or pressure. A bundle of periosteal fibers, for example, can exert tension on a bone surface, but that same surface can also be under a compressive influence from other sources, such as a flexure pressure effect on a concave curvature. Pressure effects can also be exerted by intercellular fluids in a region otherwise classified as under tension. An osteogenic cell located between collagenous fibers under tension actually receives a direct pressure effect. Moreover, compressive effects on the hard part of the bone itself can have an osteoblastic trigger effect, while compressive effects on blood vessels can have an osteoclastic effect. The old, greatly oversimplified, and inaccurate concept that one-to-one tension-deposition and pressure-resorption relationships exist is no longer acceptable, as described in Chapter 12. The overall growth control system is much more complex, and is incompletely understood at present.

nitude of compression is such that it cannot exceed capillary pressure, which is a "light" force of about 25 gm/cm^2.

The degree of vascular flow is affected by the amount and type of mechanical force acting on a soft tissue, and this is directly involved in initiating either chondrogenesis or osteogenesis. More extreme levels of hypoxia caused by higher levels of pressure are known to stimulate formation of chondroblasts leading to nonvascular cartilage, rather than osteoblasts, from undifferentiated connective tissue cells. For all of these various reasons, two basic modes of bone growth thus exist, one (intramembranous) is adapted to a localized environment of tension (or at least levels of pressure less than that of capillary pressure), and the other (endochondral) to more extreme compressive forces.

Soft tissues, in general, grow (1) by increasing the **number** of cells (as in epithelia); (2) by increasing the **size** of cells (as in skeletal muscle); or (3) by increasing the amount of **matrix** between cells (as in loose connective tissue). Many tissue types combine two or all three of these different modes of growth (as in cartilage). All are interstitial systems of growth because they involve expansive changes of tissue components already present. Bone, because it is calcified, must necessarily grow by a process of adding new cells and new matrix onto the existing **surfaces** of previously formed generations of bone tissue. It cannot, of course, expand interstitially by division and proliferation of osteocytes because the cells have no place to divide to; they and their genes are locked into their calcified, nonexpanding matrix. Bone **must**, therefore, grow in relationship to a covering or lining membrane. It is the bone surface, either periosteal or endosteal, that is the site of growth activity. This type of growth is termed "appositional," in contrast to "interstitial" expansion. All bone that is fully calcified grows in this manner regardless of its mode of osteogenesis (endochondral or intramembranous).

Where **compression** is involved that exceeds the connective tissue membrane's threshold level of capillary pressure, as mentioned above, the intramembranous growth mechanism (which is dependent upon vascular membranes, as the name indicates) does not have the capacity to function. Thus, a growth cartilage grows **toward** the site of compression. Epiphyseal plates, synchondroses, and other "growth cartilages" provide for the linear enlargement of bones that have pressure contacts at their ends. The cartilage grows interstitially and/or by apposition on one side as the older part of the cartilage on the other side is removed and replaced by bone. The cartilage functions essentially as a kind of advance ram that shields the sensitive endosteal bone membrane beneath it and, importantly, **also provides for the growth elongation of the bone at the same time**. The **other** areas of the bone grow intramembranously.

During active growth, a depository bone surface is constantly changing because of new additions; any given point within the compact substance of bone, however deep, **used** to be an actual exposed surface, either periosteal or endosteal. If a **metallic implant marker** or **vital dye** (such as alizarin, or tetracycline, or the procion dyes) is used in a living bone, growth changes that occur after the marker is implanted or the dye is administered can be determined. Such markers and the lines formed by the vital dyes become covered over wherever subsequent surface deposition occurs. (Note: Vital dyes stain only that bone actively being laid down during the period in which the dye is in the bloodstream. Thus, one injection forms a thin, colored line on all the active surfaces of the bone. Subsequently formed bone deposits are not colored.) Metallic implants (tiny tantalum bits) can be injected into the cortex of a growing bone by means of a special "gun." These radiopaque markers can then be seen in x-ray films taken days, weeks, or even years later in order to determine where and how much a bone has been **remodeled** by deposition and resorption relative to the markers. **Displacement** movements of whole bones can also be determined by noting the directions and amounts of separation among implants previously inserted into two or more separate bones.

Bone **deposition** is only part of the overall process of bone enlargement; it is one phase of a multiphase growth system. **Resorption** is another part, and this is just as important and necessary as deposition (Fig. 16–1). Ordinary resorption associated with growth is not "pathologic," although beginning students sometimes mistakenly view it as evil because resorption is a destructive process or because it can also be involved in some diseases. Resorption **must** accompany deposition, and deposition on one side of a cortical plate (or cancellous trabecula) with resorption from the other brings about the growth movement ("relocation") of the part. Thus, deposition on the periosteal side with resorption on the endosteal surface of a cortex moves the whole cortex outward and at the same time proportionately increases its thickness. Note, that a surface implant (Fig. 16–1) becomes translocated from one side to the other by this process. The implant itself does not move; rather, the remodeling bone moves around the implant. As pointed out in Chapter 2, **remodeling** also takes place everywhere throughout an entire bone because the bone does not simply expand by generalized external deposition and internal resorption.

Remodeling (Fig. 16–2) involves various combinations of deposition (*1* and *3*) and resorption (*2* and *4*) on different periosteal and endosteal surfaces in order to **move** (relocate) a part of a growing bone into a new

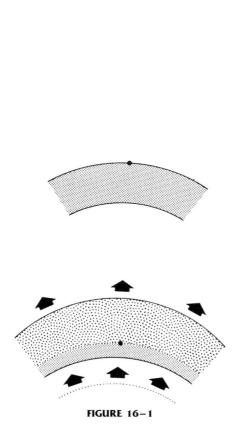

FIGURE 16–1

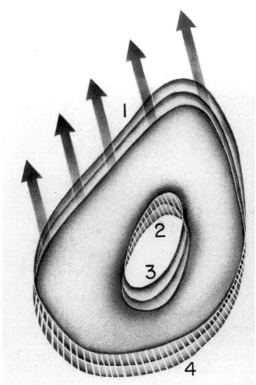

FIGURE 16–2. (From Enlow, D. H.: *Principles of Bone Remodeling.* Springfield, Ill., Charles C Thomas, 1963, with permission.)

location (see Chapter 2). The process of relocation shapes and sizes a bone continuously as a basic part of the growth mechanism.

Surface depository activity is by the osteoblasts of the innermost cellular layer of the thick periosteum or the very thin endosteum. The latter is only about one cell thick and lacks a thick, fibrous layer because muscles, tendons, and other such force-adapted tissues are not attached to it. Vessels enclosed within endosteal circumferential layers of bone characteristically enter at a right angle because the endosteum is not under tension and its vessels, therefore, are not drawn out toward the long axis of the bone. Periosteal "slippage" over a bone surface is involved in the periosteum in relation to the forces acting on it as it grows, and this causes the periosteal vessels to become enclosed at much more acute angles. The old notion of perpendicular "Volkmann" canals entering the bone from the outer periosteum needs to be forgotten. (See Enlow, 1963, for an in-depth, early historical account of bone as a tissue.)

As new bone is progressively laid down, the covering periosteal membrane **grows** in an outward direction. The outer membrane grows inward if the periosteal surface is resorptive. However, these membranes do not simply "move" as they bring about the cortical movement. They are not merely pushed or pulled or somehow migrate into their new positions. Rather, the membranes each **grow** from the one location to the other. It is the growth movement of the outer and inner membranes that produces the growth movement (remodeling) of the bony cortex located between these "genic" membranes. The membrane has its own internal, interstitial growth process. Just as the bone **remodels** during growth, the periosteum also undergoes its own internal remodeling process. Remember that the membrane itself paces the bone changes, and that the "fields" of growth activity (described in Chapter 2) reside in this membrane and the other soft tissues, rather than within or on the bone itself.

As collagenous fibers and ground substances are laid down by the osteoblasts (*g* in Fig. 16–3), this new layer of **osteoid** almost simultaneously undergoes calcification to become bone tissue (*x* in Fig. 16–4). Some of the osteoblasts are enclosed to become new osteocytes, and some of the periosteal blood vessels contiguous with the bone surface are also incorporated. The anastomosing vessels then lie within a network of **vascular canals** as bone is formed around them. Note that the fibers of attachment (Sharpeys fibers) become more deeply embedded as new bone is formed

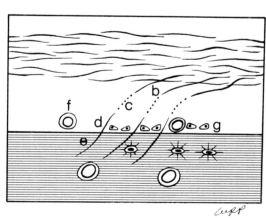

FIGURE 16–3

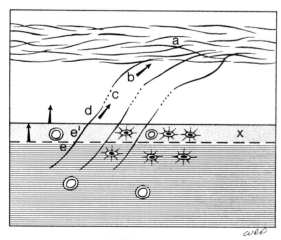

FIGURE 16–4

around the collagenous fibers in the innermost layer of the periosteum (*d*). The periosteal fibers now, themselves, **grow** and lengthen by their own remodeling outward. Fiber segment *d* thus lengthens on the outside while it is being enclosed by new bone on the inside (*e'* in Fig. 16–4). It does this by **conversion** of segment *c* into a new addition onto *d*, which elongates by this process. Segment *c* is a special **precollagenous** fibril. It is a very thin fibril that requires special staining methods (see Kraw and Enlow, 1967). Many such fibrils (i.e., "linkage" fibrils) form a distinctive zone within the periosteal membrane. Under the control of the rich population of fibroblasts, these slender fibrils become remodeled by coalescence into the thick collagenous fibers that form the lengthening segments of *d*. This is done by binding with ground substance (proteoglycans).

Segment *c* now lengthens in a direction away from the bone surface. It is not presently known whether this is done by a remodeling conversion from segment *b* through enzymatic removal of the binding ground substance to release its numerous, slender precollagenous fibrils, or whether new precollagenous lengths are added directly to *c* by the fibroblasts in this zone. As these changes occur, however, new *b* segments are being formed by fibroblastic activity as they join the expanding outer, dense "fibrous" layer of the periosteum (*a*). The entire periosteum thus **relocates** outward as the bone surface correspondingly drifts in the same direction. If the periosteal surface is **resorptive**, rather than depository, the sequence of operations is the same, but the direction is reversed. That is, the periosteum and its fibers develop **toward**, rather than away from, the bone surface, which is moving inward, rather than outward.

How does a muscle or tendon maintain continuous attachment onto a bone surface that is **resorptive**? Moreover, how does a muscle **migrate** over a bone surface (whether resorptive or depository) as the bone lengthens? For example, the muscle shown in Figures 16–5 and 16–6 **moves** its insertion. It must also sustain constant attachment on a mixed remodeling surface, part of which is undergoing progressive resorption and part deposition. The other muscle shown in Figure 16–6 attaches entirely onto a resorptive surface. Bone resorption is customarily regarded as a process that results in total destruction of the bone tissue, including as well its anchoring fibers of attachment In many non–stress-bearing locations, this can be true. In some (not all) areas involving muscle, tendon, ligament, and periodontal attachments, however, there are several histogenic means by which fibrous attachment is sustained. First, although not common, the process of fiber destruction is not necessarily complete. Some of the fibers in the ordinary bone matrix are not removed by the resorptive process, especially when aligned in the direction of strain. These fibers become

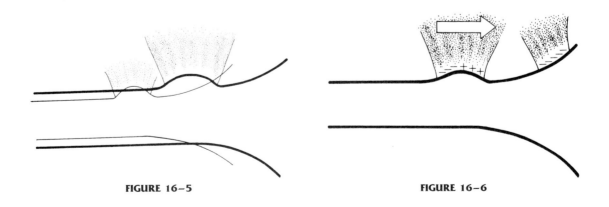

FIGURE 16–5   **FIGURE 16–6**

uncovered as the remainder of the bone matrix around them is resorbed, and they are then freed to function as fibers of the **periosteum** while retaining continuity with the fibers in the bone of which they were once a part. A second and much more commonly seen histogenetic mechanism involves an "adhesive" mode of attachment in which certain fibroblast-like cells secrete proteoglycans onto a naked resorptive surface (Kurihara and Enlow, 1980b and c). New precollagenous fibrils are then formed as the adhesive secretion of proteoglycans continues. The new fibrils then link to the more mature fibers in the periosteum, the proteoglycans serving as the binding agent (Fig. 16–7). If new bone is subsequently deposited by the periosteum, the calcified adhesive interface then becomes a "reversal line." (Note: A comparable process also occurs in periodontal attachments on remodeling alveolar bone.) This cycles over and over as the process continues.

In other stress-bearing locations, another separate mechanism is seen that provides for continuous fibrous attachments on resorptive, remodeling, and relocating bone surfaces. This involves a reconstruction of the bone **deep** to the resorptive surface in order to provide uninterrupted fibrous anchorage. "Undermining" resorption takes place, in which resorption canals are formed well below the surface of the inward-advancing resorptive periosteal front. New bone is then laid down with these deeper, protected spaces, and it is this attachment that provides additional fibrous anchorage while the outside bone surface itself is undergoing resorptive removal. Thus, as periosteal surface is resorbed, a large number of resorptive spaces are formed (in histologic sections, many appear as cut-off canals). These spaces anastomose with each other. The fibers in the new bone subsequently deposited in them are continuous by relinking with the remodeling fibers of the periosteum, and anchorage is thereby maintained (Fig. 16–8). The structural result is a generation of haversian systems (secondary osteons) **deep** to the surface. The fibrous matrix of each osteon and its connection by labile linkage fibrils to the inward-moving resorptive

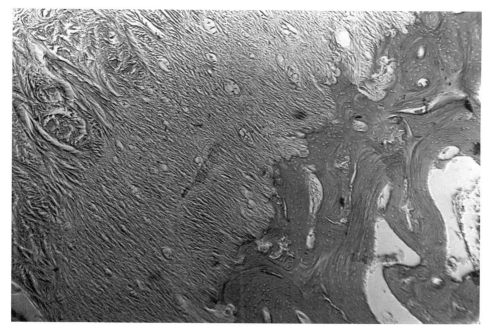

FIGURE 16–7

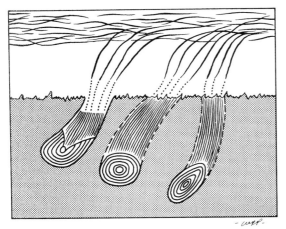

FIGURE 16-8

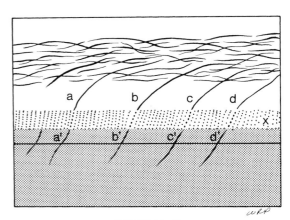

FIGURE 16-9

periosteum are protected from resorption until the resorptive front reaches them. However, new waves of haversian systems are constantly being formed in advance of the resorptive front, so that new deeper osteons replace, in turn, those that become exposed as they reach the resorptive periosteal surface. Moreover, a muscle moves and migrates along a bone surface by this same process of haversian formation, as well as by lateral reconnections of the labile linkage fibrils (x) in the intermediate part of the periosteum (or equivalent areas for direct tendon insertions). Thus, the precollagenous linkage fibrils connecting with fiber a in the outer part of the periosteum (Figs. 16–9 and 16–10) become recombined with the precollagenous fibrils of fiber b' in the inner part of the periosteum, and so on. This progression moves the entire muscle along the bone surface to keep pace with the elongation of the entire growing bone. Separations of fiber bundles by enzymatic removal of the ground substance binding, together with precollagenous fibril regroupings by new ground substance formation, are believed to carry this out. See also Figure 16–20.

Sutures have an osteogenic process comparable to periosteal bone growth. The suture is an inward reflection of the periosteal membrane, and the fibrous, linkage, and osteoblastic zones are directly continuous from one to the other (Figs. 16–11 and 16–12). As a new layer of bone is

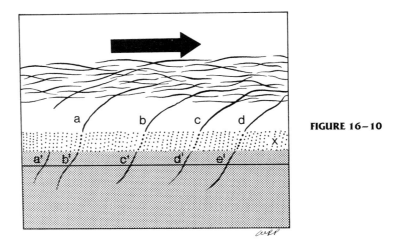

FIGURE 16-10

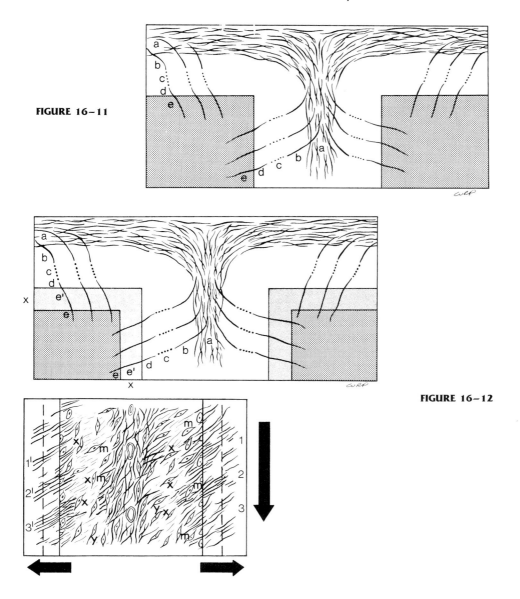

FIGURE 16–11

FIGURE 16–12

added (x), inner collagenous fibers d become embedded to form new attachment fibers (e') in the bone matrix. The d fibers, however, lengthen
by conversion from the labile linkage fibers (c) just as previously described
for the periosteum, and d fibers converted, in turn, into lengthening c
fibers (or fibroblastic activity may bring about direct lengthening of c, as
in the periosteum). As new bone is added to the sutural contact surfaces,
the bones are simultaneously displaced away from one another (see Chapter 2 for a discussion of the physical forces that cause this displacement).
Many sutures have three basic layers (on each side), as indicated here
(Fig. 16–13). Some sutural types, however, have another layer of loosely
arranged fibers located within the center of the dense-fibered capsular
layer dividing the two sides. The basic plan of growth and remodeling,
however, is the same. When the process of growth ceases, the suture becomes essentially a mature ligament, and the precollagenous linkage fibrils are no longer present.

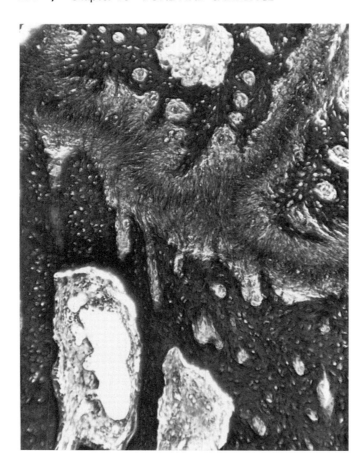

FIGURE 16-13. (From Enlow, D. H.: *The Human Face.* New York, Harper & Row, 1968, p. 96, with permission.)

Importantly, the source of the propulsive force that produces the "downward and forward" displacement movement of the nasomaxillary complex at its various sutures has long been a subject of controversy. It has recently been suggested that the abundant population of actively contractile fibroblasts ("myofibroblasts," *m* cells in Fig. 16–12) within the linkage zone of the sutural membrane provide, at least in part, a contractile force that exerts tension on the fibrous framework. This, in turn, presumably pulls one bone along its sutural interface with another bone or at least contributes to the moving, relinking placements of the fibers as some other propulsive force causes the bone movements. The bone thus "slides" along the suture as new bone tissue, at the same time, is laid down on the sutural edges. The midface is thereby **pulled** forward and downward along its multiple sutural surfaces. Special collagen-degrading and collagen-producing fibroblasts (*x* and *y*) provide the fiber remodeling and ground substance relinkage changes also involved. Fibers at level *1*, which were formerly linked with fibers at level *1'*, have become relinked with fibers at *2'*, and so on. (See Azuma et al., 1975.) Refer to pages 86 and 92.

BONE TISSUE TYPES RELATED TO DEVELOPMENT AND FUNCTION

Histology textbooks teach that the haversian system (secondary osteon) is the structural "unit" of bone. This is quite incorrect. In the bone of the young, growing child, the haversian system is **not** a major structural feature. (Most vertebrate groups and species lack haversian systems altogether. See Enlow, 1963.) This old haversian system notion not only has misled students of dentistry and medicine, but also has concealed an important concept. There are other, much more widespread kinds of bone in the child's growing skeleton. The concept is this: different functional and developmental circumstances and conditions exist, and there is a specific histologic type of bone tissue for each. Some bone types are fast growing, others slow growing. Some bone types grow inward, others outward. Some are associated with muscles, tendon, or periodontal attachments; others are not. Some bone types form a thick cortex; others, a thin cortex. Some relate to a dense vascular supply; others, to scant vascularization—and so on. "Haversian systems" could not do all this. These are important points because a basic feature of bone is its developmental versatility and adaptability as a tissue.

    Primary vascular bone tissue (Figs. 16–14 and 16–17) is the principal type of periosteal cortical bone in the growing skeleton of the child. The vessels are enclosed within canals as new bone is laid down around each vessel in the osteogenic part of the periosteum. These canals are not derived from precursor secondary resorption spaces. If the bone is fast growing, many vessels and their canals characteristically become enclosed. If it is slower growing, fewer or even no canals are incorporated within the compact bone substance. **Compacted coarse cancellous** bone (Fig. 16–15) is the principal cortical type formed by the endosteum. One half to two thirds of all the cortical bone in the body is composed of this important, distinctive structural type. It is formed by the inward growth of the cortex

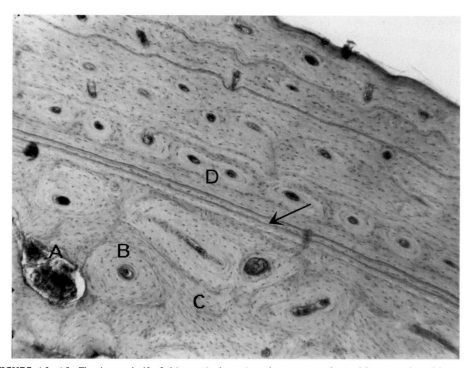

FIGURE 16–14. The lower half of this cortical section shows an endosteal layer replaced by secondary osteons. The upper half is a periosteal layer composed of a layered mix of lamellar and non-lamellar bone containing primary vascular canals and primary osteons. (From Enlow, D. H.: *Principles of Bone Remodeling.* Springfield, Ill, Charles C Thomas, 1963, with permission.)

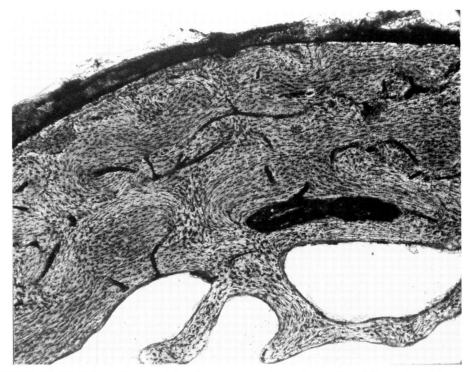

FIGURE 16–15. This section was taken from an inward-growing region of the cortex. It is compacted cancellous bone produced by endosteal deposition and periosteal resorption. The large spaces between the coarse cancellous trabeculae have been filled with lamellar bone. (From Enlow, D. H.: A study of the postnatal growth and remodeling of bone. Am. J. Anat., 110:79, 1962, with permission.)

into the medulla (i.e., periosteal resorption and endosteal deposition). Medullary cancellous bone is converted into cortical compact bone by filling the spaces until they are reduced to vascular canal size (Figs. 16–16, and 16–17). Although a major and widespread bone tissue type, standard histology texts have yet to recognize it, just as with the primary vascular type just described.

Fine cancellous bone (Fig. 16–18) is one of the fastest growing types. It is formed throughout the fetal skeleton and also occurs in rapidly enlarging parts of all postnatal bones. This type of cortical bone tissue is characterized by spaces that are larger than ordinary vascular canals, but smaller than the coarse cancelli of the medulla. **Nonlamellar** (also called "fibrous") bone is also a rapid-growing type, and it occurs in conjunction with fine cancellous bone formation, although "compact" areas of a fast-growing cortex may also be nonlamellar. (See Enlow, 1963 and 1990 for further details.)

Bundle bone is characterized by dense inclusions of attachment fibers from the periodontal membrane (see Fig. 7–3). This bone type is formed only on the depository sides of the alveolar socket. The resorptive side is usually composed of compacted coarse cancellous (endosteal) bone or, if the alveolar plate is very thin, of bundle bone formed on the depository side, but translated over to the resorptive side as alveolar drift proceeds. **Chondroid** bone is found at the apex of the alveolar rim and other rapidly forming areas throughout the skeleton (such as the apex of growing tuberosities where tendons attach). This bone tissue type resembles cartilage because of the large, rounded appearance of its crowded osteocytes sur-

FIGURE 16–16. The wide end of a bone grows in a longitudinal direction by deposition on the endosteal side and resorption from the periosteal side. This is because the **inside** surface actually faces toward the direction of growth. Medullary bone is converted into cortical bone by cancellous compaction. In areas where cancellous trabeculae are no longer present, however, inward growth involves deposition of inner circumferential bone (arrow). The inward mode of growth also serves to reduce the wide part into the more narrow part (diaphysis) as the whole bone lengthens. In the diaphysis, the direction of growth reverses, and periosteal bone is laid down. (From Enlow, D. H.: *Principles of Bone Remodeling.* Springfield, Ill. Charles C Thomas, 1963, with permission.)

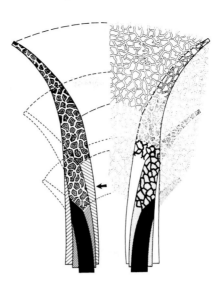

rounded by a nonlamellar, basophilic matrix. Because it undergoes internal metaplasia into **other** bone tissues types, chondroid bone is perhaps the only kind of bone tissue that actually has what might be regarded as an interstitial mode of growth.

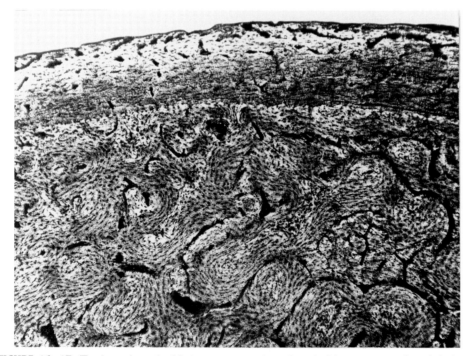

FIGURE 16–17. The inner layer in this transverse section of cortical bone was produced during a period of inward (endosteal) growth and was formed by the process of cancellous compaction. After outward reversal, a periosteal layer of primary vascular bone was subsequently laid down. Note the reversal front between these two zones. (From Enlow, D. H.: A study of the postnatal growth and remodeling of bone. Am. J. Anat., 110:79, 1962, with permission.)

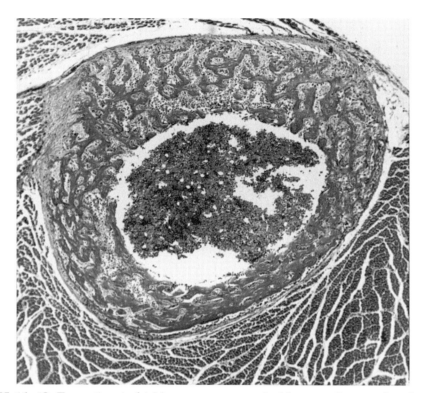

FIGURE 16–18. The cortices in fetal bones are composed of fine cancellous, nonlamellar bone tissue. Note the relatively small connective tissue-filled spaces. Areas of very fast growth in postnatal bones can also be fine cancellous in structure. (From Enlow, D. H.: A study of the postnatal growth and remodeling of bone. Am. J. Anat. 110:79, 1962, with permission.)

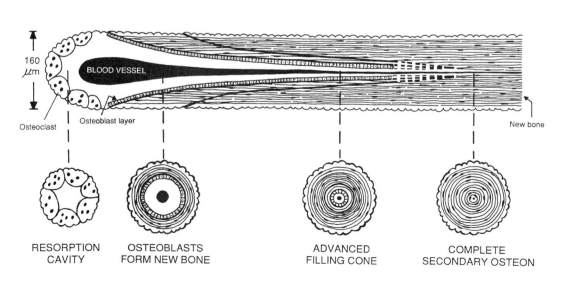

FIGURE 16–19. Schematic diagram of a cutting and filling cone. (Adapted from Roberts, W. E., P. K. Turley, N. Brezniak, and P. J. Fielder: Bone physiology and metabolism. Calif. Dent. Assoc. J., 15(10):54–61, 1987, with permission.)

Haversian Systems

When haversian (secondary) replacement of bone occurs, several functional reasons are involved, in addition to that already described, and relate to conditions that develop in the older skeleton. First, during childhood growth, generalized remodeling during growth provides a constant **turnover** of bone tissue so long as growth continues. The bone is not present long enough for any marked extent of osteocyte aging and necrosis to develop. (Bone cells have a finite life period.) Moreover, the histologic types of childhood bone are more highly vascular because they are mostly rapid forming, as just seen. This favors osteocyte survival. As a child matures and growth slows, however, slower forming bone types become more widespread, and these tend to be less dense in vascular distribution, which promotes earlier onset of osteocyte necrosis. Because "growth remodeling" no longer replaces bone in the adult, "haversian remodeling" then becomes operative to provide vital, new bone by internal cortical reconstruction. Resorption canals followed by concentric deposition of Haversian lamellae within them thus replaces old, dying, or dead cortical bone, and the result is a secondary osteon. This reconstruction process **also** contributes to min-

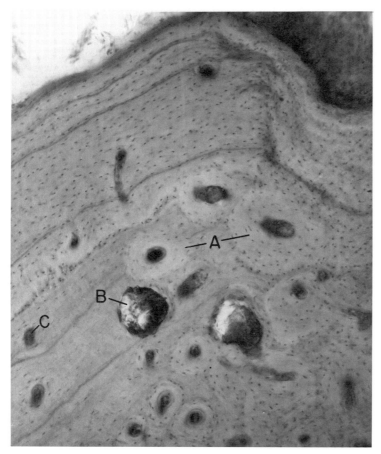

FIGURE 16–20. These secondary osteons are located in a tuberosity that is undegoing a remodeling movement. The shifting of the attached muscle involves the continued formation of haversian systems. A primary vascular canal (*C*) is enlarged into a resorption canal (*B*), and concentric lamellae subsequently deposited within the resorption spaces result in fully formed secondary osteons (*A*). (From Enlow, D. H.: Functions of the haversian system. Am. J. Anat., 110:269, 1962, with permission.)

eral homeostasis in older individuals, since more aged bone is less labile in surface ion exchanges. Another function of haversian reconstruction is to provide replacement for bone that has experienced extensive structural fatigue involving extensive "microfracture" accumulation over time.

These are important factors leading to osseointegration of dental implants. The implant is placed by the surgeon and the bone adjacent to the implant undergoes necrosis. Cutting and filling cones (See Fig. 16–19) then sequentially replace the bone contiguous with the implant, resulting in an implant that is "part" of the bone (osseointegrated).

In summary, thus, the continuous renewal of childhood bone by the growth (remodeling) process becomes largely discontinued in the adult. But, a different form of the same remodeling mechanisms (resorption and deposition) takes over in a way that does not change the size and shape of the skeleton; that is, haversian (secondary) reconstruction within the existing bone.

An interesting point is that the haversian system is a visible example of a basic biologic concept, which is the principle of the "tissue cylinder." **All** vascular tissues, soft as well as hard, involve a relationship which states, simply, that there is a cylinder of tissue supplied by blood vessels centrally positioned within that cylinder. The radius of the cylinder is the extent to which physiologic transfers can occur from the center to and from the cells resident within the cylinder. In bone, this universal tissue relationship is quite graphically demonstrated, since the secondary osteon is, itself, a functional tissue cylinder.

In conjunction with muscle migrations and continuous reattachments along a growing bone's surface (see above), a limited distribution of **haversian systems** is formed in some areas of muscle attachment on resorptive or remodeling surfaces of a bone in the child (Fig. 16–20), but otherwise, secondary osteons are not a principal feature of the young skeleton. Most haversian systems develop and accumulate much later in life and are concerned with the secondary reconstruction of the original primary cortical bone.

Lamellar bone is a slower growing type found throughout most parts of the adult's skeleton and slower forming areas of the child's skeleton. Depending on location, they may be termed periosteal circumferential, endosteal circumferential, cortical, coarse-cancellous, or haversian lamellae. **Primary osteons** (in contrast to the secondary osteon) are relative small structures in which concentric lamellae are laid down in the fine-cancellous spaces of non-lamellar bone, as seen in Figure 16–14.

Bibliography

Ackerman, J. L., Y. Tagaki, W. R. Proffit, and M. J. Baer: Craniofacial growth and development in cebocephalia Oral Surg., 19:543, 1965.

Adams, D., and M. Harkness: Histological and radiographic study of the spheno-occipital synchondrosis in cynomolgus monkeys, *Macaque irus*. Anat. Rec., 172:127, 1972.

Aduss, H.: Form, function, growth, and craniofacial surgery. Otolaryngol. Clin. North Am., 14:939, 1981.

Anderson, J. H., L. Furstman, and S. Bernick: The postnatal development of the rat palate. J. Dent Res., 46:366, 1967.

Angle, E. H.: Bone growing. Dent. Cosmos., 52:261, 1910.

Atkinson, P. J., and C. Woodhead: Changes in human mandibular structure with age. Arch. Oral Biol., 13:1453, 1968.

Avery, J. K.: Children with cleft lips and cleft palate: Embryological basis for defects of the face and palate. In: *Handicapped Children—Problems, Programs, Services in Michigan*. University of Michigan Educational Series, No. 93. Ann Arbor, University of Michigan, 1961.

Avery, J. K., and R. K. Devine: The development of the ossification centers in the face and palate of normal and cleft palate human embryos. Cleft Palate Bull., 9:25, 1959.

Avis, V.: The relation of the temporal muscle to the form of the coronoid process. Am. J. Phys. Anthropol., 17:99, 1959.

Azuma, M.: Study of histologic changes of periodontal membrane incident to experimental tooth movement. Tokyo Med. Dent. Univ., 17:149, 1970.

Azuma, M., and D. H. Enlow: Fine structure of fibroblasts in the periodontal membrane and their possible role in tooth drift and eruption. Jpn. J. Orthod., 36:1, 1977.

Azuma, M., D. H. Enlow, R. G. Frederickson, and L. G. Gaston: A myofibroblastic basis for the physical forces that produce tooth drift and eruption, skeletal displacement at sutures, and periosteal migration. In: *Determinants of Mandibular Form and Growth*. Ed. by J. A. McNamara, Jr. Ann Arbor, University of Michigan, Center for Human Growth and Development, 1975.

Babula, W. J., G. R. Smiley, and A. D. Dixon: The role of the cartilaginous nasal septum in midfacial growth. Am. J. Orthod., 58:250, 1970.

Baer, M. J.: Patterns of growth of the skull as revealed by vital staining. Hum. Biol., 26:80, 1954.

Baer, M. J., and J. A. Gavan: Symposium on bone growth as revealed by *in vitro* markers. Am. J. Phys. Anthropol., 29:155, 1968.

Bahreman, A. A., and J. E. Gilda: Differential cranial growth in rhesus monkeys revealed by several bone markers. Am. J. Orthod., 53:703, 1967.

Bang, S., and D. H. Enlow: Postnatal growth of the rabbit mandible. Arch. Oral Biol., 12:993, 1967.

Bassett, C. A. L.: Electro-mechanical factors regulating bone architecture. In: *Proceedings of the Third European Symposium on Calcified Tissues*. Davos, Switzerland, New York: Springer-Verlag, 1966.

Bassett, C. A. L.: Biologic significance of piezoelectricity. Calcif. Tissue Res., 1:252, 1968.

Baughan, B., and A. Demirjian: Sexual dimorphism in the growth of the cranium. Am. J. Phys. Anthropol., 49:383, 1978.

Baume, L. J.: The postnatal growth activity of the nasal cartilage septum. Helv. Odont. Acta, 5:9, 1961b.

Baume, L. J.: Ontogenesis of the human temporomandibular joint. I. Development of the condyles. J. Dent. Res., 41:1327, 1962.

Baume, L. J.: Cephalofacial growth patterns and the functional adaptation of the temporomandibular joint structures. Eur. Orthod. Soc. Trans., 1969: 79, 1970.

Baumrind, S.: Reconsideration of the propriety of the "pressure-tension" hypothesis. Am. J. Orthod., 55:12, 1969.

Baumrind, S., F. H. Moffett, and S. Curry: The geometry of three-dimensional measurement from paired coplanar x-ray images. Am. J. Orthod., 84: 313, 1983.

Baumrind, S., E. L. Korn, Y. Ben-Basset, and E. E. West: Quantitation of maxillary remodeling. 2. Masking of remodeling effects when an "anatomical" method of superimposition is used in the absence of metallic implants. Am. J. orthod. Dentofacial Orthop., 91:463, 1987.

Becker, R. O., C. A. L. Bassett, and C. H. Bachman: The bioelectric factors controlling bone structure. In: *Bone Biodynamics*. Boston, Little, Brown, 1964.

Beersten, W.: Migration of fibroblasts in the periodontal ligament of the mouse incisor as revealed by autoradiography. Arch. Oral Biol., 20:659, 1975.

Behrents, R. G.: Déjà vu: Neurotropism and the regulation of craniofacial growth. In: *Factors Affecting the Growth of the Midface*. Ed. by J. A. McNamara, Jr. Ann Arbor, University of Michigan, Center for Human Growth and Development, 1979.

Behrents, R. G.: *Atlas of Growth in the Aging Craniofacial Skeleton*. Monograph 18. Craniofacial Growth Series. Ed. by D. S. Carlson and K. A. Ribbens. Ann Arbor, University of Michigan, Center for Human Growth and Development, 1986.

Behrents, R. G., and L. E. Johnston: The influence of the trigeminal nerve on facial growth and development. Am. J. Orthod., 85:199, 1984.

Behrents, R. G., D. S. Carlson, and T. Abdelnour: *In vivo* analysis of bone strain about the sagittal suture in *Macaca mulatta* during masticatory movements. J. Dent. Res., 57:904, 1978.

Beresford, W. A.: *Chondroid Bone, Secondary Cartilage and Metaplasia*. Baltimore, Urban & Schwarzenberg, 1981.

Berkowitz, S.: State of the art in cleft palate orofacial growth and dentistry: A historical perspective. Am. J. Orthod., 74:564, 1978.

Bhat, M., and D. H. Enlow: Facial variations related to headform type. Angle Orthod., 55:269, 1985.

Biggerstaff, R. H., R. C. Allen, O. C. Tuncay, and J. Berkowitz: A vertical cephalometric analysis of the human craniofacial complex. Am. J. Orthod., 72:397, 1977.

Bimler, H. P.: Physiologic and pathologic variants of the mandible in form, position and size. Fortschr. Kieferorthop., 46:261, 1985.

Bishara, S. E., P. Burkey, and J. Karouf: Dental and facial asymmetries: A review. Angle Orthod., 64:324, 1994.

Bjork, A.: The use of metallic implants in the study of facial growth in children: Method and application. Am. J. Phys. Anthropol., 29:243, 1968.

Bjork, A., and V. Skieller: Growth of the maxilla in three dimensions as revealed radiographically by the implant method. Br. J. Orthod., 4:53, 1977.

Bjork, A., and V. Skieller: Normal and abnormal growth of the mandible. A synthesis of longitudinal cephalometric implant studies over a period of 25 years. Eur. J. Orthod., 5:1, 1983.

Blackwood, H. J.: Growth of the mandibular condyle of the rat studied with tritiated thymidine. Arch. Oral Biol., 11:493, 1966.

Bloore, J. A., L. Furstman, and S. Bernick: Postnatal development of the cat palate. Am. J. Orthod., 56:505, 1969.

Bookstein, F. L.: Looking at mandibular growth: Some new geometric methods. In: *Craniofacial Biology*. Ed. by D. S. Carlson. Ann Arbor, University of Michigan, Center for Human Growth and Development, 1981.

Bookstein, F. L.: On the cephalometrics of skeletal change. Am. J. Orthod., 82:177, 1982.

Bosma, J. F.: Form and function in the mouth and pharynx of the human infant. In: *Control Mechanisms in Craniofacial Growth*. Ed. by J. A. McNamara, Jr. Ann Arbor, University of Michigan, Center for Human Growth and Development, 1975.

Brash, J. C.: Some problems in the growth and development mechanics of bone. Edinb. Med. J., 41:305, 1934.

Brin, I., D. Hom, and D. Enlow: Correlation between nasal width and maxillary incisal alveolar width in postnatal facial development. Eur. J. Orthod., 12:185, 1990.

Brin, I., M. B. Kelley, J. L. Ackerman, and P. A. Green: Molar occlusion and mandibular rotation: A longitudinal study. Am. J. Orthod., 8:397, 1982.

Broadbent, B. H.: A new x-ray technique and its application to orthodontia. Angle Orthod., 1:45, 1931.

Broadbent, B. H.: The face of the normal child. Angle Orthod., 7:183, 1937.

Broadbent, B. H., B. H. Broadbent, Jr., and W. H. Golden: *Bolton Standards of Dentofacial Developmental Growth*. St. Louis, C. V. Mosby, 1975.

Brodie, A. G.: Facial patterns: A theme on variation. Angle Orthod., 16:75, 1946.

Brodie, A. G.: Late growth changes in the human face. Angle Orthod., 23:146, 1953.

Brodie, A. G.: The behavior of the cranial base and its components as revealed by serial cephalometric roentgenograms. Angle Orthod., 25:148, 1955.

Bromage, T. G.: Mapping remodeling reversals with the aid of the scanning electron microscope. Am. J. Phys. Anthropol., 81:314, 1982.

Bromage, T. G.: Interpretation of scanning electron microscopic images of abraded forming bone surfaces. Am. J. Phys. Anthropol., 64:161, 1984a.

Bromage, T. G.: Surface remodelling studies on fossil bone. J. Dent. Res., 63:491, 1984b.

Bromage, T. G.: Taung facial remodeling: A growth and development study. In: *Hominid Evolution: Past, Present, and Future*. Ed. by P. V. Tobias. New York, Alan R. Liss, 1985.

Bromage, T. G.: The ontogeny of *Pan troglodytes* craniofacial architectural relationships and implications for early hominids. J. Hum. Evol., 23:235, 1992.

Burdi, A. R.: Sagittal growth of the naso-maxillary complex during the second trimester of human prenatal development. J. Dent. Res., 44:112, 1965.

Burdi, A. R.: Early development of the human basicranium: its morphogenic controls, growth patterns and relations. In: *Development of the Basicranium*. Ed. by J. F. Bosma. DHEW Pub. 76:989, NIH, Bethesda, Md., 1976.

Burdi, A. R.: Biological forces which shape the human midface before birth. In: *Factors Affecting the Growth of the Midface*. Ed. by J. A. McNamara, Jr. Ann Arbor, University of Michigan, Center for Human Growth and Development, 1976.

Burdi, A. R., and K. Faist: Morphogenesis of the palate in normal embryos with special emphasis of the mechanisms involved. Am. J. Anat., 120:149, 1967.

Burdi, A. R., and M. N. Spyropoulos: Prenatal growth patterns of the human mandible and masseter muscle complex. Am. J. Orthod., 74:380, 1978.

Burstone, C. J.: Biomechanics of tooth movement. In: *Vistas in Orthodontics*. Ed. by B. T. Kraus and R. A. Riedel. Philadelphia, Lea & Febiger, 1962.

Carlson, D. S.: Patterns of morphological variation in the human midface and upper face. In: *Factors Affecting the Growth of the Midface*. Ed. by J. A. McNamara, Jr. Ann Arbor, University of Michigan, Center for Human Growth and Development, 1976.

Carlson, D. S.: Condylar translation and the function of the superficial masseter muscle in the rhesus monkey (*M. mulatta*). Am. J. Phys. Anthropol., 47:53, 1977.

Carlson, D. S.: Growth of the masseter muscle in rhesus monkeys (*Macaca mulatta*). Am. J. Phys. Anthropol., 60:401, 1983.

Carlson, D. S., J. A. McNamara, Jr., and D. H. Jaul: Histological analysis of the mandibular condyle in the rhesus monkey (*Macaca mulatta*). Am. J. Anat., 151:103, 1978.

Carlson, D. S., E. E. Ellis III, and P. C. Dechow: Adaptation of the suprahyoid muscle complex to mandibular advancement surgery. Am. J. Orthod. Dentofacial Orthop., 92:134, 1987.

Castelli, W. A., P. C. Ramirez, and A. R. Burdi: Effect of experimental surgery on mandibular growth in Syrian hamsters. J. Dent. Res., 50:356, 1971.

Cederquist, R., and A. Dahlberg: Age changes in facial morphology of an Alaskan Eskimo population. Int. J. Skeletal Res., 6:39, 1979.

Chaconas, S. J., and J. D. Bartroff: Prediction of normal soft tissue facial changes. Angle Orthod., 45: 12, 1975.

Charlier, J. P., A. Petrovic, and J. Herrmann: Déterminisme de la croissance mandibulaire: Effets de l'hyperpulsion et de l'hormone somatotrope sur la croissance condylienne de jeunes rats. Orthod. Fr., 39:567, 1968.

Charlier, J. P., A. Petrovic, and J. Herrmann-Stutzmann: Effects of mandibular hyperpulsion on the prechondroblastic zone of young rat condyle. Am. J. Orthod., 55:71, 1969a.

Charlier, J. P., A. Petrovic, and G. Linck: La fronde mentonnière et son action sur la croissance mandibulaire. Recherches experimentales chez la rat. Orthod. Fr., 40:99, 1969b.

Cheng, M., D. Enlow, M. Papsidero, H. Broadbent, Jr., O. Oyen, and M. Sabat: Developmental effects of impaired breathing in the face of the growing child. Angle Orthod., 58:309, 1988.

Choi, Y.-C. C.: A study of classification of Class III malocclusion in Korean children according to the craniofacial skeleton. KyungHee Dental J., 15: 1993.

Christiansen, R. L., and C. J. Burstone: Centers of rotation within the periodontal space. Am. J. Orthod., 55:353, 1969.

Cleall, J. F.: Growth of the craniofacial complex in the rat. Am. J. Orthod., 60:368, 1971.

Cleall, J. F.: Growth of the palate and maxillary dental arch. J. Dent. Res., 53:1226, 1974.

Cochran, G. V. B., R. J. Pawluk, and C. A. L. Bassett: Stress generated electric potentials in the mandible and teeth. Arch. Oral Biol., 12:917, 1967.

Cohen, M. M., Jr.: Dysmorphic growth and development and the study of craniofacial syndromes. J. Craniofac. Genet. Dev. Biol., 1:251, 1985.

Cohen, M. M., Jr.: Children, birth defects and multiple birth defects. Ann. R. Coll. Phys. Surg. Can. Part 1, 19:375, 1986; Part 2, 19:465, 1986.

Cohen, S. E.: Growth concepts. Angle Orthod., 31: 194, 1961.

Conklin, J. L., D. H. Enlow, and S. Bang: Methods for the demonstration of lipid as applied to compact bone. Stain Technol., 40:183, 1965.

Copray, J. C., J. M. H. Dibbets, and T. Kantomaa: The role of condylar cartilage in the development of the temporomandibular joint. Angle Orthod., 58:369, 1988.

Cousin, R. P., and R. Fenart: La rotation globale de la mandibule infantile envisagée dans sa variabilité. Étude en orientation vestibulaire. Orthod. Fr., 42:225, 1971.

Dahlberg, A. A.: Evolutionary background of dental and facial growth. J. Dent. Res., 44(Suppl.): 151, 1965.

Dale, J. G., A. M. Hunt, G. Pudy, and D. Wagner: Autoradiographic study of the developing temporomandibular joint. Can. Dent. Assoc. J., 29:27, 1963.

Davidovitch, Z., M. D. Finkelson, S. Steigman, J. L. Shanfeld, P. C. Montgomery, and E. Korostaff: Electric currents, bone remodeling, and orthodontic tooth movement. Part I. The effect of electric currents on periodontal cyclic nucleotides. Am. J. Orthod., 77:14, 1980a.

Davidovitch, Z., M. D. Finkelson, S. Steigman, J. L. Shanfeld, P. C. Montgomery, and E. Korostaff: Electric currents, bone remodeling, and orthodontic tooth movement. Part II. Increase in rate of tooth movement and periodontal cyclic nucleotide levels by combining force and electric current. Am. J. Orthod., 77:33, 1980b.

De Angelis, V.: Autoradiographic investigation of calvarial growth in the rat. Am. J. Anat., 123:359, 1968.

DeCoster, L.: Une nouvelle ligne de référence pour l'analyse des télé-radiographics sagittales en orthodontie. Rev. Stomatol., 11:937, 1951.

Delaire, J.: La croissance des os de la voute du crane: Principes generaux. Rev. Stomatol., 62:518, 1961.

Delaire, J.: Considérations sur la croissance faciale (en particulier de maxillaire supérieur). Déductions thérapeutiques. Rev. Stomatol., 72:57, 1971.

Delaire, J.: The potential role of facial muscles in monitoring maxillary growth and morphogenesis. In: *Muscle Adaptation in the Craniofacial Region*. Ed. by D. S. Carlson and J. A. McNamara, Jr. Ann Arbor, University of Michigan, Center for Human Growth and Development, 1976.

Delattre, A., and R. Fenart: L'hominisation de crane. Éditions due Centre National de la Recherche Scientifique, Paris, 1960.

Dempster, W. T., and D. H. Enlow: Osteone organization and the demonstration of vascular canals in the compacta of the human mandible. Anat. Rec., 133:268, 1959.

Diamond, M.: Posterior growth of the maxilla. Am. J. Orthod., 32:359, 1946.

Dibbets, J. M. H.: Juvenile temporomandibular joint dysfunction and craniofacial growth. Thesis, Dept. Orthod., Univ. of Groningen, 1977.

Dibbets, J. M. H., and L. van der Weele: Orthodontic treatment in relation to symptoms attributed to dysfunction of the temporomandibular joint: A 10-year report on the University of Groningen Study. Am. J. Orthod., 91:193, 1987.

Dibbets, J. M. H., L. van der Weele, and G. Boering: Craniofacial morphology and temporomandibular joint dysfunction in children. In: *Development Aspects of Temporomandibular Joint Disorders*. Edited by D. S. Carlson, J. A. McNamara, and K. A.

Ribbens. Ann Arbor, University of Michigan, Center for Human Growth and Development, 1985a.

Dibbets, J. M. H., L. van der Weele, and A. Uildriks: Symptoms of TMJ dysfunction: Indicators of growth patterns. J. Pedodont., 9:265, 1985b.

Dibbets, J. M. H., R. de Bruin, and L. van der Weele: Shape change in the mandible during adolescence. In: *Craniofacial Growth during Adolescence.* Ed. by D. S. Carlson, and K. A. Ribbens. Ann Arbor, University of Michigan, Center for Human Growth and Development, 1987.

Diewart, V. M.: A quantitative coronal plane evaluation of craniofacial growth and spatial relations during secondary palate development in the rat. Arch. Oral Biol., 23:607, 1978.

Diewert, V. M.: Differential changes in cartilage cell proliferation and cell density in the rat craniofacial complex during secondary palate development. Anat. Rec., 198:219, 1980.

Diewert, V. M.: Contributions of differential growth of cartilages to changes in craniofacial morphology. Prog. Clin. Biol. Res., 101:229, 1982.

DiPalma, D. M.: A morphometric study of orthopedic and functional therapy for the hyperdivergent skeletal pattern. Thesis, Case Western Reserve University School of Dentistry, 1983.

Dixon, A. D.: The early development of the maxilla. Dent. Pract., 33:331, 1953.

Dixon, A. D.: The development of the jaws. Dent. Pract., 9:10, 1958.

Dorenbos, J.: Morphogenesis of the spheno-occipital and the presphenoidal synchondrosis in the cranial base of the fetal Wistar rat. Acta Morphol. Neerl. Scand., 11:63, 1973.

Downs, W. B.: Analysis of the dento-facial profile. Angle Orthod., 26:191, 1956.

Du Brul, E. L., and D. M. Laskin: Preadaptive potentialities of the mammalian skull: An experiment in growth and form. Am. J. Anat., 109:117, 1961.

Du Brul, E. L., and H. Sicher: *The Adaptive Chin.* Springfield, Ill., Charles C Thomas, 1954.

Dullemeijer, P.: Comparative ontogeny and craniofacial growth. In: *Cranio-facial Growth in Man.* Ed. by R. E. Moyers and W. M. Krogman. Oxford, Pergamon Press, 1971.

Durkin, J. R.: Secondary cartilage: A misnomer? Am. J. Orthod., 62:15, 1972.

Durkin, J. F., J. D. Heeley, and J. T. Irving: The cartilage of the mandibular condyle. Oral Sci. Rev., 2:29, 1973.

Duterloo, H. S., and D. H. Enlow: A comparative study of cranial growth in *Homo* and *Macaca.* Am. J. Anat., 127:357, 1970.

Duterloo, H. S., and H. W. B. Jansen: Chondrogenesis and osteogenesis in the mandibular condylar blastema. Eur. Orthod. Soc. Trans., 1969:109, 1970.

Duterloo, H. S., and H. Vilmann: Translative and transformative growth of the rat mandible. Acta Ondontol. Scand., 36:25, 1978.

Duterloo, H. S., G. Kragt, and A. M. Algra: Holographic and cephalometric study of the relationship between craniofacial morphology and the initial reactions to high-pull headgear traction. Am. J. Orthod., 88:297, 1985.

Elgoyhen, J. C., R. E. Moyers, J. A. McNamara, Jr., and M. L. Riolo: Craniofacial adaptation of pro-

trusive function in young rhesus monkeys. Am. J. Orthod., 62:469, 1972.

Engle, M. B., and A. G. Brodie: Condylar growth and mandibular deformities. Surgery, 22:975, 1947.

Engstrom, C., S. Killiardis, and B. Thilander: The relationship between masticatory function and craniofacial morphology. II. A histological study in the growing rat fed a soft diet. Swed. Dent. J., 36:1, 1986.

Enlow, D. H.: Functions of the haversian system. Am. J. Anat., 110:269, 1962a.

Enlow, D. H.: A study of the postnatal growth and remodeling of bone. Am. J. Anat., 110:79, 1962b.

Enlow, D. H.: *Principles of Bone Remodeling.* Springfield, Ill., Charles C Thomas, 1963.

Enlow, D. H.: *The Human Face: An Account of the Postnatal Growth and Development of the Craniofacial Skeleton.* New York, Harper & Row, 1968b.

Enlow, D. H.: Wolff's law and the factor of architectonic circumstance. Am. J. Orthod., 54, 803, 1968.

Enlow, D. H.: Mandibular rotations during growth. In: *Determinants of Mandibular Form and Growth.* Ed. by J. A. McNamara, Jr. University of Michigan, Center for Human Growth and Development, 1975.

Enlow, D. H.: Morphologic factors involved in the biology of relapse. J. Charles Tweed Foundation, 8:16, 1980.

Enlow, D. H.: Role of the TMJ in facial growth and development. In: *President's Conference on Examination, Diagnosis, and Management of Temporomandibular Disorders.* Ed. by D. Laskin, et al. American Dental Association, Chicago, 1983.

Enlow, D. H.: Normal and abnormal patterns of craniofacial growth. In: *Scientific Foundations and Surgical Treatment of Craniosynostosis.* Ed. by J. A. Persing, M. T. Edgerton, and J. Jane. Baltimore, Williams & Wilkins, 1989.

Enlow, D. H.: Facial Growth, Third Ed., Philadelphia, W. B. Saunders, 1990.

Enlow, D. H., and S. Bang: Growth and remodeling of the human maxilla. Am. J. Orthod., 51:446, 1965.

Enlow, D. H., and D. B. Harris: A study of the postnatal growth of the human mandible. Am. J. Orthod., 50:25, 1964.

Enlow, D. H., and R. E. Moyers: Growth and architecture of the face. J.A.D.A., 82:763, 1971.

Enlow, D. H., T. Kuroda, and A. B. Lewis: The morphological and morphogenetic basis for craniofacial form and pattern. Angle Orthod., 41:161, 1971a.

Enlow, D. H., E. Harvold, R. Latham, B. Moffett, R. Christiansen, and H. G. Hausch: Research on control of craniofacial morphogenesis: An NIDR Workshop. Am. J. Orthod., 71:509, 1977.

Enlow, D. H., C. Pfister, and E. Richardson: An analysis of Black and Caucasian craniofacial patterns. Angle Orthod., 52:279, 1982.

Enlow, D. H., D. DiGangi, J. A. McNamara, and M. Mina: Morphogenic effects of the functional regulator as revealed by the counterpart analysis. Eur. J. Orthod., 10:192, 1988.

Epker, B. N., and H. M. Frost: Correlation of bone resorption and formation with the physical behavior of loaded bone. J. Dent. Res., 44:33, 1965.

Evans, C. A., and R. L. Christiansen: Facial growth associated with a cranial base defect: A case report. Angle Orthod., 49:44, 1979.

Evans, F. G.: *Stress and Strain in Bones*. Springfield, Ill., Charles C Thomas, 1957.

Fastlicht, J.: Crowding of mandibular incisors. Am. J. Orthod., 58:156, 1970.

Fenart, R.: L'hominisation du crane. Bull. Acad. Dent. (Paris), 14:33, 1970.

Fishman, L. S.: Chronological versus skeletal age, an evaluation of craniofacial growth. Angle Orthod., 49:181, 1979.

Ford, E. H.: Growth of the human cranial base. Am. J. Orthod., 44:498, 1958.

Frankel, R.: Biomechanical aspects of the form/function relationship in craniofacial morphogenesis: A clinician's approach. In: *Clinical Alteration of the Growing Face*. Ed. by J. A. McNamara, Jr., K. A. Ribbens, and R. P. Howe. Monograph 14. Craniofacial Growth Series. Ann Arbor, University of Michigan, Center for Human Growth and Development, 1983.

Frankel, R.: Concerning recent articles on Frankel appliance therapy. Am. J. Orthod., 85:441, 1984.

Frankel, R., and C. Frankel: *Orofacial orthopedics with the Function Regulator*. Basel, Karger, 1989.

Fraser, F. C.: Etiology of cleft lip and palate. In: *Cleft Lip and Palate*. Ed. by W. C. Grabb, S. W. Rosenstein, and K. R. Bzoch. Boston, Little, Brown, 1971.

Freeman, E., and A. R. Ten Cate: Development of the periodontium: An electron microscopic study. J. Periodont., 42:387, 1971.

Friedi, H., B. Johanson, J. Ahlgren, and B. Thilander: Metallic implants as growth markers in infants with craniofacial anomalies. Acta Odont. Scand., 35:265, 1977.

Frost, H. M.: Micropetrosis. J. Bone Joint Surg., 42:144, 1960.

Fukada, E., and I. Yasuada: On the piezoelectric effect of bone. J. Physiol. Soc. Jpn., 12:1158, 1957.

Furstman, L.: The early development of the human mandibular joint. Am. J. Orthod., 49:672, 1963.

Gans, G. J., and B. G. Sarnat: Sutural facial growth of the *Macaca* rhesus monkey: A gross and serial roentgenographic study by means of metallic implants. Am. J. Orthod., 37:827, 1951.

Garn, S. M.: The secular trend in size and maturational timing and its implications for nutritional assessment. J. Nutr., 117:17, 1987.

Garn, S. M., B. H. Smith, and R. E. Moyers: Structured (patterned) dimensional and developmental asymmetry. Proc. Finn. Dent. Soc., 77:33, 1981.

Garn, S. M., B. H. Smith, and M. LaVelle: Applications of patterns profile analysis to malformations of the head and face. Radiology, 150:683, 1984.

Gasser, R. F.: Early formation of the basicranium in man. In: *Development of the Basicranium*. Ed. by J. F. Bosma. DHEW Pub. 76:989, NIH, Bethesda, Md., 1976.

Gasson, N., and J. Lavergne: The maxillary rotation: Its relation to the cranial base and the mandibular corpus. An implant study. Acta Odont. Scand., 35:89, 1977.

Gianelly, A. A., and H. M. Goldman: *Biologic Basis of Orthodontics*. Philadelphia, Lea & Febiger, 1971.

Gianelly, A. A., and C. F. A. Moorrees: Condylectomy in the rat. Arch. Oral Biol., 10:101, 1965.

Gianelly, A. A., P. Brosnan, M. Martignoni, and L. Bernstein: Mandibular growth, condyle position

and Frankel appliance therapy. Angle Orthod., 53, 131, 1983.

Giles, W. B., C. L. Phillips, and D. R. Joondeph: Growth in the basicranial synchondroses of adolescent *Macaca mulatta*. Anat. Rec., 199:259, 1981.

Gillooly, C. J., Jr., R. T. Hosley, J. R. Mathews, and D. L. Jewett: Electric potentials recorded from mandibular alveolar bone as a result of forces applied to the tooth. Am. J. Orthod., 54:649, 1968.

Goldberg, G., and D. H. Enlow: Some anatomical characteristics of the craniofacial skeleton in several syndromes of the head as revealed by the counterpart analysis. J. Oral Surg., 39:489, 1981.

Gorlin, R. J., M. M. Cohen, Jr., and L. S. Levin: *Syndromes of the Head and Neck*, 3rd Ed. New York, Oxford University Press, 1990.

Graber, T. M.: Clinical cephalometric analysis. In: *Vistas of Orthodontics*. Ed. by B. S. Kraus, and R. A. Reidel. Philadelphia, Lea & Febiger, 1962.

Graber, T. M.: A study of cranio-facial growth and development in the cleft palate child from birth to six years of age. In: *Early Treatment of Cleft Lip and Palate*. Ed. by R. Hotz. Berne, Switzerland, Hans Huber, 1964.

Graber, T. M.: Extrinsic control factors influencing craniofacial growth. In: *Control Mechanisms in Craniofacial Growth*. Ed. by J. A. McNamara, Jr. Ann Arbor, University of Michigan, Center for Human Growth and Development, 1975.

Grant, D., and S. Bernick: Formation of the periodontal ligament. J. Periodontol., 43:17, 1972.

Gregory, W. K.: *Our Face from Fish to Man*. New York, Putnam, 1929.

Greulich, W. W., and S. I. Pyle: *Radiographic Atlas of Skeletal Development of the Hand and Wrist*, 2nd Ed. Stanford, Stanford University Press, 1959.

Griffiths, D. L., L. Furstman, and S. Bernick: Postnatal development of the mouse palate. Am. J. Orthod., 53:757, 1967.

Hall, B. K.: *Development and Cellular Skeletal Biology*. New York, Academic Press, 1978b.

Hall, B. K.: How is mandibular growth controlled during development and evolution? J. Craniofac. Genet. Dev. Biol., 2:45, 1982a.

Hall, B. K.: Mandibular morphogenesis and craniofacial malformations. J. Craniofac. Genet. Dev. Biol., 2:309, 1982b.

Hans, M. G., and D. Enlow: Age related differences in mandibular ramus growth: A histologic study. Angle Orthod., 65:335, 1995.

Harvold, E. P.: Neuromuscular and morphological adaptations in experimentally induced oral respiration. In: *Naso-respiratory Function and Craniofacial Growth*. Ed. by J. A. McNamara, Jr. Ann Arbor, University of Michigan, Center for Human Growth and Development, 1979.

Harvold, E. P., and K. Vargervik: Morphogenic response to activator treatment. Am. J. Orthod., 60:478, 1970.

Harvold, E. P., K. Vargervik, and G. Chierici: Primate experiments on oral sensation and dental malocclusion. Am. J. Orthod., 63:494, 1973.

Haskell, B. S.: The human chin and its relationship to mandibular morphology. Angle Orthod., 49:153, 1979.

Hellman, M.: The face in its developmental career. Dent. Cosmos., 77:685, 1935.

Herovici, C.: A polychrome stain for differentiating precollagen from collagen. Stain Technol., 38:204, 1963.

Hinton, R. J., and D. S. Carlson: Temporal changes in human temporomandibular joints' size and shape. Am. J. Phys. Anthropol., 50:325, 1979.

Hinton, W. L.: Form and function in the temporo-mandibular joint. In: *Craniofacial Biology*. Ed. by D. S. Carlson. Ann Arbor, University of Michigan, Center for Human Growth and Development, 1981.

Hirschfeld, W. J., and R. E. Moyers: Prediction of craniofacial growth: The state of the art. Am. J. Orthod., 60:435, 1971.

Hirschfeld, W. J., R. E. Moyers, and D. H. Enlow: A method of deriving subgroups of a population: A study of craniofacial taxonomy. Am. J. Phys. Anthropol., 39:279, 1973.

Hixon, E. H.: Prediction of facial growth. Eur. Orthod. Soc. Rep. Congr., 44:127, 1968.

Horowitz, S. L.: The role of genetic and local environmental factors in normal and abnormal morphogenesis. Acta Morphol. Neerl. Scand., 10:59, 1972.

Horowitz, S. L., and R. Osborne: The genetic aspects of cranio-facial growth. In: *Cranio-facial Growth in Man*. Ed. by R. E. Moyers, and W. M. Krogman. Oxford, Pergamon Press, 1971.

Houghton, P.: Rocker jaws. Am. J. Phys. Anthropol., 47:365, 1977.

Houpt, M. I.: Growth of the craniofacial complex of the human fetus. Am. J. Orthod., 58:373, 1970.

Houston, W. J. B.: The current status of facial growth prediction: A review. Br. J. Orthod., 6:11, 1978.

Houston, W. J., and W. A. B. Brown: Family likeness as a basis for facial growth prediction. Eur. J. Orthod., 2:13, 1980.

Hoyte, D. A. N.: Mechanisms of growth in the cranial vault and base. J. Dent. Res., 50:1447, 1971a.

Hoyte, D. A. N.: The modes of growth of the neurocranium: The growth of the sphenoid bone in animals. In: *Cranio-facial Growth in Man*. Ed. by R. E. Moyers, and W. M. Krogman. Oxford, Pergamon Press, 1971b.

Hoyte, D. A. N.: A critical analysis of the growth in length of the cranial base. In: *Morphogenesis and Malformation of Face and Brain*. Ed. by D. Bergsma, J. Langman, and N. W. Paul. National Foundation—March of Dimes. Birth Defects Original Article Series, Vol. 11, No. 7. New York, Alan R. Liss, 1975.

Hoyte, D. A. N.: Contributions of the spheno-ethmoidal complex to basicranial growth in the rabbit. In: *Development of the Basicranium*. Ed. by J. F. Bosma. DHEW Pub. 76:989, NIH, Bethesda, Md., 1976.

Hoyte, D. A. N., and D. H. Enlow: Wolff's law and the problem of muscle attachment on resorptive surfaces of bone. Am. J. Phys. Anthropol., 24:205, 1966.

Humphrey, T.: Reflex activity in the oral and facial area of the human fetus. In: *Second Symposium on Oral Sensation and Perception*. Ed. by J. Bosma. Springfield, Ill. Charles C Thomas, 1970.

Hunter, W. S.: The dynamics of mandibular arch perimeter change from mixed to permanent dentitions. In: *Craniofacial Biology*. Ed. by J. A. McNamara, Jr. Ann Arbor, University of Michigan,

Center for Human Growth and Development, 1977.

Hunter, W. S., and S. Garn: Evidence for a secular trend in face size. Angle Orthod., 39:320, 1969.

Hunter, W. S., and S. M. Garn: Differential secular increase in the progeny of small faced parents. J. Dent. Res., 52:212(abstr. 613), 1973.

Hunter, W. S., D. R. Balbach, and D. E. Lamphiear: The heritability of attained growth in the human face. Am. J. Orthod., 58:128, 1970.

Hylander, W. L.: Patterns of stress and strain in the macaque mandible. In: *Craniofacial Biology*. Ed. by D. S. Carlson. Ann Arbor, University of Michigan, Center for Human Growth and Development, 1981.

Hylander, W. L.: Stress and strain in the mandibular symphysis of primates: A test of competing hypotheses. Am. J. Phys. Anthrop., 64:1, 1984.

Ingerslev, C. H., and B. Solow: Sex differences in craniofacial morphology. Acta Odont. Scand., 33:85, 1975.

Ingervall, B., and E. Helkimo: Masticatory muscle force and facial morphology in man. Arch. Oral Biol., 23:203, 1978.

Ingervall, B., and B. Thilander: The human spheno-occipital synchondrosis. I. The time of closure appraised macroscopically. Acta Odont. Scand., 30:349, 1972.

Isaacson, R. J., R. J. Zapfel, F. W. Worms, and A. G. Erdman: Effect of rotational jaw growth on the occlusion and profile. Am. J. Orthod., 72:276, 1977.

Isaacson, R. J., A. G. Erdman, and B. W. Hultgren: Facial and dental effects of mandibular rotation. In: *Craniofacial Biology*. Ed. by D. S. Carlson. Ann Arbor, University of Michigan, Center for Human Growth and Development, 1981.

Isotupa, K., K. Koski, and L. Makinen: Changing architecture of growing cranial bones at sutures as revealed by vital staining with alizarin red S in the rabbit. Am. J. Phys. Anthropol., 23:19, 1965.

Israel, H.: The dichotomous pattern of craniofacial expansion during aging. Am. J. Phys. Anthropol., 47:47, 1977.

Jane, J. A.: Radical reconstruction of complex cranioorbitofacial abnormalities. In: *Morphogenesis and Malformation of Face and Brain*. Ed. by D. Bergsma, J. Langman, and N. W. Paul. National Foundation—March of Dimes. Birth Defects Original Article Series, Vol. 11, No. 7. New York, Alan R. Liss, 1975.

Johnson, P. A., P. J. Atkinson, and W. J. Moore: The development and structure of the chimpanzee mandible. J. Anat., 122:467, 1976.

Johnston, L. E.: A statistical evaluation of cephalometric prediction. Angle Orthod., 38:284, 1968.

Johnston, L. E.: The functional matrix hypothesis: Reflections in a jaundiced eye. In: *Factors Affecting the Growth of the Midface*. Ed. by J. A. McNamara, Jr. Ann Arbor, University of Michigan, Center for Human Growth and Development, 1976.

Johnston, M. C.: The neural crest in abnormalities of the face and brain. In: *Morphogenesis and Malformation of Face and Brain*. Ed. by D. Bergsma, J. Langman, and N. W. Paul. National Foundation—March of Dimes. Birth Defects

Original Article Series, Vol. 11, No. 7. New York, Alan R. Liss, 1975.

Johnston, M. C., et al.: An expanded role of the neural crest in oral and pharyngeal development. In: *Oral Sensation and Perception: Development in the Fetus and Infant*. Ed. by J. Bosma. Washington, D. C., DHEW Pub. No. 73-546, 1973.

Joho, J. P.: Changes in form and size of the mandible in the orthopaedically treated *Macacus irus* (an experimental study). Eur. Orthod. Soc. Trans. 1968:161, 1969.

Joondeph, D. R., and L. E. Wragg: Facial growth during the secondary palate closure in the rat. Am. J. Orthod., 6:88, 1966.

Kanouse, M. C., S. P. Ranfjord, and C. E. Nasjleti: Condylar growth in rhesus monkeys. J. Dent. Res., 48:1171, 1969.

Kantomaa, T.: Role of the mandibular condyle in facial growth. Proc. Finn. Dent. Soc., 81:111, 1985.

Kean, M. R., and P. Houghton: The role of function in the development of human craniofacial form: A perspective. Anat. Rec., 218:107, 1987.

Kier, E. L.: Phylogenetic and ontogenetic changes of the brain relevant to the evolution of the skull. In: *Development of the Basicranium*. Ed. by J. F. Bosma. DHEW Pub. 76:989, NIH, Bethesda, Md., 1976.

Koski, K.: Cranial growth centers: Facts or fallacies? Am. J. Orthod., 54:566, 1968.

Koski, K.: Some characteristics of cranio-facial growth cartilages. In: *Cranio-facial Growth in Man*. Ed. by R. E. Moyers, and W. M. Krogman. Oxford, Pergamon Press, 1971.

Koski, K., and O. Rönning: Growth potential of subcutaneously transplanted cranial base synchondroses of the rat. Acta Odont. Scand., 27:343, 1969.

Koski, K., and Rönning: Growth potential of intracerebrally transplanted cranial base synchondroses in the rat. Arch. Oral Biol., 15:1107, 1970.

Koski, K., and J. Varrela: The trigeminal nerve and the facial skeleton. Craniofacial Growth Series, Center for Human Growth and Development, Ann Arbor, University of Michigan, 1991.

Koskinen-Moffett, L., and B. Moffett: Influence of prenatal jaw functions on human facial development. Birth Defects, 20:47, 1984.

Koskinen-Moffett, L., R. McMinn, K. Isotupa, and B. Moffett: Migration of craniofacial periosteum in rabbits. Proc. Finn. Dent. Soc., 77:83, 1981.

Kraw, A. G., and D. H. Enlow: Continuous attachment of the periodontal membrane. Am. J. Anat., 120:133, 1967.

Kremanak, C. R., Jr.: Circumstances limiting the development of a complete explanation of craniofacial growth. Acta Morphol. Neerl. Scand., 10: 127, 1972.

Krogman, W. M.: Craniofacial growth and development: An appraisal. Yearbook Phys. Anthropol., 18:31, 1974.

Krogman, W. M., and V. Sassouni: *Syllabus in Roentgenographic Cephalometry*. Philadelphia, Philadelphia Center for Research in Child Growth, 1957.

Kurihara, S., and D. H. Enlow: Remodeling reversals in anterior parts of the human mandible and maxilla. Angle Orthod., 50:98, 1980a.

Kurihara, S., and D. H. Enlow: An electron microscopic study of attachments between periodontal fibers and bone during alveolar remodeling. Am. J. Orthod., 77:516, 1980b.

Kurihara, S., and D. H. Enlow: A histochemical and electron microscopic study of an adhesive type of collagen attachment on resorptive surfaces of alveolar bone. Am. J. Orthod., 77:532, 1980c.

Kurisu, K., J. D. Niswander, M. C. Johnston, and M. Mazaheri: Facial morphology as an indicator of genetic predisposition to cleft lip and palate. Am. J. Hum. Genet., 26:702, 1974.

Kuroda, T.: A longitudinal cephalometric study on the craniofacial development in Japanese children. Presented at the Annual Meeting of the Int. Assoc. Dent. Res., New York, 1970, Abstr. 32.

Kuroda, T., F. Miura, T. Nakamura, and K. Noguchi: Cellular kinetics of synchondroseal cartilage in organ culture. Proc. Finn. Dent. Soc., 77:89, 1981.

Kvinnsland, S.: The sagittal growth of the foetal cranial base. Acta Odontol. Scand., 29:699, 1971.

Laitman, J. T., and E. S. Crelin: Postnatal development of the basicranium and vocal tract region in man. In: *Development of the Basicranium*. Ed. by J. F. Bosma. DHEW Pub. 76:989, NIH, Bethesda, Md., 1976.

Latham, R. A.: The sliding of cranial bodies at sutural surfaces during growth. J. Anat., 102:593, 1968.

Latham, R. A.: Maxillary development and growth: The septopremaxillary ligament. J. Anat., 107: 471, 1970.

Latham, R. A.: The development, structure, and growth pattern of the human mid-palatal suture. J. Anat., 108:1, 31—41, 1971.

Latham, R. A.: The different relationship of the sella point to growth sites of the cranial base in fetal life. J. Dent. Res., 51:1646, 1972.

Latham, R. A., and J. H. Scott: A newly postulated factor in the early growth of the human middle face and the theory of multiple assurance. Arch. Oral Biol., 15:1097, 1970.

Lauritzen, C., J. Lilja, and J. Jaristedt: Airway obstruction and sleep apnea in children with craniofacial anomalies. Plastic Reconstr. Surg., 77:1, 1986.

Lavelle, C. L. B.: An analysis of foetal craniofacial growth. Ann. Hum. Biol., 1:3, 269, 1974.

Lavelle, C.: An analysis of basicranial axis form. Anat. Anz., 164:169, 1987.

Lavelle, C. L. B., R. P. Shellis, and D. F. G. Poole: *Evolutionary Changes to the Primate Skull and Dentition*. Springfield, Ill., Charles C Thomas, 1977.

Lavergne, J., and N. Gasson: A metal implant study of mandibular rotation. Angle Orthod., 46:144, 1976.

Lavergne, J., and N. Gasson: The influence of jaw rotation on the morphogenesis of malocclusion. Am. J. Orthod., 73:658, 1978.

Lewis, A. B., and A. F. Roche: Late growth changes in the craniofacial skeleton. Angle Orthod., 58: 127, 1988.

Linder-Aronson, S.: Naso-respiratory function and craniofacial growth. In: *Naso-respiratory Function and Craniofacial Growth*. Ed. by J. A. McNamara, Jr. Ann Arbor, University of Michigan, Center for Human Growth and Development, 1979.

Linder-Aronson, S.: The relation between nasorespiratory function and dentofacial morphology. Am. J. Orthod., 83:443, 1983.

Linder-Aronson, S.: Nasorespiratory considerations in orthodontics. In: *Orthodontics State of the Art Essence of the Science*. Ed. by L. W. Graber, 116, 1986.

Linge, L.: Tissue reactions in facial sutures subsequent to external mechanical influences. In: *Factors Affecting the Growth of the Midface*. Ed. by J. A. McNamara, Jr. Ann Arbor, University of Michigan, Center for Human Growth and Development, 1976.

Maj, G., and C. Luzi: Analysis of mandibular growth on 28 normal children followed from 9 to 13 years of age. Eur. Orthod. Soc. Trans., 1962.

Manson, J. D.: *A Comparative Study of the Postnatal Growth of the Mandible*. London, Henry Kimpton, 1968.

Markus, A. F., J. Delaire, and W. Smith: Facial balance in cleft lip and palate. 1. Normal development and cleft palate. Br. J. Oral Maxillofac. Surg., 30:287, 1992.

Mars, M., and W. Houston: A preliminary study of facial growth and morphology in unoperated male unilateral cleft lip and palate subjects over 13 years of age. Cleft Palate J., 27:7, 1990.

Martone, V. D., D. Enlow, M. Hans, B. H. Broadbent, and O. Oyen: Class I and Class III malocclusion sub-groupings related to headform type. Angle Orthod., 62:35, 1992.

Mathews, J. R., and W. H. Ware: Longitudinal mandibular growth in children with tantalum implants. Am. J. Orthod., 74:633, 1978.

Maxwell, L. C., D. S. Carlson, J. A. McNamara, Jr., and J. A. Faulkner: Effect of shortening or lengthening of the mandible upon the characteristics of masticatory muscle fibers in rhesus monkeys. In: *Craniofacial Biology*. Ed. by D. S. Carlson. Ann Arbor, University of Michigan, Center for Human Growth and Development, 1981.

McNamara, J. A., Jr.: *Neuromuscular and Skeletal Adaptations to Altered Orofacial Function*. Monograph 1. Craniofacial Growth Series. Ann Arbor, University of Michigan, Center for Human Growth and Development, 1972.

McNamara, J. A., Jr.: Procion dyes as vital markers in rhesus monkeys. J. Dent. Res. 52:634, 1973.

McNamara, J. A., Jr.: Functional determinants of craniofacial size and shape. In: *Craniofacial Biology*. Ed. by D. S. Carlson. Ann Arbor, University of Michigan, Center for Human Growth and Development, 1981.

McNamara, J. A., Jr.: Influence of respiratory pattern on craniofacial growth. Angle Orthod., 51: 269, 1981.

McNamara, J. A., Jr., and L. W. Graber: Mandibular growth in the rhesus monkey (*Macaca mulatta*). Am. J. Phys. Anthropol., 42:15, 1975.

McNamara, J. A., Jr., and M. L. Riolo, and D. H. Enlow: Growth of the maxillary complex in the rhesus monkey (*Macaca mulatta*). Am. J. Phys. Anthropol., 44:15, 1976.

McWilliam, J., and S. Linder-Aronson: Hypoplasia of the middle third of the face: A morphological study. Angle Orthod., 46:260, 1976.

Mednick, L. W., and S. L. Washburn: The role of the sutures in the growth of the braincase of the infant pig. Am. J. Phys. Anthropol., 14:175, 1956.

Meikle, M. C.: The role of the condyle in the postnatal growth of the mandible. Am. J. Orthod., 64: 50, 1973.

Meikle, M. C.: Remodeling. In: *The Temporomandibular Joint*, 3rd Ed. Ed. by B. G. Sarnat, and D. M. Laskin. Springfield, Ill., Charles C Thomas, 1980.

Melsen, B.: Computerized comparison of histological methods for the evaluation of craniofacial growth. Acta Odont. Scand., 29:295, 1971a.

Melsen, B.: The postnatal growth of the cranial base in *Macaca* rhesus analyzed by the implant method. Tandlaegebladet, 75:1320, 1971b.

Melsen, B.: Histological analysis of the postnatal development of the nasal septum. Angle Orthod., 47: 83, 1977.

Melsen, B., F. Melsen, and M. L. Moss: Postnatal development of the nasal septum studied on human autopsy material. In: *Craniofacial Biology*. Ed. by D. S. Carlson. Ann Arbor, University of Michigan, Center for Human Growth and Development, 1981.

Mew, J. R.: Factors influencing mandibular growth. Angle Orthod., 56:31, 1986.

Michejda, M.: The role of the basicranial synchondroses in flexure processes and ontogenetic development of the skull base. Am. J. Phys. Anthropol., 37:143, 1972a.

Michejda, M.: Significance of basiocranial synchondroses in nonhuman primates and man. *Medical Primatology*. Proc. 3rd Conf. Exp. Med. Surg. Primates, Lyon, Vol. 1. Basel, S. Karger, 1972b.

Miller, A. J., and G. Chierici: Concepts related to adaptation of neuromuscular function and craniofacial morphology. Birth Defects, 18:21, 1982.

Miller, A. J., and K. Vargervik: Neuromuscular changes during long-term adaptation of the rhesus monkey to oral respiration. In: *Naso-Respiratory Function and Craniofacial Growth*. Ed. by J. A. McNamara, Jr. Craniofacial Growth Series. Ann Arbor, University of Michigan, Center for Human Growth and Development, 1979.

Miller, A. J., K. Vargervik, and G. Chierici: Experimentally induced neuromuscular changes during and after nasal airway obstruction. Am. J. Orthod., 85:385, 1984.

Miura, F., N. Inoue, and S. Kazuo: The standards of Steiner's analysis for Japanese. Bull. Tokyo Med. Dent. Univ., 10:387, 1963.

Miura, F., N. Inoue, M. Azuma, and G. Ito: Development and organization of periodontal membrane and physiologic tooth movements. Bull. Tokyo Med. Dent. Univ., 17:123, 1970.

Moffett, B., and L. Koskinen-Moffett: A biologic look at mandibular growth rotation. In: *Craniofacial Biology*. Ed. by D. S. Carlson. Ann Arbor, University of Michigan, Center for Human Growth and Development, 1981.

Moffett, B. C., Jr.: The prenatal development of the human temporomandibular joint. Contrib. Embryol. Carneg. Inst. 36:19, 1957.

Moffett, B. C., Jr., L. C. Johnson, J. B. McCabe, and H. C. Askew: Articular remodeling in the adult human temporomandibular joint. Am. J. Anat., 115:119, 1964.

Mongini, F., G. Preti, P. M. Calderale, and G. Barberi: Experimental strain analysis on the mandibular condyle under various conditions. Med. Biol. Eng. Comput., 19:521, 1981.

Moore, A. W.: Head growth of the macaque monkey as revealed by vital staining, embedding, and undecalcified sectioning. Am. J. Orthod., 35:654, 1949.

Moore, A. W.: Observations on facial growth and its clinical significance. Am. J. Orthod., 45:399, 1959.

Moore, R. N., and C. Phillips: Sagittal craniofacial growth in the fetal Macaque monkey *Macaca nemestrina*. Arch. Oral Biol., 25:19, 1980.

Moore, W. J.: Masticatory function and skull growth. J. Zool., 146:123, 1965.

Moore, W. J.: The influence of muscular function on the growth of the skull. Scientia, 103:333, 1968.

Moore, W. J.: Associations in the hominoid facial skeletal. J. Anat., 123:111, 1977.

Moore, W. J., and C. L. B. Lavelle: *Growth of the Facial Skeleton in the Hominoidea*. New York, Academic Press, 1974.

Moorrees, C. F. A.: *Dentition of the Growing Child, A Longitudinal Study of Dental Development Between 3 and 18 Years of Age*. Cambridge, Harvard University Press, 1959.

Moorrees, C. F. A.: Register of longitudinal studies of facial and dental development. International Society of Craniofacial Biology, Washington, D.C., 1967.

Moorrees, C. F. A.: Patterns of dental maturation. In: *Craniofacial Biology*. Ed. by J. A. McNamara, Jr. Ann Arbor, University of Michigan, Center for Human Growth and Development, 1977.

Moorrees, C. F., S. Efstratiadis, and E. Kent, Jr.: The mesh diagram of facial growth. Proc. Finn. Dent. Soc., 7:33, 1991.

Moss, M. L.: Genetics, epigenetics and causation. Am. J. Orthod., 36:481, 1950.

Moss, M. L.: The primary role of functional matrices in facial growth. Am. J. Orthod., 55:566, 1969.

Moss, M. L.: Neurotropic processes in orofacial growth. J. Dent. Res., 50:1492, 1971.

Moss, M. L.: Beyond roentgenographic cephalometry—what? Am. J. Orthod., 84:77, 1983.

Moss, M. L.: The application of the finite element method to the description of craniofacial skeletal growth and form comparison. In *Human Growth: A Multidisciplinary Review*. Ed. by A. Demirjian, and M. Dubuc. London and Philadelphia, Taylor and Francis, 1986.

Moss, M. L., and L. Moss-Salentijn: The muscle-bone interface: An analysis of a morphological boundary. In: *Muscle Adaptation in the Craniofacial Region*. Ed. by D. S. Carlson, and J. A. McNamara, Jr. Ann Arbor, University of Michigan, Center for Human Growth and Development, 1978.

Moss, M. L., and L. Salentijn: The primary role of functional matrices in facial growth. Am. J. Orthod., 55:566, 1969a.

Moss, M. L., and L. Salentijn: The capsular matrix. Am. J. Orthod., 56:474, 1969b.

Moss, M. L., and L. Salentijn: The logarithmic growth of the human mandible. Acta Anat., 77:341, 1970.

Moss, M. L., H. Vilmann, G. Dasgupta, and R. Skalak: Craniofacial growth in space-time. In: *Craniofacial Biology*. Ed. by D. S. Carlson. Ann Arbor, University of Michigan, Center for Human Growth and Development, 1981.

Motohashi, N., and K. Kuroda: Morphological analysis of congenital craniofacial malformations. Kokubyo Gakkai Zasshi, 49:698, 1982.

Moyers, R. E.: The infantile swallow. Trans. Eur. Othod. Soc., 40:180, 1964.

Moyers, R. E.: Development of occlusion. Dent. Clin. North Amer., 13:523, 1969.

Moyers, R. E.: Postnatal development of the orofacial musculature. In: *Patterns of Orofacial Growth and Development*. Report 6. Washington, D.C., American Speech and Hearing Association, 1971.

Moyers, R. E.: *Handbook of Orthodontics*, 4th Ed. Chicago, Year Book Medical Publ., 1988.

Moyers, R. E., and F. L. Bookstein: The inappropriateness of conventional cephalometrics. Am. J. Orthod., 75:599, 1979.

Moyers, R. E., and F. Muira: The use of serial cephalograms to study racial differences in development. I. and II. Trans. VIII Congress of Anthrop. and Ethnol. Sci., Tokyo, 284, 1968.

Moyers, R. E., J. Elgoyhen, M. Riolo, J. McNamara, and T. Kuroda: Experimental production of Class III in rhesus monkeys. Eur. Orthod. Soc. Trans., 46:61, 1970.

Moyers, R. E., F. Bookstein, and K. E. Guire: The concept of pattern in craniofacial growth. Am. J. Orthod., 76:136, 1979.

Mugnier, A., and M. Schouker-Jolly: Physiopathologic des malocclusions dento-maxillaires moyens prophylactiques et thérapeutiques précoces. Pédod. Fr., 5:101, 1973.

Nanda, R., and B. Goldin: Biomechanical approaches to the study of alterations in facial morphology. Am. J. Orthod., 78:213, 1980.

Nanda, R. S., H. Meng, S. Kapila, and J. Goorhuis: Growth changes in the soft tissue profile. Angle Orthod., 60:177, 1990.

Nielsen, I. L.: Facial growth during treatment with the function regulator appliance. Am. J. Orthod., 85:401, 1984.

Norton, L. A.: Implications of bioelectric growth control in orthodontics and dentistry. Angle Orthod., 45:34, 1975.

Odegaard, J.: Mandibular rotation studied with the aid of metal implants. Am. J. Orthod., 58:448, 1970.

Odegaard. J., and A. G. Brodie: On the growth of the human head from birth to the third month of life. Anat. Rec., 103:311, 1949.

O'Higgins, P. O., T. Bromage, D. Johnson, W. Moore, and P. McPhie: A study of facial growth in the sooty mangabey *Cercocebus atys*. Folia Primatol., 56:86, 1991.

Oudet, C., and A. G. Petrovic: Variations in the number of sarcomeres in series in the lateral pterygoid muscle as a function of the longitudinal deviation of the mandibular position produced by the postural hyperpropulsor. In: *Muscle Adaptation in the Craniofacial Region*. Ed. by D. S. Carlson and J. A. McNamara, Jr. Ann Arbor, University of Michigan, Center for Human Growth and Development, 1978.

Oyen, O. J.: Analyses of postnatal bone growth in long bones versus the craniofacial skeleton and the formation of explanatory models of growth. Am. J. Phys. Anthropol., 75:256, 1988.

Oyen, O. J., and D. H. Enlow: Structural-functional relationships between masticatory biomechanics, skeletal biology, and craniofacial development in primates. Anthrop. Contemp., 3(2):251, 1980.

Oyen, O. J., and P. E. Lestrel: A stereometric analysis of skull growth in *P. cynocephalus anubis*. Biostereometrics '82, 361:330, 1982.

Oyen, O. J., and R. W. Rice: Supraorbital development in chimpanzees (Pan), macaques (*Macaca*), and baboons (*Papio*). J. Med. Primatol. (Lond.), 9: 161, 1980.

Oyen, O. J., and M. D. Russell: Histogenesis of the craniofacial skeleton and models of facial growth. In: *The Effect of Surgical Intervention on Craniofacial Growth*. Ed. by J. A. McNamara, Jr., D. S. Carlson, and K. A. Ribbens. Craniofacial Growth Series. Ann Arbor, University of Michigan, Center for Human Growth and Development, 1982.

Oyen, O. J., A. C. Walker, and R. W. Rice: Craniofacial growth in the olive baboon (*Papio cynocephalus anubis*): Browridge formation. Growth, 43: 174, 1979.

Oyen, O. J., R. W. Rice, and D. H. Enlow: Cortical surface patterns in human and non-human primates. Am. J. Phys. Anthropol., 54:415, 1981.

Pancherz, H., A. Winnberg, and P. Westesson: Masticatory muscle activity and hyoid bone behavior during cyclic jaw movements in man. A synchronized electromyographic and videofluorographic study. Am. J. Orthod., 89:122, 1986.

Pancherz, H., and Anehus-Pancherz, M.: Facial profile changes during and after Herbst appliance treatment. Eur. J. Orthod., 16:275, 1994.

Perry, H. T.: The temporomandibular joint. Am. J. Orthod., 52:399, 1966.

Persson, M., and W. Roy: Suture development and bony fusion in the fetal rabbit palate. Arch. Oral Biol., 24:283, 1979.

Persson, M., B. C. Magnusson, and B. Thilander: Sutural closure in rabbit and man: A morphological and histochemical study. J. Anat., 125:313, 1978.

Petit-Maire, N.: Morphogenèse du crane de primates. L'Anthropologie, 75:85, 1971.

Petrovic, A.: Recherches sur les mécanismes histophysiologiques de la croissance osseuse craniofaciale, Ann. Biol., 9:63, 1970.

Petrovic, A. G., and J. Stutzmann: New ways in orthodontic diagnosis and decision-making: Physiologic basis. J. Jpn. Orthod. Soc., 51:3, 1992.

Petrovic, A., J. Stutzmann, and C. Oudet: Condylectomy and mandibular growth in young rats. A quantitative study. Proc. Finn. Dent. Soc., 77:139, 1981a.

Petrovic, A. G., J. J. Stutzmann, and N. Gasson: The final length of the mandible: Is it genetically predetermined? In: *Craniofacial Biology*. Ed. by D. S. Carlson. Ann Arbor, University of Michigan, Center for Human Growth and Development, 1981b.

Phelps, A. E.: A comparison of lower face changes. Angle Orthod., 48:283, 1978.

Popovich, F., G. W. Thompson, and S. Saunders: Craniofacial measurements in siblings of the Burlington Growth Center sample. J. Dent. Res., 56: A113, 1977.

Poswillo, D.: Hemorrhage in development of the face. In: *Morphogenesis and Malformation of Face and Brain*. Ed. by D. Bergsma, J. Langman, and N. W. Paul. National Foundation—March of Dimes. Birth Defects Original Article Series, Vol. 11, No. 7. New York, Alan R. Liss, 1975.

Poswillo, D. E.: Etiology and pathogenesis of first and second branchial arch defects: The contribution of animal studies. In: *Symposium on Diagnosis and Treatment of Craniofacial Anomalies*.

Ed. by J. M. Converse, J. G. McCarthy, and D. Wood-Smith. St. Louis, C. V. Mosby Co., 1979.

Poswillo, D. E.: Congenital malformations: Prenatal experimental studies. In: *The Temporomandibular Joint*, 3rd Ed. Ed. by B. G. Sarnat, and D. M. Laskin. Springfield, Ill., Charles C Thomas, 1980.

Precious, D. S.: Function: The basis of facial esthetics. J. Can. Dent. Assoc., 58:463, 1992.

Precious, D., and J. Delaire: Balanced facial growth: a schematic interpretation. Oral. Surg. Oral Med. Oral Pathol., 63:637, 1987.

Pritchard, J. J., J. H. Scott, and F. G. Girgis: The structure and development of cranial and facial sutures. J. Anat., 90:73, 1956.

Proffit, W. R.: The facial musculature in its relation to the dental occlusion. In: *Muscle Adaptation in the Craniofacial Region*. Ed. by D. S. Carlson, and J. A. McNamara, Jr. University of Michigan, Center for Human Growth and Development, 1978.

Pruzansky, S.: Anomalies of face and brain. In: *Morphogenesis and Malformation of Face and Brain*. Ed. by D. Bergsma, J. Langman, and N. W. Paul. National Foundation, 11:7, 1975.

Rabine, M.: The role of uninhibited occlusal development. Am. J. Orthod., 74:51, 1978.

Rangel, R. D., O. Oyen, and M. Russell: Changes in masticatory biomechanics and stress magnitude that affect growth and development of the facial skeleton. Prog. Clin. Biol. Res., 187:281, 1985.

Reitan, K.: Bone formation and resorption during reversed tooth movement. In: *Vistas in Orthodontics*. Ed. by B. T. Kraus, and R. A. Riedel. Philadelphia, Lea & Febiger, 1962.

Reitan, K.: Biomechanical principles and reactions. In: *Current Orthodontic Concepts and Techniques*. Ed. by T. M. Graber, Philadelphia, W. B. Saunders, 1969.

Richardson, E. R.: Racial differences in dimensional traits of the human face. Angle Orthod., 50:301, 1980.

Ricketts, R. M.: A principle of arcial growth of the mandible. Angle Orthod., 42:368, 1972a.

Ricketts, R. M.: A four-step method to distinguish orthodontic changes from natural growth. J. Clin. Orthod., 9:208, 1975b.

Ricketts, R. M.: The interdependence of the nasal and oral capsules. In: *Naso-respiratory Function and Craniofacial Growth*. Ed. by J. A. McNamara, Jr. Ann Arbor, University of Michigan, Center for Human Growth and Development, 1979.

Ricketts, R. M., R. W. Bench, J. J. Hilgers, and R. Schulhof: An overview of computerized cephalometrics. Am. J. Orthod., 61:1, 1972.

Riedel, R.: A review of the retention problem. Angle Orthod., 30:179, 1960.

Riolo, M. L.: Growth and remodeling of the cranial floor: A multiple microfluoroscopic analysis with serial cephalometrics. M. S. Thesis, Georgetown University, Washington, D.C., 1970.

Riolo, M. L., and J. A. McNamara, Jr.: Cranial base growth in the rhesus monkey from infancy to adulthood. J. Dent. Res., 52:249, 1973.

Riolo, M. L., R. E. Moyers, J. A. McNanara, and W. S. Hunter: *An Atlas of Craniofacial Growth: Cephalometric Standards from the University School Growth Study, The University of Michigan*. Monograph 2. Craniofacial Growth Series. Ann Arbor, University of Michigan, Center for Human Growth and Development, 1974.

Roberts, G. J., and J. J. Blackwood: Growth of the cartilages of the mid-line cranial base: A radiographic and histological study. J. Anat., 36:307, 1983.

Roche, A. F., and A. B. Lewis: Late growth changes in the cranial base. In: *Development of the Basicranium*. Ed. by J. F. Bosma. DHEW Pub. 76:989, NIH, Bethesda, Md., 1976.

Roche, A. F., W. C. Chumlea, and D. Thissen: *Assessing the Skeletal Maturity of the Hand-Wrist: Fels Method*. Springfield, Ill., Charles C Thomas, 1988.

Rönning, O.: Observations on the intracerebral transplantation of the mandibular condyle. Acta Odont. Scand., 24:443, 1966.

Rönning, O., and K. Koski: The effect of periostomy on the growth of the condylar process in the rat. Proc. Finn. Dent. Soc., 70:28, 1974.

Ross, R. B.: Lateral facial dysplasia (first and second branchial arch syndrome, hemifacial microsomia). In: *Morphogenesis and Malformation of Face and Brain*. Ed. by D. Bergsma, J. Langman, and N. W. Paul. National Foundation—March of Dimes, New York, Alan R. Liss, 11:7, 1975.

Ross, R. B., and M. C. Johnston: *Cleft Lip and Palate*. Baltimore, Williams & Wilkins, 1972.

Rubin, R. M.: Mode of respiration and facial growth. Am. J. Othod., 78:504, 1980.

Salentijn, L., and M. L. Moss: Morphological attributes of the logarithmic growth of the human face: Gnomic growth. Acta Anat., 78:185, 1971.

Salyer, K. E., I. R. Munro, L. A. Whitaker, and I. Jackson: Difficulties and problems to be solved in the approach to craniofacial malformations. In: *Morphogenesis and Malformation of Face and Brain*. Ed. by D Bergsma, J. Langman, and N. W. Paul. National Foundation—March of Dimes, New York, Alan R. Liss, 11:7, 1975.

Sarnat, B. G.: The postnatal maxillary-nasal-orbital complex: Experimental surgery. In: *Factors Affecting the Growth of the Midface*. Ed. by J. A. McNamara, Jr. Ann Arbor, University of Michigan, Center for Human Growth and Development, 1976.

Sarnat, B. G.: Growth pattern of the mandible: Some reflections. Am. J. Orthod. Dentofacial Orthop., 90:221, 1986.

Sarnat, B. G., and M. R. Wexler: Growth of the face and jaws after resection of the septal cartilage in the rabbit. Am. J. Anat., 118:755, 1966.

Sarnat, B. G., J. A. Feigenbaum, and W. M. Krogman: Adult monkey coronoid process after resection of trigeminal nerve motor root. Am. J. Anat., 150:129, 1977.

Sassouni, V.: *The Face in Five Dimensions*. Philadelphia, Philadelphia Center for Research in Child Growth, 1960.

Sassouni, V.: *Heredity and Growth of the Human Face*. Pittsburgh, University of Pittsburgh, 1965.

Saunders, S. R.: Surface and cross-sectional comparisons of bone growth remodeling. Growth, 49:105, 1985.

Savara, B. S., and I. J. Singh: Norms of size and annual increments of seven anatomical measures of maxillae in boys from three to sixteen years of age. Angle Orthod., 38:104, 1968.

Schouker-Jolly, M.: Utilisation d'appareillages extra-oraux récents dans le prognathisme mandi-

bulaire, associe à une hypoplasie maxillaire. Méd. Infant., 6:479, 1972.

Schudy, F. F.: Vertical growth vs. anteroposterior growth as related to function and treatment. Angle orthod., 34:75, 1964.

Schumacher, G. H.: Factors influencing craniofacial growth. Prog. Clin. Biol. Res., 187:3, 1985.

Scott, J. H.: The cartilage of the nasal septum. Br. Dent. J., 95:37, 1953.

Scott, J. H.: Growth at facial sutures. Am. J. Orthod., 42:381, 1956.

Shah, S. M., and M. R. Joshi: An assessment of asymmetry in the normal craniofacial complex. Angle Orthod., 48:141, 1978.

Shapiro, P. A.: Responses of the nonhuman maxillary complex to mechanical forces. In: *Factors Affecting the Growth of the Midface*. Ed. by J. A. McNamara, Jr. Ann Arbor, University of Michigan, Center for Human Growth and Development, 1976.

Shapiro, G. G., and P. Shapiro: Nasal airway obstruction and facial development. Clin. Rev. Allergy, 2:225, 1984.

Shaw, R. E., L. Mark, D. Jenkins, and E. Mingolla: A dynamic geometry for predicting growth of gross craniofacial morphology. Prog. Clin. Biol. Res., 101:423, 1982.

Shore, R. C., and B. K. B. Berkovitz: An ultrastructural study of periodontal ligament fibroblasts in relation to their possible role in tooth eruption and intracellular collagen degradation in the rat. Am. J. Orthod., 24:155, 1979.

Sicher, H., and J. P. Weinmann: Bone growth and physiologic tooth movement. Am. J. Orthod. Oral Surg., 30:109, 1944.

Siegel, M. I.: The facial and dental consequences of nasal septum resections in baboons. Med. Primatol., 1972:204, 1972.

Sirianni, J. E., and A. L. Van Ness: Postnatal growth of the cranial base in *Macaca nemestrina*. Am. J. Phys. Anthropol., 49:329, 1978.

Sirianni, J. E., A. L. Van Ness, and D. R. Swindler: Growth of the mandible in adolescent pigtailed macaques (*Macaca nemestrina*). Hum. Biol., 54:31, 1982.

Smahel, Z., and Z. Mullerova: Facial growth and development in unilateral cleft lip and palate: A longitudinal study. J. Craniofac. Genet. Dev. Biol., 14:57, 1994.

Smith, B. H., S. M. Garn, and W. S. Hunter: Secular trends in face size. Angle Orthod., 56:196, 1986.

Solow, B.: Factor analysis of cranio-facial variables. In: *Cranio-facial Growth in Man*. Ed. by R. E. Moyers, and W. M. Krogman. Oxford, Pergamon Press, 1971.

Solow, B., and E. Greve: Craniocervical angulation and nasal respiratory resistance. In: *Nasorespiratory Function and Craniofacial Growth*. Ed. by J. A. McNamara, Jr. Ann Arbor, University of Michigan, Center for Human Growth and Development, 1979.

Solow, B., and A. Tallgren: Head posture and craniofacial morphology. Am. J. Phys. Anthropol., 44:417, 1976.

Spyropoulos, M. N.: The morphogenetic relationship of the temporal muscle to the coronoid process in human embryos and fetuses. Am. J. Anat., 150:395, 1977.

Stenstrom, S. J., and B. L. Thilander: Effects of nasal septal cartilage resections on young guinea pigs. Plast. Reconstr. Surg., 45:160, 1970.

Storey, A. T.: Physiology of a changing vertical dimension. J. Prosthet. Dent., 1:912, 1962.

Stutzmann, J., and A. Petrovic: Particularités de croissance de la suture palatine sgaittale de jeune rat. Bull. Assoc. Anat. (Nancy), 148:552, 1970.

Stutzmann, J. J., and A. G. Petrovic: Experimental analysis of general and local extrinsic mechanisms controlling upper jaw growth. In: *Factors Affecting the Growth of the Midface*. Ed. by J. A. McNamara, Jr. Ann Arbor, University of Michigan, Center for Human Growth and Development, 1976.

Stutzmann, J., and A. Petrovic: Intrinsic regulation of the condylar cartilage growth rate. Eur. J. Orthod., 1:41, 1979.

Subtelny, J. D.: Longitudinal study of soft tissue facial structures and their profile characteristics defined in relation to underlying skeletal structures. Am. J. Orthod., 45:481, 1959.

Subtelny, J. D.: Oral respiration: Facial maldevelopment and corrective dentofacial orthopedics. Angle Orthod., 50:147, 1980.

Swindler, D. R., J. E. Sirianni, and L. H. Tarrant: A longitudinal study of cephalofacial growth in *Papio cynocephalus and Macaca nemestrina* from three months to three years. IVth International Congress of Primatology, Vol. 3, *Craniofacial Biology of Primates*. Basel, S. Karger, 1973.

Symons, N. B. B.: The development of the human mandibular joint. J. Anat., 86:326, 1952.

Tallgren, A., and B. Solow: Hyoid bone position, facial morphology and head posture in adults. Eur. J. Orthod., 9:1, 1987.

Ten Cate, A. R.: Development of the periodontium. In: *Biology of the Periodontium*. Ed. by A. H. Melcher, and W. H. Bowen. New York, Academic Press, 1969.

Ten Cate, A. R., E. Freeman, and J. B. Dicker: Sutural development: Structure and its response to rapid expansion. Am. J. Orthod., 71:622, 1977.

Tessier, P. J.: Ostéotomies totales de la face: syndrome de Crouzon, syndrome d'Apert., oxycéphalies, scaphocáephalies, turriecéphalies. Ann. Chir. Plast., 12:273, 1967.

Tessier, P., J. Delaire, J. Billet, and H. Landais: Considérations sur le développement de l'orbite: Ses incidences sur la croissance faciale. Rev. Stomatol., 63:1–2, 27–39, 1964.

Thilander, B., and B. Ingervall: The human spheno-occipital synchondrosis. II. A histological and microradiographic study of its growth. Acta Odont. Scand., 31:323, 1973.

Thilander, B., G. E. Carlsson, and B. Ingervall: Postnatal development of the human temporomandibular joint. I. A histological study. Acta Odont. Scand., 34:117, 1976.

Thimaporn, J., J. Goldberg, and D. Enlow: Effects of premature fusion of the zygomaxillary suture on the growth of the rat nasomaxillary complex. J. Oral Maxillofac. Surg., 48:835, 1990.

Tommasone, D., R. Rangel, S. Kurihara, and D. Enlow: Remodeling patterns in the facial and cranial skeleton of the human cleft palate fetus. Kalevi Koski Festschrift, Proc. Finnish Dent. Soc. (Special Issue), 77:171, 1981.

Trenouth, M. J.: Asymmetry of the human skull during fetal growth. Anat. Res., 211:205, 1985.

Treuenfels, H.: Head position, atlas position and breathing in open bite. Fortschr. Kieferothop., 45: 111, 1984.

Trouten, J. C., D. H. Enlow, M. Rabine, A. E. Phelps, and D. Swedlow: Morphologic factors in open bite and deep bite. Angle Orthod., 53:192, 1983.

Tuncay, O. C., J. Haselgrove, P. Frasca, C. Piddington, and I. Shapiro: Scanning microfluorometric F1 measurements of redox 35(2): 1990.

Tuncay, O. C., D. Ho, and M. Banks: Oxygen tension regulates osteoblast function. Am. J. Orthod. Dentofac. Orthoped., 105(5): 1994.

Turpin, D. L.: Growth and remodeling of the mandible in the *Macaca mulatta* monkey. Am. J. Orthod., 54:251, 1968.

Tweed, C. H.: The Frankfort-mandibular incisor angle (FMIA) in orthodontic diagnosis, treatment planning and prognosis. Angle Orthod., 24:121, 1954.

van der Beek, M. C., J. Hoeksma, and B. Prahl-Andersen: Vertical facial growth: A longitudinal study from 7 to 14 years of age. Eur. J. Orthod., 13:202, 1991.

van der Klaauw, C. J.: Size and position of the functional components of the skull (conclusion). Arch. Neerl. Zool., 9:369, 1952.

van der Linden, F. P. G. M.: Changes in the dentofacial complex during and after orthodontic treatment. Eur. J. Orthod., 1:97, 1979.

van der Linden, F. P.: Bone morphology and growth potential: A perspective of postnatal normal bone growth. Prog. Clin. Biol. Res., 187:181, 1985.

van der Linden, F., and H. S. Duterloo: *Development of the Human Dentition*. Hagerstown, Md., Harper & Row, 1976.

van der Linden, F. P. G. M., and D. H. Enlow: A study of the anterior cranial base. Angle Orthod., 41:119, 1971.

van Limborgh, J.: A new view on the control of the morphogenesis of the skull. Acta Morphol. Neerl. Scand., 8:143, 1970.

van Limborgh, J.: The role of genetic and local environmental factors in the control of postnatal craniofacial morphogenesis. Acta Morphol. Neerl. Scand., 10:37, 1972.

Vargervik, K., and E. Harvold: Experiments on the interaction between orofacial function and morphology. Ear Nose Throat J., 66:201, 1987.

Vargervik, K., and A. J. Miller: Observations on the temporal muscle in craniosynostosis. Birth Defects, 18:45, 1982.

Vidic, B.: The morphogenesis of the lateral nasal wall in the early prenatal life of man. Am. J. Anat., 130:121, 1971.

Vig, P. S.: Respiratory mode and morphological types: Some thoughts and preliminary conclusions. In: *Naso-Respiratory Function and Craniofacial Growth*. Ed. by J. A. McNamara, Jr. Ann Arbor, University of Michigan, Center for Human Growth and Development, 1979.

Vig, P. S., and A. B. Hewitt: Asymmetry of the human facial skeleton. Angle Orthod., 45:125, 1975.

Vig, P. S., D. M. Sarver, D. J. Hall, and D. W. Warren: Quantitative evaluation of nasal airflow in relation to facial morphology. Am. J. Orthod., 79: 263, 1981.

Vilmann, H.: Growth of the cranial base in the rat. In: *Development of the Basicranium*. Ed. by J. F. Bosma. DHEW Pub. 76-989, NIH, Bethesda, Md., 1976.

Vinkla, H., L. Odent, D. Odent, K. Koski, and J. A. McNamara: Variability of the craniofacial skeleton. III. Radiographic cephalometry of juvenile *Macaca mulatta*. Am. J. Orthod., 68:1, 1975.

Walker, G.: A new approach to the analysis of craniofacial morphology and growth. Am. J. Orthod., 61:221, 1972.

Walker, G., and C. J. Kowalski: A two-dimensional coordinate model for the quantification, description, analysis, prediction and simulation of craniofacial growth. Growth, 35:119, 1971.

Walker, G., and C. J. Kowalski: On the growth of the mandible. Am. J. Phys. Anthropol., 36:111, 1972.

Washburn, S. L.: The relation of the temporal muscle to the form of the skull. Anat. Rec., 99:239, 1947.

Weidenreich, F.: The brain and its role in the phylogenetic transformation of the human skull. Trans. Am. Phil. Soc., 31:321, 1941.

Whitaker, L. A., and J. A. Katowitz: Nasolacrimal apparatus in craniofacial deformity. In: *Symposium on Diagnosis and Treatment of Craniofacial Anomalies*. Ed. by J. M. Converse, J. G. McCarthy, and D. Wood-Smith. St. Louis, C. V. Mosby, 1979.

Williams, S., and B. Melsen: The interplay between sagittal and vertical growth factors: An implant study of activator treatment. Am. J. Orthod., 8: 327, 1982.

Winnberg, A., and H. Pancherz: Head posture and masticatory muscle function: An EMG investigation. Eur. J. Orthod., 5:209, 1983.

Wisth, P. J.: Nose morphology in individuals with angle Class I, II, or III occlusions. Acta Odont. Scand., 33:53, 1975.

Woo, J. K.: Ossification and growth of the human maxilla, premaxilla and palate bones. Anat. Rec., 105:737, 1949.

Woodside, D. G., A. Metaxas, and G. Altuna: The influence of functional appliance therapy on glenoid fossa remodeling. Am. J. Orthod. Dentofacial Orthop., 92:181, 1987.

Wright, D. M., and B. C. Moffett: The postnatal development of the human temporomandibular joint. Am. J. Anat., 141:235, 1974.

Young, R. W.: The influence of cranial contents on postnatal growth of the skull in the rat. Am. J. Anat., 105:383, 1959.

Youdelis, R. A.: The morphogenesis of the human temporomandibular joint and its associated structures. J. Dent. Res., 45:182, 1966.

Zengo, A. N., C. A. L. Bassett, R. J. Pawluk, and G. Prountzos: *In vivo* bioelectric potentials in the dentoalveolar complex. Am. J. Orthod., 66:130, 1974.

Zins, J., Kusiak, L. Whitaker, and D. H. Enlow: Influence of recipient site on bone grafts to the face. J. Plast. Reconstr. Surg., 73:371, 1984.

Zuckerman, S.: Age changes in the basicranial axis of the human skull. Am. J. Phys. Anthropol., 13: 521, 1955.

Zwarych, P. D., and M. B. Quigley: The intermediate plexus of the periodontal ligament: History and further investigations. J. Dent. Res., 44:383, 1965.

INDEX

Note: Page numbers in *italics* indicate illustrations; page numbers followed by t indicate tables.

295

Cortical bone, 69
Counterpart(s), Enlow analysis of, 254–258, *257*
  imbalances in, 41
  in facial patterns, 173
  principle of, 40–41, *41*
Cradling, headform and, 128
Cranial base, Bolton, 261
Cranial base angle, 180, *181*
Cranial fossa
  anterior, brachycephalic *vs.* dolichocephalic, 126, *127*
    counterparts of, 40
    growth field boundaries of, 158–159, *159*
    growth of, 107–108, *108*
    in facial growth, 49–50, *50*
    of child, 143
    orbital cavity and, *109,* 109–110
    palate as projection of, 126
  Class II *vs.* Class III, 188
  counterpart of, 40, 48
  growth of, 106–108, *108*
  in facial growth, 45–46, *46,* 48
  inclination of, *176–177,* 179–180
  ramus and, in mandibular remodeling, 73–74
Cranial index, headform and, *125*
Cranial nerve(s), basicranial growth and, 103
  fetal, 222, 224–225
Craniofacial level(s), 14
Craniostat, 261
Crouzon syndrome, 4
Crying infant, 235
Cupid's bow, *140,* 142
Curve of Spee, 186–187

Dacryon, 261
Dental arch, positioning of, 34
Dentition. See also *Tooth (teeth).*
  developmental adjustments in, 213–214
Dentoalveolar compensation, 184–186, *185–186*
Dentoalveolar curve (of Spee), 186–187
Deposition, of bone, process of, 5–6, *6–7,* 268, *268*
  surface for, 21, *21*
Dick Tracy nose, 124–125, *125,* 174
Dieting, facial features after, 135
Dinaric headform, 128–129, 174
  ears in, *125,* 129
  malocclusion tendencies of, 129, 215
  nose in, 129
  of mandible. See *Mandible, displacement of.*
  of maxilla. See *Maxilla, displacement of.*
  of palate, 52–53
Displacement. See *Bone(s), displacement of.*
Dolichocephalic headform, 11, *12*
  cranial index of, *125*
  facial features with, 123–126, *124–125,* 194, *194–195*
    aging and, 136
    sexual dimorphism of, 132–133
  malocclusion tendencies in, Class II, 166–167, *167–168,* 177, 188, 194
    Class III, 189
  nose in, 124–125, *125*
Drift, vertical. See *Vertical drift.*

Ear(s), dinaric, *125,* 129
  fetal, 224, *224*
  of infant and child, 137
  variations in, *141*

Endochondral bone, 67, 105
Endocranial fossa, 99
Endosteal bone, 21, *21*
Enlow, counterpart analysis of, 254–256, *257*
Epithelial pearl(s), 227
Ethmoidal sinus, 143. See also *Sinus(es).*
Ethnicity. See also entries related to specific ethnic group, e.g., *Caucasian face.*
  facial patterns and, 174, 193–199
  headform and, 126, 128, 174
  malocclusion tendencies in, 169–170
Euryprosopic facial type, 123, 125
Eye(s), of child, 137
  of infant, 138
Eyeball(s), brachycephalic *vs.* dolichocephalic, 126
Eyelid(s), variations in, *139*

Face. See also *Facial* entries.
  bones of, 21, *21*
  human, *vs.* other mammals, 146–147, 153, *153*
  normal, 262
  shape of, variations in, *141*
  vertical alignment of, 158
  width of, in humans *vs.* other mammals, 153, *153*
  wrinkling of, 135
Facial angle, 261
Facial expression. See also *Facial pattern.*
  in infant, 237
Facial growth, airway in, 12–13, *13*
  anterior cranial fossa and forehead in, 49–50, *50*
  anteroposterior (frontal) axis of, 260–261
  brain and basicranium configuration in, 11–12, *12*
  calvaria bones in, 49
  cephalometric landmarks in. See *Cephalometrics, landmarks in.*
  changing features in, 136–139, *137–142,* 141–145
  control processes in, 200–219
  counterparts in. See *Counterpart(s).*
  cranial floor imbalance in, 34
  direction of, 7
  displacement in. See *Bone(s), displacement of.*
  fetal, 220–232
  frontozygomatic, 55, *56*
  levels in, 14
  malar area in, 55–56, *56*
  matching maxillar and mandibular protrusion in, 49
  maxillary tuberosity in, 42
    backward growth of, 41, *42*
  middle cranial fossa in, 45–46, *46,* 48
  nasal septum in, 85, 205–206
  nasomaxillary complex in, *46,* 46–47
  neuromuscular function and, 239–240
  of infant, 136–137, *137–138*
  oral region and, 13–14
  overbite in, *54,* 54–55
  ramus in. See also *Ramus.*
    backward growth of, 43–44, *44*
    horizontal growth of, 48, *48*
    remodeling of, 42–43, *44*
  remodeling in. See *Bone(s), remodeling of.*
  resorptive, 32
  rotation in, 21, 34, 216
  sexual dimorphism in, 250, *251,* 252t, *253*
  sinuses in, 143
  superimposed headfilm tracings in, *36,* 36–38
  suture displacement in, 51

Growth (*Continued*)
  of face. See *Facial growth.*
  of soft tissue, 267
  of sutures, 272–273, *273–274*
    basicranial growth and, *101*, 102, 107–108, *108*
  process of. See *Growth process.*
  working with, 1, 14
    remodeling fields and, 23
    tooth movement and, 111
    vertical drift in, 88
Growth axis, lateral, 262
Growth cartilage, 265–266
  compression of, 267
Growth control. See *Growth process.*
Growth field, 15, 156
  boundary(ies) of, 156–161, *158–165*, 163–164
    brain and basicranium sharing of, 156–157
    degeneration and, 156
    for anterior cranial fossa, 158–159, *159*
    for brain, 157–158, *158*
    for nasomaxillary complex, 158–159, 161
    lingual tuberosity as, 160
    rebound and, 156, 164–165
  facial configuration variations and, 23
  mandibular, 23
  remodeling and, 23
  three-dimensional, 24
Growth movement. See also *Bone(s), displacement of;*
    Bone(s), remodeling of.
  biologic processes underlying, 53
  kinds of, 5, *5*, 15, 214
  non-biologic material and, 7–8
Growth process, 3. See also *Facial growth.*
  activating signals in, 13
  balance in, 1–2, 17, 39–40, 212–213
  bioelectric signals in, 208–209
  biomechanical forces in, 204, 209–210
  clinical intervention in, 217–218
  compensatory, 2, 4, 13–14, 40, 84–85, 183–184
    dentoalveolar, 184–186, *185–186*
    intervention in, 217–218
  composite explanations of, 206–207
  condyles in, 204–205
  control messengers in, 1, 207–208
  counterpart principle in. See *Counterpart(s).*
  determinants of, 2
  differential progression in, 211–212
  directions of, 41, *42*
  drift in. See *Vertical drift.*
  feedback interrelationships in, 210–211
  functional matrix in, 85, 205–206
    contradiction in, 218
  genetic, 202–204
  goodness of anatomic fit in, 10, 212–213
  headform in, 214–215. See also *Headform.*
  histogenic tissues in, 9
  interdependence of, 4–5, 10–11, *11*, 17, 211–213, 219
  nasal septum theory of, 83–84
  neurotropic factor in, 209
  occlusal curve in, 213
  piezo factor in, 208–210
  pterygomaxillary fissure movement in, 41–42, *42*
  rebound in, 2, 4, 94
    growth field boundaries and, 156, 164–165
  regional control of, 10–11, *11*
  regional imbalances in, 212–213
  structural and functional equilibrium in, 212
  sutures in, 204–205

Growth process (*Continued*)
  synchondroses in, 204–205
  timing and duration of, 9
  triggers in, 209–210
  vectors in, 9
Growth remodeling. See also *Bone(s) remodeling of.*
  definition of, 19
  enlargement in, 27
  relocation and, 26, *27*
Growth rotation(s), 21, 34, 216
Growth site(s), mandibular condyle as, 23
Growth spurt, circumpubertal, 252t

Haversian system, 274–275, *279*, 279–280
Headfilm tracing(s), superimposed, *36*, 36–38, 163, *164*
Headform, Alpine, 128, 196
  appliances and, 129
  as growth control factor, 214–215
  brachycephalic. See *Brachycephalic headform.*
  cradling and, 128
  dinaric, 128–129, 174
    malocclusion tendencies in, 129, 215
  dolichocephalic. See *Dolichocephalic headform.*
  ethnicity and, 126, 128, 174
  facial pattern and. See specific headform, e.g.,
      Dolichocephalic headform, facial features with.
  malocclusion tendencies and, 166–170, *167–169*, *177*, 188, 215
  mesocephalic, 126
  population groupings and, 126, 128
  sleeping habits and, 128–129, *129*, 157
Height, facial, 261
Histogenic tissue, 9
Howship lacuna, 117
Hyoid bone, fetal, *223, 225*

Implant marker, in remodeling, 24
Incisor inferius, 262
Incisor superius, 262
Infant. See also *Child;* Neonate.
  basicranium of, 144
  cheekbone of, 142
  chin of, 136, 143
  crying, 235
  dental battery of, *138*, 144–145
  ears of, 137
  face of, expression on, 237
    growth of, 136–137, *137–138*
    proportions of, 15, *16*
  fontanelles of, 144
  gag reflex of, 235
  gonial angle of, 144
  jaw position of, neural regulation of, 238–239
  mastication by, 236–237
  mastoid process of, 144
  maxillary arch of, 144
  nose of, 139
  orbital rim of, 139, 141
  speech development in, 237–238
  suckling by, 234–235
  swallowing by, 234–235, 238
Infradentale, definition of, 262
Inion, definition of, 262
Interincisal angle, 262
Interstitial growth, 267